Current Topics in
Microbiology
264/II # and Immunology

Editors

R.W. Compans, Atlanta/Georgia
M. Cooper, Birmingham/Alabama · Y. Ito, Kyoto
H. Koprowski, Philadelphia/Pennsylvania · F. Melchers, Basel
M. Oldstone, La Jolla/California · S. Olsnes, Oslo
M. Potter, Bethesda/Maryland
P.K. Vogt, La Jolla/California · H. Wagner, Munich

Springer
Berlin
Heidelberg
New York
Barcelona
Hong Kong
London
Milan
Paris
Tokyo

Pathogenicity Islands and the Evolution of Pathogenic Microbes

Volume II

Edited by J. Hacker and J.B. Kaper

With 24 Figures and 12 Tables

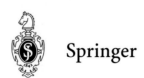 Springer

Professor Dr. Jörg Hacker
Universität Würzburg
Institut für Molekulare Infektionsbiologie
Röntgenring 11
97070 Würzburg
Germany
e-mail: j.hacker@mail.uni-wuerzburg.de

Professor Dr. James B. Kaper
University of Maryland School of Medicine
Center for Vaccine Development
685 W. Baltimore Street
21201 Baltimore, MD
USA
e-mail: jkaper@umaryland.edu

Cover Illustration: Distribution of chromosomal alterations among different pathogenic *E. coli* isolates. The individual chromosomes are displayed in equal length in the following order, from outwards to inwards: 536 (UPEC), IHE3034 (MENEC), 4797/97 (EHEC), E2348/69 (EPEC), C9221a (ETEC), EDL1284 (EIEC), and DPA065 (EAEC). Missing ORFs are marked by *vertical lines* in the individual chromosomes. The position of the deleted ORFs refers to the *E. coli* MG1655 chromosome (*outer circle*). The positions of tRNA genes frequently used as chromosomal insertion sites of horizontally acquired DNA elements are marked within the map of the *E. coli* strain MG1655. (Data from Dobrindt et al. 2001b).

ISSN 0070-217X
ISBN 3-540-42682-5 Springer-Verlag Berlin Heidelberg New York

Springer-Verlag Berlin Heidelberg New York
a member of BertelsmannSpringer Science + Business Media GmbH

http://www.springer.de

© Springer-Verlag Berlin Heidelberg 2002
Library of Congress Catalog Card Number 15-12910
Printed in Germany

Cover Design: *design & production GmbH*, Heidelberg
Typesetting: Scientific Publishing Services (P) Ltd, Madras
Printed on acid-free paper   SPIN: 10847860   27/3020 - 5 4 3 2 1 0

Preface

In the year 1972 the famous evolutionary biologist Theodor Dobzhansky wrote that "nothing makes sense in biology except in the light of evolution". This sentence holds true even for the new developments in molecular biology: recombinant DNA technology, cloning of prokaryotic and eukaryotic genes, establishment of whole genome sequences, and reprogramming of cellular processes following transfer of chromosomes.

The evolutionary aspects of modern biology are of particular importance when interpreting the results from the different genome sequencing projects. As of the year 2001 more than 45 bacterial genomes have been sequenced, including more than 30 genomes of pathogenic bacteria such as *Helicobacter pylori*, *Pseudomonas aeruginosa*, and *Staphylococcus aureus*, or pathogenic variants of the species *Escherichia coli*. The interpretion of these sequences reveal that the Darwinian laws of evolution – establishment of genetic variability, formation of new phenotypes, and natural selection of the newly formed variants – are also true for both pathogenic and nonpathogenic microbes. The ongoing genome sequencing projects as well as genetic studies performed over the last 10–15 years, however, also provided new insights into the mechanisms which led to the generation of new genetic variants. It became clear that, in addition to the generation of point mutations and the processes of genetic rearrangements, horizontal gene transfer plays a tremendous role in the evolution of prokaryotes and, presumably, also in the development of eukaryotic organisms. This volume of *Current Topics in Microbiology and Immunology* entitled "Pathogenicity Islands and the Evolution of Pathogenic Microbes" also focuses on these general mechanisms of the evolution of prokaryotes. The genetic processes which drive the evolution of bacteria are summarized in the first chapter of the book "Evolution of Prokaryotic Genomes", written by W. Arber.

A few years ago one of the great pioneers of molecular pathogenesis research, S. Falkow, postulated that lateral gene transfer processes in bacteria lead to "evolution in quantum

leaps". Our publication aims to summarize the current knowledge on the impact of lateral gene transfer in the evolution of
pathogenic microbes, with a particular focus on new genetic
elements, termed pathogenicity islands (PAI). PAIs were first
described more than 10 years ago for pathogenic variants of the
species *Escherichia coli*. PAIs have now been described for more
than 30 species of pathogenic microbes and the ongoing discussion of the definition of PAIs and their significance in microbial
evolution is also reflected in our book. From our point of view,
PAIs represent formerly transferred or still mobile genetic elements which encode virulence factors and are present in pathogenic bacteria, but not present in related nonpathogenic
specimens. PAIs are often flanked by particular boundary regions
(direct repeat sequences, IS elements); they are often located near
tRNA genes and often unstable. PAIs encode so-called virulence-
associated genes, which are parts of PAIs together with "mobility
genes" encoding transposases, integrases, or other enzymes active
in genetic recombination. As the first PAIs have been described in
pathogenic strains of *Escherichia coli*, the two chapters by Redford and Welch and by Torres and Kaper, entitled "Extraintestinal *Escherichia coli* As a Model System for the Study of
Pathogenicity Islands" and "Pathogenicity Islands of Intestinal
E. coli" summarize our knowledge on the occurrence and
distribution of PAI in extraintestinal and intestinal *E. coli*. The
newly established DNA sequence of the enterohemorrhagic
E. coli O157:H7 isolate also contributes to the discussion on PAIs
in pathogenic *E. coli*.

It has been known for a number of years that not only PAIs
but also plasmids and bacteriophages are able to carry genes
whose products are involved in pathogenic processes. Accordingly, such elements and their products play an important role in
pathogenesis due to intestinal *E. coli* as well due to *Shigella*. The
role of PAIs in shigellosis is summarized in the article "Pathogenicity Islands of *Shigella*" by Ingersoll et al. Besides *E. coli* and
the closely related species of the *Shigella* group, additional
members of the enterobacteria such as *Yersinia*, *Salmonella*, and
Erwinia are described in various contributions. Thus, in the article by Kingley and Bäumler "Pathogenicity Islands and Host
Adaptation of *Salmonella* Serovars" the different genetic elements leading to the various variants of *Salmonella* are discussed.
In this respect it seems useful to distinguish between larger "islands" which exhibit a number of specific features (see above) and
smaller genetic regions termed "islets". PAI and islets as well as
bacteriophages and even plasmids all play a role in the formation
of lipopolysaccharides (LPS) of gram-negative bacteria and

capsules, which are produced by a variety of bacteria, both gram-negative and gram-positive. While Reeves and Wang describe the genomic organization of LPS-specific loci in their chapter, the one by Barrett et al. deals with the genomic structure of capsular determinants. Both describe common structures of LPS and capsules in different pathogens but also focus on the differences among various species and the genetic basis of these cell surface components. In both of these chapters, LPS and capsular-specific gene clusters are considered as "genetic modules" which have the capacity to recombine new variants of the cell surface. Vogel and Frosch in their contribution "The Genus *Neisseria*: Population, Structure, Genome Plasticity and Evolution of Pathogenicity" consider the respective loci as part of plasticity regions in the genomes of pathogenic *Neisseria* which may be introduced into new recipients by transformation rather than by transduction with phages or by plasmid-driven conjugation.

Another interesting aspect which is reflected in various chapters is that genomes evolve by acquisition of new pieces of DNA following gene transfer, and also by genome reduction. Different mechanisms include the deletion of sequences or the elimination of functions by the accumulation of point mutations or rearrangements. In the contribution by Carniel "Plasmids and Pathogenicity Islands of *Yersinia*" the importance of mobile genetic elements for the pathogenic phenotypes of *Yersinia* is described. Here, a reduction of functions is considered to be a prerequisite for the evolution of the very dangerous bacterial species *Yersinia pestis* from *Y. pseudotuberculosis* over the last 2000–10,000 years. In addition, the genomes of pathogenic shigellae exhibit deleted regions compared to those of *E. coli*, termed "black holes", whose absence is required for a fully virulent phenotype. In their chapter "Phylogenetic Relationships and Virulence Evolution in the Genus *Bordetella*" von Wintzingerode and coworkers provide evidence that the genome of the causative agent of whooping caugh, *Bordetella pertussis*, is 100kb smaller than the genome of the less pathogenic species *Bordetella bronchiseptica*, another example of genome evolution by reduction.

It has been known for a long time that the occurrence of bacteriophages and plasmids is not restricted to pathogenic bacteria. Rather such genetic elements are quite widespread in the prokaryotic world. The same holds true for elements which exhibit a general composition which is similar to that of PAI. Thus, J. Rood in the contribution "Genomic Islands of *Dichelobacter nodosus*" describes the genome structure of an animal pathogen, in which he was able to identify DNA elements very similar to PAIs, but with unknown pathogenic properties. In addition,

Labig et al. in their chapter "Pathogenicity Islands and PAI-like Structures in *Pseudomonas* Species" describe genomic islands in various species of the *Pseudomonas* group, where their products may contribute to the pathogenic potency of *Pseudomonas aeruginosa*, but also to the metabolic diversity of nonpathogenic *Pseudomonas* species such as *Pseudomonas putida*. Furthermore, the chapter by Dobrindt et al.. "Genome Plasticity of Pathogenic and Nonpathogenic Enterobacteria" demonstrates that symbiotic bacteria may also carry elements which correspond to genomic islands. Kim and Alfano demonstrate in their work "Pathogenicity Islands and Virulence Plasmids of Bacterial Plant Pathogens" that plant pathogens also carry such genetic elements.

The general mechanism of the type III secretion system of delivering molecules from bacteria to host cells is not restricted to pathogens either. Thus, type III-specific secretion systems are produced by pathogens such as intestinal *E. coli*, *Yersinia*, *Shigella*, and *Salmonella* but also by different plant pathogens and by symbiotic *Pseudomonas* bacteria. Furthermore, type IV pathways are expressed by *Helicobacter pylori*, *Legionella pneumoniae*, and *Agrobacterium tumefaciens*. The chapters by Odenbreit and Hass "*Helicobacter pylori*: Impact of Gene Transfer and the Role of the cag Pathogenicity Island for Host Adaptation and Virulence" and Heuner et al. "Genome Structure and Evolution of *Legionella* Species" present examples of the occurrence, structure, and function of type IV secretion systems in various human pathogens. As demonstrated by Kim and Alfano, similar systems exist in the plant pathogen *Agrobacterium tumefaciens* which has the capacity to transfer DNA from bacteria to plant cells. This mechanism reflects another essential mechanism in the evolution of host–pathogen relationship.

Another function that is mediated by horizontal gene transfer is antibiotic resistance. As shown in the chapters "Phages and Other Mobile Virulence Elements in Gram-positive pathogens" by Gentry-Weeks et al. and "Impact of Integrons and Transposons on the Evolution of Resistance and Virulence" by Rowe- Magnus et al. various genetic elements, such as plasmids, "islands", transposons, integrons and "super integrons" play a role in the distribution of resistance determinants. In particular cases, resistance- and virulence-specific genes can be part of the same genetic entity, which speaks for a co-evolution of the two properties.

The fact that PAIs and PAI-like elements such as plasmids and phages are constitutive parts of the genomes of gram-positive pathogens is supported by the data given in the chapter by Gentry-Weeks and also by the contributions "Pathogenicity

Islands and Other Virulence Elements in *Listeria*" by Kreft et al. and "Genome Structure and Evolution of the *Bacillus cereus* Group" by Kolsto et al.. Both groups of organisms, *Listeria* and *Bacillus*, comprise pathogenic as well as nonpathogenic members and the respective genetic elements – phages, plasmids, and islands – truly behave as pathogens or as commensals of the normal microbial flora. Furthermore, we propose that genetic elements such as genomic islands may also be present in euka-ryotes. Köhler et al. in "Genome Structure of Pathogenic Fungi" discuss new data which support this view.

In this volume of *Current Topics in Microbiology and Im-munology* a number of genome structures of pathogenic microbes are presented. It will be our future task to understand the func-tions of the known genes and their products and to identify new ones as more sequence information becomes available. This will enable us to speculate on the processes of natural selection, which, in consequence, lead to the development of new species and pathotypes. The Darwianin laws will need to be considered when new data on these processes are obtained in order to demonstrate that PAIs and other genetic elements really "make sense in the light of evolution".

J. HACKER and J.B. KAPER

List of Contents

List of Contents
of Companion Volume 264/I

List of Contributors

(Their addresses can be found at the beginning of their respective chapters.)

List of Contributors
of Companion Volume 264/I

ARBER, W. 1

BARRETT, B. 137

BÄUMLER, A.J. 67

CARNIEL, E. 89

DOBRINDT, U. 157

EBAH, L. 137

GERLACH, G. 177

GROISMAN, E.A. 49

GROSS, R. 177

HACKER, J. 157

HENTSCHEL, U. 157

INGERSOLL, M. 49

KAPER, J.B. 31, 157

KIEWITZ, C. 201

KINGSLEY, R.A. 67

LARBIG, K. 201

REDFORD, P. 15

REEVES, P.P. 109

ROBERTS, I.S. 137

SCHNEIDER, B. 177

TORRES, A.G. 31

TÜMMLER, B. 201

VON WINTZINGERODE, F.
  177

WANG, L. 109

WELCH, R.A. 15

ZYCHLINSKY, A. 49

Helicobacter pylori: Impact of Gene Transfer and the Role of the *cag* Pathogenicity Island for Host Adaptation and Virulence

S. Odenbreit and R. Haas

1 Introduction

Helicobacter pylori (*Hp*) causes one of the most common bacterial infections in humans, affecting approximately half of the population worldwide. *Hp* is the cause of chronic active gastritis and peptic ulceration (Blaser 1992), and is associated

Max von Pettenkofer Institut für Hygiene und Medizinische Mikrobiologie, Pettenkoferstrasse 9a, 80336 München, Germany with the development of gastric carcinoma and mucosa-associated lymphoid tissue (MALT) lymphoma (FORMAN et al. 1993; STOLTE and EIDT 1993). The chronic infection is usually acquired early in childhood and can persist in the stomach of patients for a lifetime, if untreated.

Hp causes acute and chronic inflammation in the stomach, but the degree of inflammation is strain- and host-dependent. Despite histological gastritis in the infected stomach mucosa, no clinical consequences are observed in the majority of individuals. However, in 20%–30% of infected persons, the long-term consequences are peptic ulceration, or even gastric cancer, which are life-threatening diseases.

In most developing countries, infection in both children and adults is very high, reaching 80%–100%. In northern Europe and the United States, however, the infection of children is rare, but adults are still infected in the range of 30%–50%. It is still unclear how *Hp* transmission occurs. A faecal–oral spread and a gastric-oral-oral mode of transmission are discussed (DORE et al. 2000). Children are often infected with the identical strain as their parents, and infection of the mother is a high risk factor for an infection of the child, especially in the first 2 years of life ROTHENBACHER et al. 1999). Once chronic infection with a certain *Hp* strain is established, infection with a second strain appears to be very rare.

Several bacterial factors contribute to the efficient colonisation and survival of *Hp* in the human stomach. To colonise, *Hp* must safely penetrate the mucus layer, passing an extremely acidic environment, the stomach lumen (pH < 2). The metalloenzyme urease and a bundle of polar sheathed flagella are both essential for this crucial step, as demonstrated by the inability of isogenic knockout mutants in the corresponding genes to colonise in animal models (EATON et al. 1991; EATON et al. 1996).

Specific adhesins are produced, which allow a tight binding of the bacteria to gastric epithelial cells. Well characterised are the membrane proteins BabA2 (blood group antigen binding adhesin A) (ILVER et al. 1998) and AlpAB (adhesion-associated lipoprotein) (ODENBREIT et al. 1999). BabA2 binds to the Lewis[b] blood group antigen (BORÉN et al. 1993), whereas the receptor for AlpAB is not known. Other potential receptors are described, but no specific adhesins have been identified (GERHARD et al. 2000). Adhesion is believed to be beneficial in reducing the risk of a bacterial elimination by mucus shedding. More important, however, might be the signalling to host epithelial cells, either directly by receptor binding, or by use of the contact dependent type IV secretion system (see below).

The vacuolating cytotoxin (VacA), encoded by the *vacA* gene, is thought to be one of the major virulence factors of *Hp* (COVER and BLASER 1992). The protein is produced as a precursor of 139–140kDa and belongs to the group of autotransporter proteins (SCHMITT and HAAS 1994; COVER et al. 1994; TELFORD et al. 1994). VacA causes degeneration of target cells by interference with the vacuolar trafficking system. Large acidic vacuoles are generated, which appear to be hybrids of late endosomal and lysosomal compartments (PAPINI et al. 1997). The mature VacA is a secreted AB-type toxin of ~95kDa (for a recent review see FISCHER and HAAS 1999).

A further *Hp* protein with a direct effect on the host is the neutrophil-activating protein (HP-NAP) (EVANS et al. 1995). It is an oligomeric protein, consisting of 10–12 monomers of a 17-kDa polypeptide with homology to iron-binding proteins (TONELLO et al. 1999). HP-NAP is chemotactic for human leukocytes, and it activates their NADPH oxidase to produce reactive oxygen intermediates (SATIN et al. 2000). Thus, HP-NAP may be involved in recruitment of neutrophils to the gastric mucosa and may contribute to the inflammatory response.

A major genetic difference between individual *Hp* isolates is the presence or the absence of the *cag* pathogenicity island (*cag*-PAI). The Cytotoxin-associated antigen A (CagA), a 128–145kDa immunodominant protein, is encoded by the *cagA* gene, located at the right border of this PAI (CENSINI et al. 1996). The CagA antigen was originally believed to be strictly co-expressed with the VacA cytotoxin, hence the name CagA, but, subsequently, it has been shown that there is not really a strict association between the expression of both genes (TUMMURU et al. 1994; XIANG et al. 1995). *Hp* strains producing CagA and VacA were designated as type I strains, without both antigens, they are classified as type II. Type I strains tend to be more associated with severe disease than type II, although expression of *cagA* is not necessarily associated with clinical symptoms (EVANS et al. 1998; PARK et al. 1998).

The development of molecular genetic techniques for *Hp* in the last 10 years, as well as the publication of two *Hp* genome sequences from two unrelated strains (TOMB et al. 1997; ALM et al. 1999), provides a basis for a better understanding of the biological processes of pathogenicity and evolution of this fascinating microorganism. Some progress has been made recently in understanding the mechanism of natural transformation, which is discussed as the basis for horizontal gene transfer in *Hp*. Furthermore, the structure and function of the *cag*-PAI has been studied extensively. In this review, we intend to discuss the data available on the role, the mechanism and the consequences of gene transfer and the presence of the *cag*-PAI for adaptation of *Hp* to its host.

2 Genetic Diversity

2.1 Early Studies Indicating Genetic Diversity in *Hp*

The first hints for genetic diversity came from restriction fragment length polymorphism (RFLP) analysis with frequently cutting enzymes like *Hind*III (LANGENBERG et al. 1986; MAJEWSKI and GOODWIN 1988) or *Hae*III (OWEN et al. 1990). Chromosomal DNA of fresh *Hp* isolates showed a unique digestion pattern. In contrast, subculturing of defined isolates did not change the pattern over a time period of up to 10 months, indicating that the DNA digestion pattern is rather stable within an individual strain. RFLP was coupled with pulsed-field gel electrophoresis (PFGE) to obtain a more defined pattern, allowing the construction of genome maps (TAYLOR et al. 1992). In further studies, random amplified poly-morphic DNA PCR fingerprinting (RAPD-PCR) and PCR-based RFLP led to similar results (AKOPYANZ et al. 1992a; AKOPYANZ et al. 1992b). Among 64 inde-pendent isolates, for instance, all strains could be distinguished by a single RAPD primer. When KANSAU et al. (1996) sequenced an internal 210bp-PCR fragment of the *ureC* gene, they found that all sequences were unique. In all these cases, however, a comparison of isolates from consecutive biopsies of the same patient could not detect any changes in DNA level. All these data together suggest that *Hp* exhibits a very high level of genetic diversity, but the genetic status in an individual strain colonizing a defined patient seems to be rather stable, at least on the level detectable by the methods described above.

2.2 Micro- and Macro-Diversity as the Driving Force of *Hp* Diversity

The genetic diversity described previously may be due to two major mechanisms: well known as micro- and macro-diversity. Micro-diversity is caused by point mutations within individual genes, which can be silent/synonymous or non-synonymous. By synonymous point mutations additional sites for restriction enzymes can occur or disappear, resulting in different restriction patterns in RFLP analysis. The same effect can be achieved by changing the gene order in the chromosome, the so-called macro-diversity of a genome. Mutational events like translocation or inversion of DNA fragments can displace present restriction sites to another locus, changing the RFLP pattern as well. Additionally, gene duplica-tions, horizontal gene transfer and homologous recombination play an important role in macro-diversity. In the following section, the contribution of micro- and macro-diversity to genetic polymorphism in *Hp* will be discussed.

2.2.1 Microdiversity in *Hp*

2.2.1.1 *Hp:* A Mutator Species?

The most important step in the evolutionary fate of a gene might be point mutations occurring by deletions or nucleotide exchanges. Apart from the RFLP analysis described above, there are few systematic approaches investigating *Hp* diversity on the DNA sequence level. A major breakthrough in this respect was the availability of the complete genome sequences of the independent *Hp* strains 26695 (TOMB et al. 1997) and J99 (ALM et al. 1999). Thus, *Hp* was the first bacterial species providing us with two complete genome sequences. As expected from the preceding studies, the sequence variation within individual genes was considerable, with the majority of exchanges in the third codon position of the genes, which implicates that most mutations are silent. Thus, the impact of mutations on the proteome is lower than expected from the DNA sequence diversity.

The main reasons for point mutations can be found in errors during replication on either intact or damaged DNA templates. WANG et al. (1999a) summarised the putative predispositions of *Hp* to an elevated mutation rate as the major cause of genetic diversity; in *Escherichia coli* the so-called *mutHLS* system is involved in DNA mismatch repair. According to the *Hp* genome sequences available, homologues of *mutH* and *mutL* are lacking, whereas a gene homologous to *mutS* is present. However, the *Hp mutS* gene seems to belong to another subfamily not involved in DNA mismatch repair (HOLLINGSWORTH et al. 1995), suggesting that such a mismatch repair system is missing in *Hp*, unless compensated by another unknown system.

Hp produces a RecA protein, which is involved in homologous recombinational repair and UV-light resistance (THOMSPSON and BLASER 1995). In *E. coli*, RecA is not only involved in homologous recombination, but it also regulates the SOS response by acting as a co-protease, cleaving the LexA repressor and the UmuD protein when activated by exposure to single-stranded DNA. A LexA binding motif upstream of the *Hp recA* gene or other SOS genes is, however, not present, and there are no homologues to *lexA* or *umuC/umuD* in the genome. This suggests that there is no SOS response and no trans-lesion synthesis pathway present in *Hp*. In comparison to *E. coli*, *Hp* is lacking some systems to prevent or repair mutagenesis events, making this species probably more prone to exogenous, mutagenic influences.

Deletion of genes encoding DNA repair proteins leads to higher mutation frequencies, so-called mutator phenotypes (HORST et al. 1999). A low level of mutator cells may be beneficial for a population in terms of rapid adaptation properties to external stress, which would not be possible in normal wild-type bacteria. Mutation frequencies in *Hp* isolates display a considerable variation, and *Hp* strains with mutation rates being even higher than in typical *E. coli* mutator strains can be isolated (M. Sjölund, personal communication). From this point of view, the classification of *Hp* as a mutator species might be justified.

2.2.1.2 *Hp*: A Panmictic Species?

The micro-diversity caused by de novo mutations generally leads to an accumulation of point mutations and the development of a clonal species. This means that a bacterium always carries the base exchanges of its ancestral cell and acquires additional mutations, resulting in a phylogenetic tree, which can discriminate between ancestor and descendant. This coupling of defined mutations is disturbed when homologous recombination between two strains takes place. In this case, defined combinations of gene sequences become uncoupled so that the resulting variant strain cannot be attributed to a distinct position in the phylogenetic tree. SUERBAUM et al. (1998) investigated the sequences of three gene fragments (*flaA*, *flaB* and *vacA*) from *Hp* isolates from different geographic regions (Germany, Canada and South Africa) for their clonality by using the homoplasy test (MAYNARD and SMITH 1998) and compatibility matrices (JAKOBSEN and EASTEAL 1996). These two methods have been developed to evaluate the recombination rate within closely related organisms and to reveal reticulate evolution. These studies suggested that *Hp* shows a sequence diversity similar to *Neisseria meningitidis*, but recombinational events are much more frequent in *Hp* than in all other bacterial species (SUERBAUM et al. 1998). The calculated homoplasy ratios of the *Hp* genes are close to 1.0, a status describing a level of free recombination, the so-called linkage equilibrium, which is the characteristic of a panmictic species. *Hp* isolates of family members could not be distinguished at any genetic locus investigated, suggesting that *Hp* clones can be transmitted within families and clonality may exist under these conditions. In the last few years, an intense discussion emerged to answer the question of which of these two mechanisms – de novo mutation or recombination – is the main driving force for genetic variation in *Hp*. As it turns out, both mechanisms might be essential to explaining the data concerning the genetic diversity in *Hp*.

2.2.2 Macro-Diversity in *Hp*

In early studies by TAYLOR et al. (1992), BUKANOV and BERG (1994) and JIANG et al. (1996), the genome maps of five independent strains were constructed by PFGE-RFLP and analysis of a cosmid library combined with cross-hybridisations and hybridisations with up to 17 specific gene probes. All five strains exhibited extensive variations of the gene arrangement in the chromosome. Among the 17 genes tested, only four were located in the same quarter of the genome (*katA*, *vacA*, *hpaA* and *pfr*), and the order of these genes was also variable (JIANG et al. 1996). The recent comparison of the genome sequences of *Hp* 26695 and J99 provided us with a detailed insight into the genome diversity on the gene arrangement level (ALM et al. 1999). About 7% of the genes in both genomes were unique, with about 50% of these genes located in a chromosomal segment, called the plasticity region. This region displays a significantly different G + C content compared with the rest of the genome, and it contains IS elements, suggesting that it might represent a pathogenicity island. To align the two chromosomes, it is necessary to introduce 10 translocations and/or inversions of DNA fragments ranging between 1 and 83kb in size. Most of the borders of these gene rearrangements contain either repeated sequence motifs or insertion elements (IS605 or IS606) or are associated with DNA-restriction/modification and outer membrane protein (*omp*) genes. Although the strains J99 and 26695 seem to be more or less closely related, it appears that the *Hp* chromosome is subjected to a permanent shuffling of genes, resulting in a huge diversity within this species.

3 Natural Transformation Competence and Gene Transfer in *Hp*

Horizontal gene transfer is an extremely efficient way for microorganisms to generate dynamic genomes and to effectively change the ecological and pathogenic character of bacterial species. As already mentioned above, *Hp* is very potent in genetic exchange, but what is the basis of this exchange? Three mechanisms of horizontal gene transfer are commonly observed in the bacterial world: natural transformation, conjugation and transduction. Although bacteriophages have been described in *Hp*, (VON HEINEGG et al. 1993) there is currently no evidence that transduction is a mechanism involved in generating genetic diversity. Furthermore, a DNase-insensitive DNA transfer between *Hp* strains in vitro has been reported (KUIPERS et al. 1998). However, proof of conjugative transfer of plasmid or chromosomal DNA between *Hp* strains, especially under colonisation conditions in vivo, is still lacking.

Natural transformation competence was reported for *Hp* several years ago (NEDENSKOV-SORENSEN et al. 1990). We described an operon consisting of four genes, *orf2*, *comB1*, *comB2* and *comB3*, identified by *blaM* transposon shuttle mutagenesis (HOFREUTER et al. 1998; HOFREUTER et al. 2000). Transposon insertions in any one of the *comB* genes drastically reduced the natural transformation competence for plasmid and chromosomal *Hp* DNA. Using a shuttle vector-based genetic complementation of the individual knockout mutant strains, we demonstrated that each of the three *comB* genes is essential for natural transformation (HOFREUTER et al. 2001). Amino acid sequence comparison revealed that ComB1, ComB2 and ComB3 are homologues of VirB8, VirB9 and VirB10, respectively, of the *Agrobacterium tumefaciens* VirB type IV secretion apparatus (see Chap. 4 for details about type IV systems). The short peptide Orf2 is a putative lipoprotein reminiscent of the *A. tumefaciens* VirB7. Thus, the ComB proteins show significant homology to the basic components of a type IV secretion system.

The *comB* genes are probably not sufficient to constitute the whole competence apparatus. Two further genes were identified in the genome sequences of *Hp* with homology to known competence genes in other bacterial species (KARUDAPURAM and BARCAK 1997), *dprA* (HP0333) and *comEC* (HP1361). A *dprA* knockout mutant in *Hp* reduces transformation efficiencies for both chromosomal and plasmid DNA about 100-fold (ANDO et al. 1999; SMEETS et al. 2000b). For ComEC, an integral membrane protein originally described in *Bacillus subtilis*, no experimental data are available for *Hp*. In addition, a novel gene essential for *Hp* competence was identified recently, termed *comH*. It seems to be restricted to *Hp*, since no significant homologues of *comH* were identified in currently available databases. The gene encodes an exported protein, which is supposed to be involved in binding or uptake of DNA (SMEETS et al. 2000a).

For several well-known transformation systems, like *Neisseria gonorrhoeae* or *B. subtilis* (FUSSENEGGER et al. 1997), type IV pilin-like molecules build a channel between the cytoplasmic and the outer membrane, or the peptidoglycan layer, respectively, which is involved in DNA uptake. In *Hp*, however, neither genes for type IV pilin-like proteins nor for a cognate type IV prepilin peptidase were found in the genome sequence (TOMB et al. 1997; ALM et al. 1999). We, therefore, postulate that in *Hp*, the type IV pilus channel is replaced by a conjugation-like type IV apparatus, originally identified for DNA and protein-export systems (HOFREUTER et al. 2001). In conjunction with natural competence, the apparatus would act as a type IV DNA import system. The putative outer membrane DNA recognition/ binding protein and the inner membrane transporter might be encoded by genes identified to be essential for natural transformation, such as *comH*, *hp0333* and possibly others, which have not been identified yet. Nevertheless, it is completely unclear whether natural transformation occurs under in vivo conditions in the human stomach. The various promising animal models should be used to clarify this question in the future.

4 The *cag*-PAI

The *cagA* gene is a marker for a large 37kb locus, consisting of 29 putative genes (CENSINI et al. 1996). The locus actually fulfils the criteria for a pathogenicity island (PAI) (HACKER et al. 1997). The sequence is only found in disease-associated strains, and the G + C content of the region (35%) differs significantly from the rest of the genome (39%). The flanking direct repeats, the presence of IS elements (IS*605*), the conserved insertion site and the tight packaging of genes associated with virulence (encoding a type IV secretion system, see below) suggested that the 37-kb region is a typical pathogenicity island. The *cag*-PAI, which was most likely acquired by horizontal gene transfer from an unknown bacterial source, is inserted at the 3′-end of the glutamate racemase gene flanked by a 31-bp direct repeat sequence (CENSINI et al. 1996). The mechanism of this transmission is unknown.

Based on the sequence data, it was speculated that the *cag*-PAI encodes a type IV secretion apparatus, able to translocate DNA or proteins into the eucaryotic host cell. Six genes with homology to operons of *Agrobacterium tumefaciens* (*virB*), *Bordetella pertussis* (*ptl*), and *E. coli* (*tra*) are scattered over the 37-kb region (COVACCI and RAPPUOLI 1998). These systems, known as type IV secretion systems (WINANS et al. 1996), are built from core components of conjugation machines. Meanwhile, the family of type IV secretion systems has been greatly expanded with the identification of additional systems involved in translocation of proteins and DNA. CHRISTIE and VOGEL (2000) suggested grouping those systems assembled from homologues of the VirB apparatus into type IVa (*A. tumefaciens virB/E. coli* pKM101, RP4α, R388, F,/*Legionella pneumophila* LvH) and those with homology to IncI/Tra, the original conjugation systems, into type IVb (*Brucella* spp. VirB/*B. pertussis*, Ptl/*Hp*, Cag/*Rickettsia prowazekii*). The *L. pneumophila* Dot/Icm and the *Shigella flexneri* IncI/Trb system would be grouped into type IVc, and other groups might follow in future.

4.1 The *cag* Type IV Secretion System

Five independent groups have shown recently that the genes of the *cag*-PAI actually encode a functional type IV secretion system and that *Hp* delivers the

CagA protein into cultured gastric epithelial cells (SEGAL et al. 1999; ODENBREIT et al. 2000; STEIN et al. 2000; BACKERT et al. 2000; ASAHI et al. 2000). CagA is immediately phosphorylated by a tyrosine residue by an as yet unidentified eucaryotic kinase, and the protein (CagA^{P-tyr}) is recruited to the membrane close to the location where the bacteria attach (SEGAL et al. 1999; ODENBREIT et al. 2000). Mutations in genes of the *cag*-PAI encoding putative components of the secretion apparatus, like the ATPase CagE, completely abolish translocation and phosphorylation, demonstrating the dependence of CagA delivery on a functional type IV secretion apparatus. A direct consequence of CagA translocation is the dephosphorylation of a complex of tyrosin-phosphorylated cellular proteins in the size of 120–130kDa (p120–130) and 80kDa (p80) (ODENBREIT et al. 2000). Comparison of independent CagA sequences reveals three putative tyrosine phosphorylation sites, one in the N-terminal region and two in the C-terminal half of the molecule. These sites are variable among different *Hp* strains, due to codon exchanges or deletions, giving rise to strains with two, one or none of these putative tyrosine-phosphorylation sites in their CagA (ODENBREIT et al. 2000). CagA is not only translocated into epithelial cells, but also into human granulocytes and macrophage cell lines. Interestingly, CagA^{P-tyr} is processed in phagocytic, but not in epithelial, cells giving rise to a tyrosine-phosphorylated 35–45kDa C-terminal fragment of CagA (ODENBREIT et al. 2001). The function of this processing and the protease involved are unknown.

4.2 Phenotypes of *Hp* Strains Carrying the *cag*-PAI

4.2.1 Chemokine Induction

In human gastric biopsy material, mRNA expression of interleukin 8 (IL-8), GRO α, ENA-78, RANTES and MCP-1, which all belong to the C-X-C group of chemokines, was found to be significantly greater in patients with *cag*A-positive *Hp*, as compared with *cag*A-negative patients (SHIMOYAMA et al. 1998). Binding of *Hp* carrying an intact *cag*-PAI to gastric epithelial cells in vitro induces the secretion of IL-8 (CRABTREE et al. 1994). *Hp* type I strains mediate gastric inflammation by activating the nuclear transcription factors kappa B (NFκB) and AP-1, which are involved in transcription of a set of proinflammatory genes in the cell. The induced signalling cascade involves the cellular stress response kinase pathway from Rho GTPases (Rac1, CDC42) via the p21-activated kinase (PAK-1) to AP-1 and NFκB activation (NAUMANN et al. 1999) (Fig. 1). CagA itself seems, however, not to be directly involved in the signalling events leading to activation of NFκB and AP-1, since isogenic mutants in *cag*A still induce IL-8 (CRABTREE et al. 1995). Interestingly, defined knockout mutations in several genes of the *cag*-PAI or a complete deletion of the PAI from the *Hp* chromosome completely abolish the activities mentioned above (MÜNZENMAIER et al. 1997; NAUMANN et al. 1999). Thus, *Hp* seems to be able to take advantage of a balanced inflammatory state in the stomach for its colonisation. A challenging question, however, is how *Hp* induces

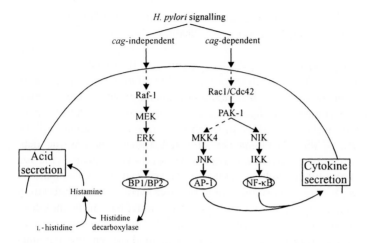

Fig. 1. Signal transduction pathways induced by *Hp*. There are two main signal transduction pathways involved in *Hp* signalling: (1) In a *cag*-dependent way, *Hp* modulates the innate immune response by activating the transcription factors AP-1 and NF-κB, which lead to an increased cytokine secretion. (2) In a *cag*-independent manner, (an) unknown *Hp* effector(s) activate(s) the transcription factors BP1 and BP2, which stimulate the histidine decarboxylase promoter. The release of histamine plays a crucial role in the activation of acid secretion in the gastric mucosa. This model has been adapted according to WESSLER et al. (2000) and FORYST-LUDWIG and NAUMANN (2000). ERK (extracellular signal-regulated kinase), MEK (mitogen-activated protein kinase/ERK kinase), MKK (mitogen-activated protein kinase kinase), JNK (c-jun N-terminal kinase), NF-κB (nuclear factor κB), NIK (NF-κB inducing kinase), IKK (IκB kinase), PAK-1 (p21-activated kinase 1), BP1/2 (gastrin-responsive element binding proteins 1/2), AP-1 (activator protein 1). *Dotted lines* correspond to indirect and *solid lines* to direct activations

the signalling cascades, whether a translocated bacterial factor besides CagA is involved, or whether binding to a cell-surface receptor, like an integrin, might transduce the signal into the cell.

4.2.2 Actin Reorganisation and Pedestal Formation

An electron microscopic study by SEGAL et al. (1996) showed that the binding of type I *Hp* strains induced an actin rearrangement and formation of cup-like pedestals, reminiscent of the situation seen with enteropathogenic *E. coli* (EPEC) (GOOSNEY et al. 1999). SU et al. (1998) reported that the Lewis[b]-independent adherence of type I, but not type II, *Hp* strains was strongly reduced by chloramphenicol and cycloheximide, inhibitors of bacterial and eucaryotic protein synthesis, respectively. They concluded that interaction might depend on one or more host cell receptors probably triggered by components of the *cag*-PAI of *Hp*. A β1 integrin-deficient cell line showed strongly reduced binding of *Hp*, as did AGS cells treated with α5- or β1-integrin-specific antibodies, as compared to the same β1-integrin-expressing transfectant (SU et al. 1999). This might indicate that β1 integrins act as receptors for the type IV secretion apparatus of *Hp*.

A further phenotype associated with the presence of CagA[P-tyr] in epithelial cells is spreading and elongated growth, the induction of lamellipodia and filapodia.

This was designated as the hummingbird phenotype (Segal et al. 1999), indicating that CagA$^{P\text{-tyr}}$ might be involved in actin reorganisation of the cell.

4.2.3 Interaction of *Hp* with Professional Phagocytes

The infection with *Hp* is chronic, and the bacteria must have evolved a mechanism whereby they can evade the attack of the immune system. The interaction of *Hp* with professional phagocytes is a topic of significant controversy. One possibility for pathogens is to avoid their own phagocytosis, a strategy that is used by *Yersinia* species, like *Y. enterocolitica* or *Y. pseudotuberculosis* (Rosqvist et al. 1988). They inject so-called Yop effector proteins (YopH) into the phagocytes to paralyse the host cell cytoskeleton, making phagocytes unable to engulf the bacteria. A similar resistance to phagocytosis by monocytes and PMNs has been reported recently for *Hp* (Ramarao et al. 2000a). The process was found to be dependent on key components of the type IV secretion system and on de novo protein synthesis in the bacteria. Binding to phagocytes induced a strong extracellular release of oxygen radicals (oxidative burst), which was, however, survived by *Hp*, due to its strong catalase activity (Ramarao et al. 2000b). In other studies, *Hp* type I strains were found to be efficiently phagocytosed by mononuclear phagocytes. Type I strains, but not type II strains, induced a so-called megasome by fusion of single phagosomal compartments and survived for a prolonged time period in this novel compartment (Allen et al. 2000). Our own studies demonstrated translocation of CagA into phagocytic cells. By comparing a wild-type and a mutant strain with a deletion of the complete *cag*-PAI, we did not find a significant difference in the number of extracellular, adherent or ingested bacteria. Furthermore, we did not observe a prolonged intracellular survival difference between groups (Odenbreit et al. 2001). Thus, our data suggest that the *cag*-PAI is neither directly involved in phagocytosis resistance nor in intracellular survival of *Hp*.

4.3 Structural Variation of the *cag*-PAI

The structure of the *cag*-PAI is extremely diverse in *Hp* strains, as indicated by comparison of complete sequences of *cag*-PAIs from independent strains and by comparison of clinical isolates by Southern hybridisation and PCR amplification (Jenks et al. 1998; Maeda et al. 1999; Slater et al. 1999) (Fig. 2). The PAI exists in certain strains as an uninterrupted unit, as found in the completely sequenced strains J99 (Alm et al. 1999) and 26695 (Tomb et al. 1997), which might represent the originally acquired form. In some strains, the PAI is, however, divided into two parts by the insertion of an IS*605* element into the middle of the gene sequence, thus generating the *cag*I and the *cag*II region (Censini et al. 1996; Tomb et al. 1997). The IS*605* element is a new type of IS-element, which carries two putative open reading frames encoding two transposases (*tnpA* and *tnpB*) (Tomb et al. 1997).

Maeda et al. (1999) addressed the question of whether the *cagA* gene is a marker for the presence of an intact *cag*-PAI in Japanese strains. The study

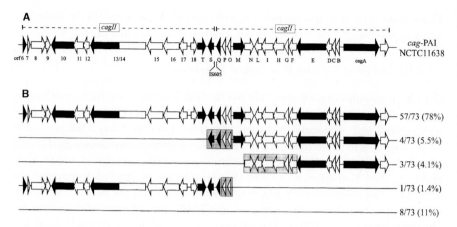

Fig. 2A,B. Variation in the structure of the *cag*-PAI. **A** Structure of the *cag*-PAI from CUGG17874 (identical to NCTC11638) as a reference. In this strain, the *cag*-PAI is interrupted by two IS605 elements and intervening chromosomal regions. **B** Detection of selected genes of the *cag*-PAI in different *Hp* isolates. Target genes were detected by PCR and/or hybridisation with specific probes. Open reading frames predicted to be present in the *cag*-PAI of the clinical isolates are indicated as *arrows*. Genes drawn in *black* hybridised to the specific probes and/or could be amplified by PCR. *Grey boxes* indicate genes of which the presence is uncertain or variable. From these data, it may be concluded that the *cag*-PAI is subject to a certain degree of variation rather than an invariable unit, the clinical significance of which cannot be evaluated so far (JENKS et al. 1998)

confirmed the high prevalence of *cagA*[+] strains in Japan (100% in this study). Only six of 63 strains did not produce the CagA protein, a similar proportion to that found in a European study (XIANG et al. 1995). Two of these strains had an intact *cag*-PAI, and induced IL-8 release from epithelial cells. The other four had sections of the *cag*-PAI missing and induced low levels of IL-8 (Fig. 2). KERSULYTE et al. (1999) investigated the fate of two strains naturally co-infecting a patient, one of which was a type I strain, whereas the other was lacking the *cag*-PAI. Interestingly, typing of the resulting hybrid strains clearly showed that the type I strain had acquired a panel of DNA-fragments from the other isolate and had lost its *cag*-PAI. Surprisingly, the sequencing of the regions flanking the *cag*-empty site revealed that the *cag*-PAI had been lost by recombination via the flanking regions rather than by excision through the direct repeats. This study suggests that at least two possible mechanisms may convert a type I strain to a *cag*⁻ strain – excision and recombination – and that this event probably occurs in the patient in vivo. Based on these data, one would argue that *cag*-PAI deletion events occurred not only distantly in evolutionary time but are an ongoing phenomenon, perhaps allowing better co-adaptation between *Hp* and its host.

4.4 Structural Variation of CagA

Not only is the *cag*-PAI diverse in its structure, but also the CagA protein itself. After the initial identification of the antigen by APEL et al. (1988), the gene was characterised on the molecular level (COVACCI et al. 1993; TUMMURU et al. 1993). They described duplications of short amino acid sequences (D1–D3) in the C-terminal part of the CagA protein. Later, YAMAOKA et al. (1998) examined 155 *cagA*-positive *Hp* isolates from Japanese patients and grouped them into types A–D, according to the nature and number of repeats at the 3′region of the gene (Fig. 3). The Japanese *cagA* genes differed markedly in the 3′-sequence from that of Western strains. Whether this structural variation of the CagA protein has some functional implications is still unresolved. Furthermore, the presence or absence of tyrosine-phosphorylation sites in CagA might be a major difference, which might have functional implications for signalling events in the cell (ODENBREIT et al. 2000). Therefore, more epidemiological studies have to be performed, and the disease outcome should be compared with the different types of CagA molecules in large controlled studies. Furthermore, we have to learn much more about the function of CagA in the eucaryotic cell.

4.5 Role of the *cag*-PAI in Colonisation

In humans there is a correlation between infection with *Hp* type I organisms and occurrence of peptic ulcers and cancer. Interestingly, in Korea and Japan 100% of the isolates are *cagA*$^+$, whereas in other parts of the world 60%–70% of isolates are reported to be *cagA*$^+$. Colonisation with type I strains has been reported to occur with higher cell densities in vivo (fourfold higher) compared with *cagA*$^-$ strains, as determined by PCR and quantitative culture from gastric biopsy

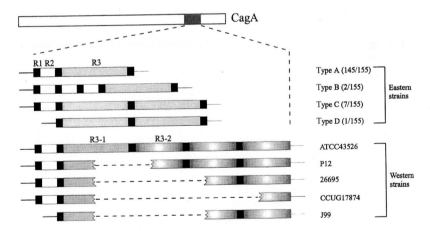

Fig. 3. Sequence variation in the C-terminal part of CagA proteins. Size variation of CagA is predominantly due to the different number of repeated amino acid units in its C-terminal region. Whereas R1 and R2 repeats are conserved among *Hp* strains, the R3 repeats are markedly different between Eastern and Western strains, suggesting some clonal grouping of strains concerning the *cagA* gene. The partial deletion of R3–1 and R3–2 repeats can lead to the fusion of both repeats. CagA sequences: Eastern strains, ATCC43526 and CCUG 17874 (YAMAOKA et al. 1998). P12 (ODENBREIT et al. 2000). 26695 (TOMB et al. 1997), J99 (ALM et al. 1999)

specimens (ATHERTON et al. 1996). In the Mongolian gerbil animal model, mutations in *cagA* and *vacA* did not abolish colonisation of *Hp*, whereas a *ureA*-negative mutant was not able to colonise (WIRTH et al. 1998). The isolation and comparison of multiple colonies from a single human gastric biopsy often reveals pairs of *cag*[+] and *cag*[−] isolates with identical fingerprints (VAN DER ENDE et al. 1996). This indicates that there might be an equilibrium of *cag*[+] and *cag*[−] bacteria in the stomach, which changes to a predominance of *cag*[+] *Hp* during acute phases of disease and switches to an overgrowth of *cag*[−] bacteria during remission phases (COVACCI et al. 1999).

5 *Hp* and Host Adaptation

5.1 Variation of the LPS Structure

5.1.1 *Hp* and Molecular Mimicry

In 1991, Negrini et al. histochemically demonstrated that specific human *Hp* antibodies and serum antibodies originating from mouse infection experiments react with the gastric mucosa. Thus, *Hp*-induced autoantibodies might influence the severity of gastritis observed upon *Hp* infection. Further studies strongly associated IgG autoantibodies with the *Hp* infection status, the degree of inflammation and the phenomenon of gastric atrophy (FALLER et al. 1996; NEGRINI et al. 1996). But what are the targets of these autoantibodies? First hints to the answer to this question came from SHERBURNE and TAYLOR (1995), who could identify the Lewis[x] structure on the surface of *Hp* reacting with autoantibodies by immuno-electron microscopy studies. This antigen, which (together with Lewis[y]) belongs to the so-called type-2 chain Lewis (=Le[x/y]) antigens (Fig. 4A), is expressed on the surface of gastric cells, adenocarcinoma and some phagocytic cells (SAKAMOTO et al. 1989). In several investigations, Le[x] and/or Le[y] was found to build up the terminal oligomeric structures of the *Hp* LPS (ASPINALL et al. 1996; ASPINALL and MONTEIRO 1996; SIMOONS-SMIT et al. 1996). In addition to Le[x/y], the presence of type I chain Le[a], Le[b] and Le[d] (H-type 1) epitopes were also found in some *Hp* isolates (MONTEIRO et al. 1998). APPELMELK et al. (1997) discussed the Lewis[x/y]-driven molecular mimicry between *Hp* and its host and the consequences for the disease. Thus, the nature of molecular mimicry is well established, but the clear impact of autoreactivity of specific *Hp* antibodies upon development of gastritis and other outcomes of disease has to be proven in more detail.

5.1.2 Slipped Strand Mispairing Regulates Expression of Fucosyltransferase Genes

From several bacterial pathogens, like pathogenic *Neisseria* species (STERN and MEYER 1987) and *Haemophilus influenzae* (WEISER et al. 1989), it is known that

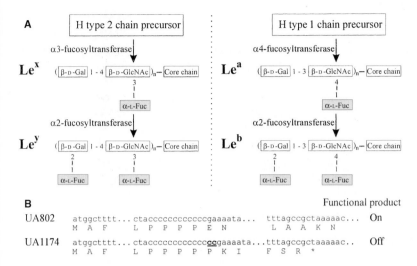

Fig. 4A,B. Variation of the *Hp* LPS pattern by switching of fucosyltransferase genes. **A** Synthesis of the different Lewis antigens starting from the respective H type chain precursor (*N*-acetyllactosamine). Alternatively, the Le^y/Le^b antigens can be synthesized by fucosylation of the mono-fucosylated H-type chains (Fucα1–2Galβ1–3GlcNAc = H type1, Fucα1–2Galβ1–4GlcNAc = H type2). **B** Switching of the α2-fucosyltransferase gene (*fucT2*) by slipped strand mispairing. The insertion of additional C-nucleotides within the poly-(C) tract by slippage of the DNA-polymerase causes a shifting of the open reading frame and the abrogation of the gene product (WANG et al. 1999b)

homopolymeric tracts of nucleotides or repeated oligonucleotides within genes or promoter regions can lead to mistakes during the replication of the chromosome. These changes in the number of such repeated sequences may cause the abrogation of an intact open reading frame or modulate the promoter activity of such a gene. This switching (on/off), which is called slipped strand mispairing (SSM) (Fig. 4B), occurs with distinct frequency and is dependent on the nature of the DNA poly-merase. The sequencing of the *Hp* genomes and the specific search for such re-peated sequences identified a panel of some 20–30 phase-variable genes (SAUNDERS et al. 1998), most of which are involved in the synthesis of LPS structures, in DNA restriction/modification systems or belong to the large outer membrane protein (Omp) family. It has been speculated that switching of the surface-exposed struc-tures might have some impact on the adaptation of *Hp* to different host structures (ALM et al. 1999).

The molecular basis of Lewis antigen expression in *Hp* is the presence of different fucosyltransferase genes, which link fucose residues to a poly-*N*-Acetyl-lactosamine core chain in specific ways. In the genome sequence of *Hp* 26695 (TOMB et al. 1997) two α3-fucosyltransferase genes (*hp379* and *hp651*) have been identified conferring the α1–3 linkage to the glucosamin residue (Le^x), genes that later were annotated as the *futA* and *futB* genes, respectively (APPELMELK et al. 1999). In addition to the α3-fucosyltransferase, for Le^y expression (α1–2 linkage to galactose) an α2-fucosyltransferase is required, which is encoded by the *fucT2* gene (WANG et al. 1999b). All three fucosyltransferase genes exhibited homopolymeric (C)-tracts in the 5′-region leading to an intact or frame-shifted gene product (APPELMELK et al. 1999; WANG et al. 1999b). For instance, whereas *Hp* NCTC11637 expressing an intact *futA* gene presents Lewis$^{x/y}$ structures on the surface, a phase variant defective in both *futA* and *futB* cannot produce any fucosylated epitopes (APPELMELK et al. 1999).

Due to the extensive possibilities of *Hp* changing its LPS structure and thus modulating its surface interaction with the host, this large pool of bacterial phenotypes might give this pathogen the chance to successively adapt to the respective niche of its host. Whether the autoimmune response challenged by Lewis-antigens provides *Hp* with any specific advantage of surviving and persistently colonising the gastric mucosa is not clear, but it must be taken into consideration that the molecular mimicry increases the degree of gastric inflammation.

5.2 Variation in Adherence Properties of *Hp*

It is believed that the adherence of *Hp* to gastric epithelium is a prerequisite for efficient colonization and provides the possibility for cross-talk between *Hp* and its host. In the *Hp* genome, some 30 genes have been classified as genes encoding outer membrane proteins (Omp), some of which are believed to be functional adhesins. The Omp proteins exhibit more or less conserved regions in the *N*-terminus and the *C*-terminus, respectively, whereas the middle region is quite variable. When the sequences of the strains J99 and 26695 were compared with each other, it became evident that most *omp* genes had a homologous counterpart in the other strain. Because of this obviously large amount of related DNA sequences, it was assumed that these genes might be targets for frequent recombination and gene shuffling, leading to a mosaic-like structure of the *omp* genes (TOMB et al. 1997). One proof for this hypothesis might be the inversion no. 6, which was necessary to align the sequences of the two *Hp* genomes (ALM et al. 1999): in a comparison of both sequences, it was stated that the so-called *babA* (*hp1243*/*jhp833*) and *babB* (*hp896*/*jhp1164*) genes (ILVER et al. 1998) had been reciprocally exchanged – maybe within their conserved C-terminal domain. It is interesting that strain 26695 is deficient in Le^b-binding (ILVER et al. 1998), whereas strain J99 produces an adherence-competent BabA protein recognizing the Le^b-antigen (T. Borén, personal communication). Other *omp* genes are closely associated with IS elements (*hp25*, *hp722* and *hp912*/*913*) or repeated sequences (*hp227*, *hp317*, *hp477*, *hp722*, *hp725*, *hp896*, *hp923*, *hp1243* and *hp1342*), which are predestined hot spots for recombination events. These examples support the presumption that genomic diversity can influence adherence and thus the colonisation properties of *Hp*.

As already discussed in the LPS section, SSM also seems to play a role in the phase variation of several *omp* genes. In contrast to the LPS biosynthesis genes, the *omp* genes usually switch by varying the number of (CT)-dinucleotide repeats. Interestingly, *hopZ*, one of the phase-variable *omp* genes (*hp9*/*jhp7*-homologous) was described as conferring in vitro-binding of *Hp* ATCC43504 (identical to NCTC11637) to the gastric carcinoma cell line AGS (PECK et al. 1999). An isogenic *hopZ* mutant was severely reduced in adhesion. Although the correlation between phase variation of *omp* genes and adherence is not statistically proven, it seems feasible to postulate that besides recombination events, SSM might be involved in changing the adhesin pattern of particular strains and might, thus, modulate the host-specific adaptation and targeting.

6 Conclusions and Perspectives

Hp is one of the most common bacterial pathogens worldwide. In terms of its chromosomal DNA sequence, *Hp* strains are very diverse, but the proteins encoded are rather conserved between different strains. This genetic variation is discussed as a result of an elevated mutation rate within the species *Hp*, combined with an extremely high frequency of horizontal gene transfer and recombination between strains. This high genetic variability might play a substantial role in modulation of gene expression and/or in generating subtle changes in protein antigenic epitopes for immune evasion or specific enzymatic functions involved in host adaptation. The *cag*-PAI encodes a functional type IV secretion system, which is involved in injection of the bacterial protein CagA into eucaryotic cells and induction of IL-8 secretion from epithelial cells. In fresh clinical isolates, the *cag*-PAI is frequently deleted, either partially or completely, indicating that the bacteria are facing situations in which the secretion system might have disadvantages for the bacteria or are just dispensable. In future, the development of new animal models should allow better understanding of the mode of action of putative *Hp* pathogenicity factors. Since the infection with *Hp* in the gerbil model induces inflammation, ulcers and gastric cancer similar to that in humans, it might be possible in future to study the impact of putative virulence factors (*cag*-PAI, Omp- and LPS-variation) on the disease outcome in vivo.

Acknowledgements. Work in the institute of the authors is mainly supported by the Deutsche Forschungsgemeinschaft (DFG) (HA 2697/2-2) and (HA 2697/1-3). We thank Dr. W. Fischer and Dr. B.P. Burns for helpful suggestions on the manuscript.

References

Akopyanz N, Bukanov N, Westblom TU, Berg DE (1992a) PCR-based RFLP analysis of DNA sequence diversity in the gastric pathogen *Helicobacter pylori*. Nucleic Acids Res 20:6221–6225
Akopyanz N, Bukanov NO, Westblom TU, Kresovich S, Berg DE (1992b) DNA diversity among clinical isolates of *Helicobacter pylori* detected by PCR-based RAPD fingerprinting. Nucleic Acids Res 20:5137–5142

18   S. Odenbreit and R. Haas

Allen LA, Schlesinger LS, Kang B (2000) Virulent strains of *Helicobacter pylori* demonstrate delayed phagocytosis and stimulate homotypic phagosome fusion in macrophages. J Exp Med 191:115–128

Alm RA, Ling LS, Moir DT, King BL, Brown ED, Doig PC, Smith DR, Noonan B, Guild BC, deJonge BL, Carmel G, Tummino PJ, Caruso A, Uria-Nickelsen M, Mills DM, Ives C, Gibson R, Merberg D, Mills SD, Jiang Q, Taylor DE, Vovis GF, Trust TJ (1999) Genomic-sequence comparison of two unrelated isolates of the human gastric pathogen *Helicobacter pylori*. Nature 397:176–180

Ando T, Israel DA, Kusugami K, Blaser MJ (1999) HP0333, a member of the *dprA* family, is involved in natural transformation in *Helicobacter pylori*. J Bacteriol 181:5572–5580

Apel I, Jacobs E, Kist M, Bredt W (1988) Antibody response of patients against a 120kd surface protein of *Campylobacter pylori*. Zentralbl Bakteriol Mikrobiol Hyg 268:271–276

Appelmelk BJ, Martin SL, Monteiro MA, Clayton CA, McColm AA, Zheng P, Verboom T, Maaskant JJ, van den Eijnden DH, Hokke CH, Perry MB, Vandenbroucke-Grauls CM, Kusters JG (1999) Phase variation in *Helicobacter pylori* lipopolysaccharide due to changes in the lengths of poly(C) tracts in alpha3-fucosyltransferase genes. Infect Immun 67:5361–5366

Appelmelk BJ, Negrini R, Moran AP, Kuipers EJ (1997) Molecular mimicry between *Helicobacter pylori* and the host. Trends Microbiol 5:70–73

Asahi M, Azuma T, Ito S, Ito Y, Suto H, Nagai Y, Tsubokawa M, Tohyama Y, Maeda S, Omata M, Suzuki T, Sasakawa C (2000) *Helicobacter pylori* CagA protein can be tyrosine phosphorylated in gastric epithelial cells. J Exp Med 191:593–602

Aspinall GO, Monteiro MA (1996) Lipopolysaccharides of *Helicobacter pylori* strains P466 and MO19: structures of the O-antigen and core oligosaccharide regions. Biochemistry 35:2498–2504

Aspinall GO, Monteiro MA, Pang H, Walsh EJ, Moran AP (1996) Lipopolysaccharide of the *Helicobacter pylori* type strain NCTC-11637 (ATCC-43504) – structure of the O-antigen chain and core oligosaccharide regions. Biochemistry 35:2489–2497

Atherton JC, Tham KT, Peek RM, Cover TL, Blaser MJ (1996) Density of *Helicobacter pylori* infection in vivo as assessed by quantitative culture and histology. J Infect Dis 174:552–556

Backert S, Ziska E, Brinkmann V, Zimny-Arndt U, Fauconnier A, Jungblut PR, Naumann M, Meyer TF (2000) Translocation of the *Helicobacter pylori* CagA protein in gastric epithelial cells by a type IV secretion apparatus. Cell Microbiol 2:155–164

Blaser MJ (1992) Hypotheses on the pathogenesis and natural history of *Helicobacter pylori*-induced inflammation. Gastroenterology 102:720–727

Borén T, Falk P, Roth KA, Larson G, Normark S (1993) Attachment of *Helicobacter pylori* to human gastric epithelium mediated by blood group antigens. Science 262:1892–1895

Bukanov NO, Berg DE (1994) Ordered cosmid library and high-resolution physical-genetic map of *Helicobacter pylori* strain NCTC11638. Mol Microbiol 11:509–523

Censini S, Lange C, Xiang ZY, Crabtree JE, Ghiara P, Borodovsky M, Rappuoli R, Covacci A (1996) Cag, a pathogenicity island of *Helicobacter pylori*, encodes type I-specific and disease-associated virulence factors. Proc Natl Acad Sci USA 93:14648–14653

Christie PJ, Vogel JP (2000) Bacterial type IV secretion: conjugation systems adapted to deliver effector molecules to host cells. Trends Microbiol 8:354–360

Covacci A, Censini S, Bugnoli M, Petracca R, Burroni D, Macchia G, Massone A, Papini E, Xiang Z, Figura N, Rappuoli R (1993) Molecular characterization of the 128-kDa immunodominant antigen of *Helicobacter pylori* associated with cytotoxicity and duodenal ulcer. Proc Natl Acad Sci USA 90:5791–5795

Covacci A, Rappuoli R (1998) *Helicobacter pylori*: molecular evolution of a bacterial quasi- species. Curr Opin Microbiol 1:96–102

Covacci A, Telford JL, Del Giudice G, Parsonnet J, Rappuoli R (1999) *Helicobacter pylori* virulence and genetic geography. Science 284:1328–1333

Cover TL, Blaser MJ (1992) Purification and characterization of the vacuolating toxin from *Helicobacter pylori*. J Biol Chem 267:10570–10575

Cover TL, Tummuru MKR, Cao P, Thompson S, Blaser MJ (1994) Divergence of genetic sequences for the vacuolating cytotoxin among *Helicobacter pylori* strains. J Biol Chem 269:10566–10573

Crabtree JE, Farmery SM, Lindley IJD, Figura N, Peichl P, Tompkins DS (1994) CagA/cytotoxic strains of *Helicobacter pylori* and interleukin-8 in gastric epithelial cell lines. J Clin Pathol 47:945–950

Crabtree JE, Xiang Z, Lindley IJD, Tompkins DS, Rappuoli R, Covacci A (1995) Induction of inter-leukin-8 secretion from gastric epithelial cells by a cagA negative isogenic mutant of *Helicobacter pylori*. J Clin Pathol 48:967–969

Dore MP, Osato MS, Malaty HM, Graham DY (2000) Characterization of a culture method to recover *Helicobacter pylori* from the feces of infected patients. Helicobacter 5:165–168

Eaton KA, Brooks CL, Morgan DR, Krakowka S (1991) Essential role of urease in pathogenesis of gastritis induced by *Helicobacter pylori* in gnotobiotic piglets. Infect Immun 59:2470–2475

Eaton KA, Suerbaum S, Josenhans C, Krakowka S (1996) Colonization of gnotobiotic piglets by *Helicobacter pylori* deficient in 2 flagellin genes. Infect Immun 64:2445–2448

Evans DG, Queiroz DM, Mendes EN, Evans DJ Jr. (1998) *Helicobacter pylori cagA* status and s and m alleles of *vacA* in isolates from individuals with a variety of *H. pylori*-associated gastric diseases. J Clin Microbiol 36:3435–3437

Evans Jr DJ, Evans DG, Takemura T, Nakano H, Lampert HC, Graham DY, Granger DN, Kvietys PR (1995) Characterization of a *Helicobacter pylori* neutrophil-activating protein. Infect Immun 63:2213–2220

Faller G, Steininger H, Eck M, Hensen J, Hahn EG, Kirchner T (1996) Antigastric autoantibodies in *Helicobacter pylori* gastritis: prevalence, in-situ binding-sites and clues for clinical relevance. Virchows Arch 427:483–486

Fischer W, Haas R (1999) *Helicobacter pylori* vacuolating cytotoxin. In: Aktories K, Just I (eds) Handbook of Experimental Pharmacology. Springer-Verlag, Berlin, pp 489–507

Forman D, Coleman M, Debacker G, Eider J, Moller H, Damotta LC, Roy P, Abid L, Tjonneland A, Boeing H, Haubrich T, Wahrendorf J, Manousos O, Tulinius H, Ogmundsdottir H, Palli D, Cipriani F, Fukao A, Tsugane S, Miyajima Y, Zatonski W, Tyczynski J, Calheiros J, Zakelj MP, Potocnik M, Webb P, Knight T, Wilson A, Kaye S, Potter J (1993) An international association between *Helicobacter pylori* infection and gastric cancer. Lancet 341:1359–1362

Foryst-Ludwig A, Naumann M (2000) PAK1 activates the NIK-IKK NF-kappaB pathway and proinflammatory cytokines in *H. pylori*-infection. J Biol Chem 15;275(50):39779–85

Fussenegger M, Rudel T, Barten R, Ryll R, Meyer TF (1997) Transformation competence and type-4 pilus biogenesis in *Neisseria gonorrhoeae* – a review. Gene 192:125–134

Gerhard M, Hirno S, Wadström T, Miller-Podraza H, Teneberg S, Karlsson K-A, Appelmelk B, Odenbreit S, Haas R, Arnquvist A, Borén T (2000) *Helicobacter pylori*, an adherent pain in the stomach. In: Achtman M, Suerbaum S (eds) *Helicobacter pylori*: Molecular and Cellular Biology. Horizon Scientific Press, Wymondham, UK

Goosney DL, de Grado M, Finlay BB (1999) Putting *E. coli* on a pedestal: a unique system to study signal transduction and the actin cytoskeleton. Trends Cell Biol 9:11–14

Hacker J, Blum-Oehler G, Muhldorfer I, Tschäpe H (1997) Pathogenicity islands of virulent bacteria: structure, function and impact on microbial evolution. Mol Microbiol 23:1089–1097

Hofreuter D, Odenbreit S, Henke G, Haas R (1998) Natural competence for DNA transformation in *Helicobacter pylori*: identification and genetic characterization of the *comB* locus. Mol Microbiol 28:1027–1038

Hofreuter D, Odenbreit S, Puls J, Schwan D, Haas R (2000) Genetic competence in *Helicobacter pylori*: mechanisms and biological implications. Res Microbiol 151:487–491

Hofreuter D, Odenbreit S, Haas R (2001) Natural transformation competence in *Helicobacter pylori* is mediated by the basic components of a type IV secretion system. Mol Microbiol 41:379–391

Hollingsworth NM, Ponte L, Halsey C (1995) MSH5, a novel MutS homolog, facilitates meiotic reciprocal recombination between homologs in *Saccharomyces cerevisiae* but not mismatch repair. Genes Dev 9:1728–1739

Horst JP, Wu TH, Marinus MG (1999) *Escherichia coli* mutator genes. Trends Microbiol 7:29–36

Ilver D, Arnqvist A, Ogren J, Frick IM, Kersulyte D, Incecik ET, Berg DE, Covacci A, Engstrand L, Borén T (1998) *Helicobacter pylori* adhesin binding fucosylated histo-blood group antigens revealed by retagging. Science 279:373–377

Jakobsen IB, Easteal S (1996) A program for calculating and displaying compatibility matrices as an aid in determining reticulate evolution in molecular sequences. Comput Appl Biosci 12:291–295

Jenks PJ, Megraud F, Labigne A (1998) Clinical outcome after infection with *Helicobacter pylori* does not appear to be reliably predicted by the presence of any of the genes of the *cag* pathogenicity island. Gut 43:752–758

Jiang Q, Hiratsuka K, Taylor DE (1996) Variability of gene order in different *Helicobacter pylori* strains contributes to genome diversity. Mol Microbiol 20:833–842

Kansau I, Raymond J, Bingen E, Courcoux P, Kalach N, Bergeret M, Braimi N, Dupont C, Labigne A (1996) Genotyping of *Helicobacter pylori* isolates by sequencing of PCR products and comparison with the RAPD technique. Res Microbiol 147:661–669

Karudapuram S, Barcak GJ (1997) The *Haemophilus influenzae dprABC* genes constitute a competence-inducible operon that requires the product of the *tfoX* (*sxy*) gene for transcriptional activation. J Bacteriol 179:4815–4820

Kersulyte D, Chalkauskas H, Berg DE (1999) Emergence of recombinant strains of *Helicobacter pylori* during human infection. Mol Microbiol 31:31–43

Kuipers EJ, Israel DA, Kusters JG, Blaser MJ (1998) Evidence for a conjugation-like mechanism of DNA transfer in *Helicobacter pylori*. J Bacteriol 180:2901–2905

Langenberg W, Rauws EA, Widjojokusumo A, Tytgat GN, Zanen HC (1986) Identification of *Campylobacter pyloridis* isolates by restriction endonuclease DNA analysis. J Clin Microbiol 24:414–417

Maeda S, Yoshida H, Ikenoue T, Ogura K, Kanai F, Kato N, Shiratori Y, Omata M (1999) Structure of *cag* pathogenicity island in Japanese *Helicobacter pylori* isolates. Gut 44:336–341

Majewski SIH, Goodwin CS (1988) Restriction endonuclease analysis of the genome of *Campylobacter pylori* with a rapid extraction method: evidence for considerable genomic variation. J Infect Dis 157:465–471

Maynard SJ, Smith NH (1998) Detecting recombination from gene trees. Mol Biol Evol 15:590–599

Monteiro MA, Chan KH, Rasko DA, Taylor DE, Zheng PY, Appelmelk BJ, Wirth HP, Yang M, Blaser MJ, Hynes SO, Moran AP, Perry MB (1998) Simultaneous expression of type 1 and type 2 Lewis blood group antigens by *Helicobacter pylori* lipopolysaccharides. Molecular mimicry between *H. pylori* lipopolysaccharides and human gastric epithelial cell surface glycoforms. J Biol Chem 273:11533–11543

Münzenmaier A, Lange C, Glocker E, Covacci A, Moran A, Bereswill S, Baeuerle PA, Kist M, Pahl HL (1997) A secreted/shed product of *Helicobacter pylori* activates transcription factor nuclear factor-kappa B. J Immunol 159:6140–6147

Naumann M, Wessler S, Bartsch C, Wieland B, Covacci A, Haas R, Meyer TF (1999) Activation of activator protein 1 and stress response kinases in epithelial cells colonized by *Helicobacter pylori* encoding the *cag* pathogenicity island. J Biol Chem 274:31655–31662

Nedenskov-Sorensen P, Bukholm G, Bovre K (1990) Natural competence for genetic transformation in *Campylobacter pylori*. J Infect Dis 161:365–366

Negrini R, Lisato L, Zanella I, Cavazzini L, Gullini S, Villanacci V, Poiesi C, Albertini A, Ghielmi S (1991) *Helicobacter pylori* infection induces antibodies cross-reacting with human gastric mucosa. Gastroenterology 101:437–445

Negrini R, Savio A, Poiesi C, Appelmelk BJ, Buffoli F, Paterlini A, Cesari P, Graffeo M, Vaira D, Franzin G (1996) Antigenic mimicry between *Helicobacter pylori* and gastric mucosa in the pathogenesis of body atrophic gastritis. Gastroenterology 111:655–665

Odenbreit S, Till M, Hofreuter D, Faller G, Haas R (1999) Genetic and functional characterisation of the *alpAB* gene locus essential for adhesion of *Helicobacter pylori* to human gastric tissue. Mol Microbiol 31:1537–1548

Odenbreit S, Püls J, Sedlmaier B, Gerland E, Fischer W, Haas R (2000) Translocation of *Helicobacter pylori* CagA into gastric epithelial cells by type IV secretion. Science 287:1497–1500

Odenbreit S, Gebert B, Püls J, Fischer W, Haas R (2001) Interaction of *Helicobacter pylori* with professional phagocytes: role of the *cag* pathogenicity island and translocation, phosphorylation and specific processing of CagA. Cell Microbiol Jan;3(1):21–31

Owen RJ, Fraser J, Costas M, Morgan D, Morgan DR (1990) Signature patterns of DNA restriction fragments of *Helicobacter pylori* before and after treatment. J Clin Pathol 43:646–649

Papini E, Satin B, Bucci C, Debernard M, Telford JL, Manetti R, Rappuoli R, Zerial M, Montecucco C (1997) The small GTP-binding protein Rab7 is essential for cellular vacuolation induced by *Helicobacter pylori* cytotoxin. EMBO J 16:15–24

Park SM, Park J, Kim JG, Cho HD, Cho JH, Lee DH, Cha YJ (1998) Infection with *Helicobacter pylori* expressing the *cagA* gene is not associated with an increased risk of developing peptic ulcer diseases in Korean patients. Scand J Gastroenterol 33:923–927

Peck B, Ortkamp M, Diehl KD, Hundt E, Knapp B (1999) Conservation, localization and expression of HopZ, a protein involved in adhesion of *Helicobacter pylori*. Nucleic Acids Res 27:3325–3333

Ramarao N, Gray-Owen SD, Backert S, Meyer TF (2000a) *Helicobacter pylori* inhibits phagocytosis by professional phagocytes involving type IV secretion components. Mol Microbiol 37:1389–1404

Ramarao N, Gray-Owen SD, Meyer TF (2000b) *Helicobacter pylori* induces but survives the extracellular release of oxygen radicals from professional phagocytes using its catalase activity. Mol Microbiol 38:103–113

Rosqvist R, Bolin I, Wolf-Watz H (1988) Inhibition of phagocytosis in *Yersinia pseudotuberculosis*: a virulence plasmid-encoded ability involving the Yop2b protein. Infect Immun 56:2139–2143

Rothenbacher D, Bode G, Berg G, Knayer U, Gonser T, Adler G, Brenner H (1999) *Helicobacter pylori* among preschool children and their parents: evidence of parent-child transmission. J Infect Dis 179:398–402

Sakamoto J, Watanabe T, Tokumaru T, Takagi H, Nakazato H, Lloyd KO (1989) Expression of lewis[a], lewis[b], lewis[x], lewis[y], sialyl-lewis[a], and sialyl-lewis[x] blood group antigens in human gastric carcinoma and in normal gastric tissue. Cancer Res 49:745–752

Satin B, Del Giudice G, Della Bianca V, Dusi S, Laudanna C, Tonello F, Kelleher D, Rappuoli R, Montecucco C, Rossi F (2000) The neutrophil-activating protein (HP-NAP) of *Helicobacter pylori* is a protective antigen and a major virulence factor. J Exp Med 191:1467–1476

Saunders NJ, Peden JF, Hood DW, Moxon ER (1998) Simple sequence repeats in the *Helicobacter pylori* genome. Mol Microbiol 27:1091–1098

Schmitt W, Haas R (1994) Genetic analysis of the *Helicobacter pylori* vacuolating cytotoxin: structural similarities with the IgA protease type of exported protein. Mol Microbiol 12:307–319

Segal ED, Cha J, Lo J, Falkow S, Tompkins LS (1999) Altered states: involvement of phosphorylated CagA in the induction of host cellular growth changes by *Helicobacter pylori*. Proc Natl Acad Sci USA 96:14559–14564

Segal ED, Falkow S, Tompkins LS (1996) *Helicobacter pylori* attachment to gastric cells induces cytoskeletal rearrangements and tyrosine phosphorylation of host cell proteins. Proc Natl Acad Sci USA 93:1259–1264

Sherburne R, Taylor DE (1995) *Helicobacter pylori* expresses a complex surface carbohydrate, Lewis[x]. Infect Immun 63:4564–4568

Shimoyama T, Everett SM, Dixon MF, Axon AT, Crabtree JE (1998) Chemokine mRNA expression in gastric mucosa is associated with *Helicobacter pylori cagA* positivity and severity of gastritis. J Clin Pathol 51:765–770

Simoons-Smit IM, Appelmelk BJ, Verboom T, Negrini R, Penner JL, Aspinall GO, Moran AP, She FF, Shi BS, Rudnica W, Savio A, Degraaff J (1996) Typing of *Helicobacter pylori* with monoclonal antibodies against lewis antigens in lipopolysaccharide. J Clin Microbiol 34:2196–2200

Slater E, Owen RJ, Williams M, Pounder RE (1999) Conservation of the *cag* pathogenicity island of *Helicobacter pylori*: associations with vacuolating cytotoxin allele and IS605 diversity. Gastroenterology 117:1308–1315

Smeets LC, Bijlsma JJ, Boomkens SY, Vandenbroucke-Grauls CM, Kusters JG (2000a) *comH*, a novel gene essential for natural transformation of *Helicobacter pylori*. J Bacteriol 182:3948–3954

Smeets LC, Bijlsma JJ, Kuipers EJ, Vandenbroucke-Grauls CM, Kusters JG (2000b) The *dprA* gene is required for natural transformation of *Helicobacter pylori*. FEMS Immunol Med Microbiol 27:99–102

Stein M, Rappuoli R, Covacci A (2000) Tyrosine phosphorylation of the *Helicobacter pylori* CagA antigen after *cag*-driven host cell translocation. Proc Natl Acad Sci USA 97:1263–1268

Stern A, Meyer TF (1987) Common mechanism controlling phase and antigenic variation in pathogenic *Neisseriae*. Mol Microbiol 1:5–12

Stolte M, Eidt S (1993) Healing gastric MALT lymphomas by eradicating *H pylori*. Lancet 342:568

Su B, Hellstrom PM, Rubio C, Celik J, Granstrom M, Normark S (1998) Type I *Helicobacter pylori* shows Lewis(b)-independent adherence to gastric cells requiring de novo protein synthesis in both host and bacteria. J Infect Dis 178:1379–1390

Su B, Johansson S, Fallman M, Patarroyo M, Granstrom M, Normark S (1999) Signal transduction-mediated adherence and entry of *Helicobacter pylori* into cultured cells. Gastroenterology 117:595–604

Suerbaum S, Smith JM, Bapumia K, Morelli G, Smith NH, Kunstmann E, Dyrek I, Achtman M (1998) Free recombination within *Helicobacter pylori*. Proc Natl Acad Sci USA 95:12619–12624

Taylor DE, Eaton M, Chang N, Salama SM (1992) Construction of a *Helicobacter pylori* genome map and demonstration of diversity at the genome level. J Bacteriol 174:6800–6806

Telford JL, Ghiara P, Dell'Orco M, Commanducci M, Burroni D, Bugnoli M, Tecce MF, Censini S, Covacci A, Xiang Z, Papini E, Montecucco C, Parente L, Rappuoli R (1994) Gene structure of the *Helicobacter pylori* cytotoxin and evidence of its key role in gastric disease. J Exp Med 179:1653–1658

Thompson SA, Blaser MJ (1995) Isolation of the *Helicobacter pylori recA* gene and involvement of the *recA* region in resistance to low pH. Infect Immun 63:2185–2193

Tomb J-F, White O, Kerlavage AR, Clayton RA, Sutton GG, Fleischmann RD, Ketchum KA, Klenk HP, Gill S, Dougherty BA, Nelson K, Quakenbush J, Zhou L, Kirkness EF, Peterson S, Loftus B, Richardson D, Dodson R, Khalak HG, Glodek A, McKenney K, Fitzegerald LM, Lee N, Adams MD, Hickey EK, Berg DE, Gocayne JD, Utterback TR, Peterson JD, Kelley JM, Cotton MD, Weidman JM, Fujii C, Bowman C, Watthey L, Wallin E, Hayes WS, Borodovsky M, Karp PD, Smith HO, Fraser CM, Venter JC (1997) The complete genome sequence of the gastric pathogen *Helicobacter pylori*. Nature 388:539–547

Tonello F, Dundon WG, Satin B, Molinari M, Tognon G, Grandi G, Del Giudice G, Rappuoli R, Montecucco C (1999) The *Helicobacter pylori* neutrophil-activating protein is an iron-binding protein with dodecameric structure. Mol Microbiol 34:238–246

Tummuru MKR, Cover TL, Blaser MJ (1993) Cloning and expression of a high-molecular-mass major antigen of *Helicobacter pylori*: evidence of linkage to cytotoxin production. Infect Immun 61:1799–1809

Tummuru MKR, Cover TL, Blaser MJ (1994) Mutation of the cytotoxin-associated *cagA* Gene does not affect the vacuolating cytotoxin activity of *Helicobacter pylori*. Infect Immun 62:2609–2613

van der Ende A, Rauws EA, Feller M, Mulder CJ, Tytgat GN, Dankert J (1996) Heterogeneous *Helicobacter pylori* isolates from members of a family with a history of peptic ulcer disease. Gastroenterology 111:638–647

von Heinegg EH, Nalik HP, Schmid EN (1993) Characterisation of a *Helicobacter pylori* phage (HP1). J Med Microbiol 38:245–249

Wang G, Humayun MZ, Taylor DE (1999a) Mutation as an origin of genetic variability in *Helicobacter pylori*. Trends Microbiol 7:488–493

Wang G, Rasko DA, Sherburne R, Taylor DE (1999b) Molecular genetic basis for the variable expression of Lewis Y antigen in *Helicobacter pylori*: analysis of the alpha (1, 2) fucosyltransferase gene. Mol Microbiol 31:1265–1274

Weiser JN, Love JM, Moxon ER (1989) The molecular mechanism of phase variation of *H. influenzae* lipopolysaccharide. Cell 59:657–665

Wessler S, Höcker M, Fischer W, Wang TC, Rosewicz S, Haas R, Wiedenmann B, Meyer TF, Naumann M (2000) *Helicobacter pylori* activates the histidine decarboxylase promoter through a mitogen-activated protein kinase pathway independent of pathogenicity island-encoded virulence factors. J Biol Chem 275:3629–3636

Winans SC, Burns DL, Christie PJ (1996) Adaptation of a conjugal transfer system for the export of pathogenic macromolecules. Trends Microbiol 4:64–68

Wirth HP, Beins MH, Yang M, Tham KT, Blaser MJ (1998) Experimental infection of Mongolian gerbils with wild-type and mutant *Helicobacter pylori* strains. Infect Immun 66:4856–4866

Xiang ZY, Censini S, Bayeli PF, Telford JL, Figura N, Rappuoli R, Covacci A (1995) Analysis of expression of CagA and VacA virulence factors in 43 strains of *Helicobacter pylori* reveals that clinical isolates can be divided into two major types and that CagA is not necessary for expression of the vacuolating cytotoxin. Infect Immun 63:94–98

Yamaoka Y, Kodama T, Kashima K, Graham DY, Sepulveda AR (1998) Variants of the 3′ region of the *cagA* gene in *Helicobacter pylori* isolates from patients with different *H. pylori*-associated diseases. J Clin Microbiol 36:2258–2263

The Genus *Neisseria*: Population Structure, Genome Plasticity, and Evolution of Pathogenicity

U. Vogel and M. Frosch

1 Introduction

The genus *Neisseria* comprises at least 20 known species (Bacterial Nomenclature Up-to-Date: http://www.dsmz.de/bactnom/nam2092.htm). Several of these were isolated from humans (*N. cinerea*, *N. elongata*, *N. gonorrhoeae*, *N. lactamica*, *N. meningitidis*, *N. mucosa*, *N. sicca*, *N. subflava*, *N. weaveri*), whereas others were recovered from guinea pigs, dogs, cats, lizards and rhesus monkeys (a detailed description of neisserial taxonomy can be obtained from the following web-site: http://www.ridom.de/). With the exception of *N. gonorrhoeae*, which is a mucosal pathogen of the urogenital tract, neisserial species colonise the nasopharynx of their hosts. The human oral cavity is autochthonously colonised by *Neisseria* spp. within the first days of life (Rotimi and Duerden 1981). Colonisation of other sites have

Institut für Hygiene und Mikrobiologie, Universität Würzburg, Josef-Schneider-Strasse 2, 97080 Würzburg, Germany

been reported in children, e.g. of the mid-ear, or of the duodenum (GORDTS et al. 2000; LLOYD STILL and SHWACHMAN 1975). *N. gonorrhoeae* (the gonococcus) causes gonorrhea with an estimated annual incidence of 62 million cases per year (WHO facts sheet, http://www.who.int/HIV_AIDS/knowledge/facsheet.html). The gonococcus most likely emerged from a nasopharyngeal ancestor and adapted to the novel urogenital niche, where it is almost sexually isolated from other neisserial species (VAZQUEZ et al. 1995). It is most likely that this nasopharyngeal ancestor is shared with meningococci (*Neisseria meningitidis*). This can be inferred from chromosomal DNA/DNA hybridisation studies, which revealed an astonishing relationship between the two species (HOKE and VEDROS 1982). Another argument is provided by the fact that the complete meningococcal and gonococcal 16S rRNA sequences are 98% identical.

Next to the gonococcus, *N. meningitidis* is of outstanding relevance as a pathogen causing sporadic cases of sepsis and meningitis in toddlers and young adults (ACHTMAN 1995; JONES 1995). In addition, about 30 major epidemics, each affecting between 50 and 100,000 people, have been reported since 1971 (WHO document WHO/EMC/BAC/98.3; http://www.who.int/emc-documents/meningitis/whoemcbac983c.html). There is a discrepancy between the high colonisation rates among humans (about 10% of Europeans) but relatively low incidence rate of disease. Therefore, the meningococcus is thought to be a commensal species, which accidentally causes disease. This point of view was refined by molecular epidemiology: most meningococcal strains are avirulent commensals of the nasopharynx, which are rarely found as disease isolates. In contrast, hypervirulent meningococcal lineages, which are infrequently isolated from carriers, account for more than 90% of cases worldwide (ACHTMAN 1997; BYGRAVES et al. 1999; CAUGANT et al. 1988; WANG et al. 1993). Besides virulence attributes, additional host factors, i.e. reduced local or systemic immunity, or a disturbed mechanical barrier of the nasopharynx epithelium caused by smoking, viral illness, or even tooth extraction (CARTWRIGHT 1995; PEDERSEN et al. 1993) contribute to the development of meningococcal disease.

Infections by so-called apathogenic *Neisseria* spp. – i.e. all but *N. gonorrhoeae* and *N. meningitidis* – are very rare, and disease reports have an anecdotal character (e.g. DENNING and GILL 1991). Among the apathogenic *Neisseriae*, *N. cinerea*, *N. polysaccharaea* and *N. lactamica* are most closely related to *N. gonorrhoeae* and *N. meningitidis*. These neisserial species share a variety of common antigens with the pathogenic *Neisseriae*, e.g. lipopolysaccharide structures and porins (DERRICK et al. 1999; KIM et al. 1989; KREMASTINOU et al. 1999; TRONCOSO et al. 2000). Therefore, it is not surprising that there is convincing epidemiological evidence suggesting that *N. lactamica*, which is most prevalent in kindergarten and primary school children (BLAKEBROUGH et al. 1982; CARTWRIGHT et al. 1987; OLSEN et al. 1991; TRONCOSO et al. 2000), protects this age group from meningococcal disease (COEN et al. 2000; GOLD et al. 1978), probably by the induction of a protective humoral immunity and inhibition of meningococcal colonisation.

The observation of intra- and inter-specific horizontal gene transfer (BOWLER et al. 1994; FEIL et al. 1996, 1999; HOLMES et al. 1999; LINZ et al. 2000; SAEZ NIETO et al. 1990; SEILER et al. 1996; SMITH et al. 1999b; VAZQUEZ et al. 1995; ZHOU et al. 1992) has resulted in the description of a gene pool of *Neisseria* spp. (MAIDEN et al. 1996). The players of this gene pool and the barriers restricting it are yet to be exactly defined. It would simplify matters to view the tremendous genetic and antigenetic variability of *Neisseriae* exclusively in the light of horizontal gene transfer. Other categories of neisserial variability have to be taken into account: mutations driven by immune selection, e.g. of genes encoding the surface exposed and immunogenic porins, must be distinguished from mutations within genes whose alleles exhibit a low ratio of non-synonymous to synonymous mutations, e.g. housekeeping genes, where there is a functional constraint to keep the frequency of non-synonymous mutations as low as possible. Furthermore, there is on/off-switching of genes and phenotypes by slipped strand mispairing, which has been described in meningococci for the *opc* gene (SAKARI et al. 1994), genes necessary for capsule expression (HAMMERSCHMIDT et al. 1996; LAVITOLA et al. 1999), and porin genes (VAN DER ENDE et al. 1995). Nevertheless, the concept of horizontal gene transfer greatly enhanced the understanding of neisserial population structures and of the neisserial species concept.

Recent advances in molecular techniques resulted in a rapid increase of knowledge both of horizontal gene transfer and of genome plasticity in *Neisseria*. The basis for multilocus sequence typing (MLST) (ENRIGHT and SPRATT 1999; MAIDEN et al. 1998), which is now the gold standard for typing of genetically variable bacteria, has been laid out using multilocus enzyme electrophoresis (CAUGANT et al. 1986, 1987, 1988). Detailed restriction mapping of meningococcal and gonococcal strains revealed the genomic organization of the species (BAUTSCH 1998; BIHLMAIER et al. 1991; DEMPSEY and CANNON 1994; GAHER et al. 1996). This approach has now been pursued in genome sequencing: two meningococcal genomes have been sequenced (PARKHILL et al. 2000; TETTELIN et al. 2000); a third is in progress at the Sanger Centre (http://www.sanger.ac.uk/Projects/N_*meningitidis*/seroC.shtml), and a gonococcal genome is currently annotated at the University of Oklahoma (http://dna1.chem.ou.edu/gono.html). Differences between strains have been followed by representational difference analysis (BART et al. 2000; CLAUS et al. 2000; KLEE et al. 2000; PERRIN et al. 1999; TINSLEY and NASSIF 1996). This technique allows a rapid analysis of differences between strains. It is conceivable that this approach will be replaced in future by the micro-array technique, which is more accurate, precise and comprehensive.

2 Horizontal Gene Transfer in *Neisseria*

The identification of neisserial mosaic genes like the *iga* genes encoding the IgA1 protease (HALTER et al. 1989) or the *pbp* genes encoding penicillin binding proteins (BOWLER et al. 1994; LUJAN et al. 1991) demonstrated that transformation promotes DNA exchange between species and genera. DNA transfer in *Neisseria* is independent of the growth phase (LORENZ and WACKERNAGEL 1994). Meningococci have been shown to pick up preferentially DNA harbouring DNA uptake signals (DUS; 5'-GCCGTCTGAA) (ELKINS et al. 1991; GOODMAN and SCOCCA 1988; SMITH et al. 1999). These DUS occur frequently in the base paired stem of transcription terminators. There are far more than 1,000 DUS per genome (SMITH et al. 1999). Although DUS greatly enhance the uptake of foreign DNA, the genomes of *Neisseria* are spiked with foreign DNA of divergent nucleotide composition (CLAUS et al. 2000; FROSCH et al. 1989; KLEE et al. 2000), which obviously did not originate from the genus *Neisseria*, suggesting that DUS-independent DNA uptake occurred during evolution. *Neisseriae* incorporate most of the extra-cellular DNA in its double-stranded form, which contrasts to other well-studied models of natural transformation (BISWAS et al. 1981; CHAUSSEE et al. 1998; STEIN 1991). This special feature raised the question of whether restriction endonucleases cleaving double-stranded DNA regulate transformation in *Neisseriae*. In accordance with this hypothesis is the recent observation in our laboratory that the restriction-modification system *Nme*BI causes a moderate inhibition of transformation of meningococci carrying *nmeBI* with chromosomal DNA of a heterologous clonal grouping lacking this restriction-modification system (CLAUS et al. 2000). Therefore, the differential distribution of restriction-modification systems in meningococcal clonal groupings (CLAUS et al. 2000) points to the interesting hypothesis that the pattern of restriction-modification systems regulates communication between strains. However, this hypothesis has not been entirely proven yet.

Under experimental conditions, not all segments of the neisserial chromosome are transformed equally well. We could previously identify genetic loci designated *hrt* (high rate of transformation), which transformed meningococci with a rate 1,000-fold higher than the controls (CLAUS et al. 1998). In one locus, *hrtA*, an elevated number of DUS was found. In seven out of eight loci, high levels of the bases G and C were observed. We assumed that the high stability of GC-base pairing promotes efficient transformation. It might, however, be possible that structural features of the chromosomal loci harbouring *hrt* genes favour their accessibility to recombination.

3 Population Structure of *Neisseria* Species

The genomes of bacteria are subject to rapid evolutionary processes due to their short generation times. Macro-evolution describes long-term changes resulting into the development of new species and genera, whereas the term micro-evolution is used for rapid processes resulting into variants of a species (MORSCHHÄUSER et al. 2000). Micro-evolution comprises point mutations, allelic exchange of genes, acquisition of new genes by horizontal gene transfer, and gene loss by chromosomal deletion. The speed by which a species diversifies depends on several parameters, e.g.:

a. The generation time
b. The effectiveness of transmission and fitness profiles of single clones

c. Environmental conditions

d. The availability of foreign DNA

e. The sensitivity of the species to transformation, transduction, and conjugation

f. The effectiveness of bottlenecks

There are phylogenetically young species in which only a single sequence type has been described. *Yersinia pestis* provides an example for rarely recombining species, which did not have enough time to diversify by micro-evolution (ACHTMAN et al. 1999b). In contrast, there are freely recombining, weekly clonal species, like *H. pylori*, with a tremendous amount of unique isolates (ACHTMAN et al. 1999a; SUERBAUM 2000; SUERBAUM and ACHTMAN 1999; SUERBAUM et al. 1998). Mathematical analysis of *H. pylori* genes by the homoplasy test revealed that this species is almost panmictic (SUERBAUM 2000).

3.1 Population Structure of Meningococci

In comparison to genes of *H. pylori*, meningococcal genes show a rather low homoplasy value, suggesting the existence of clonality (SUERBAUM et al. 1998; SUERBAUM 2000). Clonality is evident, although meningococci frequently recombine (FEIL et al. 1999; HOLMES et al. 1999) and are supplied in the oral cavity with huge amounts of bacterial DNA, either isogenic or from other genera. Meningococcal clonality evolves from effective bottlenecks limiting the distribution of meningococcal variants generated during micro-evolution. In addition, variants with increased fitness tend to expand rapidly (SPRATT and MAIDEN 1999). For example, the sequence type 11 has been isolated worldwide for decades (WANG et al. 1993) and remained almost unchanged with respect to sequences of seven housekeeping genes (see the MLST web-site: http://mlst.zoo.ox.ac.uk/), which argues for rapid expansion due to increased fitness. Despite very frequent recombination, the population structure of meningococci, therefore, exhibits a relatively limited number of successful recombinant clones and clonal groupings. It should be noted that a complete picture of the population structure of meningococci will be provided in future by multilocus sequence analysis of large carriage studies, which are currently being undertaken in several laboratories including our own. Collections of carried meningococci are almost ideal for population analysis because there is no sampling bias towards hypervirulent disease isolates (SPRATT and MAIDEN 1999). With our current knowledge, however, meningococci should be placed somewhere in the middle between *Y. pestis* and *H. pylori* with regard to the dichotomy of clonality and panmixis (Fig. 1).

3.2 Clonal Groupings of Meningococci and Genetic Isolation

Most cases of meningococcal disease are caused by a few subgroups of serogroup A meningococci, electrophoretic type (ET)-5 complex meningococci, the lineage 3, the

Clonal   Panmictic

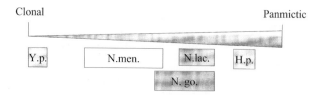

Fig. 1. Schematic illustration of the population structures of neisserial species in comparison to *Yersinia pestis* (*Y.p.*, clonal), and *Helicobacter pylori* (*H.p.*, frequently recombining, weakly clonal) on a hypothetical scale starting with clonality and ending with panmixis. *N.men.*, (*N. meningitidis*); *N.lac.*, (*N. lactamica*); *N.go.*, (*N. gonorrhoeae*)

ET-37 complex, and the cluster A4, the latter four lineages being responsible for most of the cases of serogroup B and C disease worldwide (ACHTMAN 1995). These clonal groupings are rarely found in healthy carriers but are over-represented among cases of meningococcal disease (CAUGANT et al. 1988). Unpublished work from our laboratory showed that a clone of the ET-37 complex, i.e. the ET-15 clone, was responsible for about 10% of the cases of meningococcal disease in the examined population but that it occurred only in 0.24% of strains recovered from healthy children and young adults (U. Vogel and M. Frosch, unpublished). Why are these clonal groupings maintained for decades in the human population without significant genomic alterations? As stated above, the isolation of single clones, such as the sequence type 11 of the ET-37 complex isolated from all continents for decades, argues for the extraordinary fitness of this clone.

Genetic isolation has been reported in naturally transformable bacteria despite horizontal gene transfer (LACKS and SPRINGHORN 1984; MAJEWSKI and COHAN 1998; MAJEWSKI et al. 2000; ZAWADZKI et al. 1995). Alleles of a gene can be genetically isolated by sequence divergence, e.g. a decline of recombination rates between *Bacillus* species correlated to sequence distances of the alleles analysed (ZAWADZKI et al. 1995). Plasmid and phage transfer has been shown to be controlled by restriction-modification systems in pneumococci (LACKS and SPRINGHORN 1984). It is intuitively understandable that ecological separation by a lack of physical contact plays a role in genetic isolation, e.g. the separation of the niches of gonococci and meningococci are responsible for very infrequent genetic exchange between these species (VAZQUEZ et al. 1995). Clonal groupings of meningococci share the same ecological niche. Sequence distances between alleles do not reach the distances by far reported in the experimental *Bacillus* model. Furthermore, different lineages occur in defined human populations simultaneously (CAUGANT et al. 1988). Nevertheless, we could observe by plasmid profiling and RDA a variety of differentially distributed and stable genetic markers occurring in defined hypervirulent lineages, but not in others (CLAUS et al. 2000; H. Claus and U. Vogel unpublished). Among those were plasmids, restriction-modification systems, and prophage DNA (Table 1). Other groups previously showed that *opcA* (ZHU et al. 1999), *tbpB* (ROKBI et al. 2000) and *porB* genes (CAUGANT et al. 1987) are differentially distributed. These examples show that despite frequent horizontal gene transfer, there are a variety of genetic markers, which rarely cross the border to

Table 1. Differential distribution of genes in hypervirulent lineages of meningococci

Locus	ET-37 complex	ET-5 complex	Reference
porB	Class 2	Class 3	Caugant et al. 1987
opcA	–	+	Zhu et al. 1999
tbpB	Isotype I	Isotype II	Rokbi et al. 2000
nmeAI	+	–	Claus et al. 2000
nmeBI	–	+	Claus et al. 2000
nmeDI	+	–	Claus et al. 2000
prophage 37/1–26[a]	+	–	Unpublished
pJS-B	+	–	Unpublished

[a] The prophage 37/1–26 has not been completely sequenced to date.

another clonal grouping, suggesting that genetic isolation is an important anta-
gonist to horizontal gene transfer in neisserial species. It has been unclear until now
whether this is restricted to hypervirulent lineages and whether genetic isolation is
only observed for certain genes or chromosomal fragments. Furthermore, the
mechanisms of genetic isolation have to be elucidated in future. One hypothesis
could be that clonal lineages are less easily transformable. It was recently shown
that in nature, ET-37 complex meningococci did not acquire DNA from apathogenic neisserial species as frequently as serogroup A meningococci (Linz et al.
2000). However, it is very easy to transform ET-37 complex meningococci in the
laboratory, and horizontal gene transfer to ET-37 meningococci has been observed
in vivo (Kertesz et al. 1998; Kriz et al. 2000). We, therefore, favour the hypothesis
that e.g. differentially distributed restriction-modification systems account for
barriers of transformation (Claus et al. 2000).

3.3 Population Structure of Gonococci and *N. lactamica*

It is well documented that gonococci are less clonal than meningococci (O'Rourke
and Spratt 1994; O'Rourke and Stevens 1993). Only one clonal lineage could be
determined by multilocus enzyme electrophoresis (MLEE), i.e. arginine-, hypo-
xanthine-, uracil-requiring isolates (AHU) (Gutjahr et al. 1997). In the report by
Gutjahr et al., it was suggested that AHU-isolates recombine but the derivatives do
not survive or that asymptomatic infections due to AHU-isolates are frequent,
which favours clonal spread of the isolates. Several studies indicated frequent
recombination also for other neisserial species (Feil et al. 1996; Lujan et al. 1991;
Zhou et al. 1992, 1997). Sequence typing of several apathogenic species by
sequence determination of four genes clearly indicated that recombination is so
frequent that the phylogenies of *Neisseria* should be demonstrated by phylogenetic
networks rather than by phylogenetic trees (Smith et al. 1999b). We recently typed
26 strains of *N. lactamica* isolated from epidemiologically related sources. We
found 17 genotypes; identical genotypes were epidemiologically linked (D. Alber
et al. unpublished). This finding shows that in *N. lactamica*, clonality can only be
detected in cases of direct transmission. A final judgement about the population

structure of *N. lactamica* is not possible at the moment but will be achieved by sequence typing of large worldwide and representative strain collections.

4 Genomic Rearrangements of *Neisseria* Species

We recently reported an epidemiological work-up of carrier strains isolated from healthy contacts of a case of serogroup C disease (VOGEL et al. 1998). Pulsed field gel electrophoresis of the nasopharyngeal isolate of the patient and its variant acquired from the blood culture of the patient revealed that during the passage of the nasopharynx the disease isolate lost 40kb of its chromosome. This finding illustrates a certain instability of meningococcal chromosomes.

A systematic analysis of genomic rearrangements of neisserial genomes came from the comparison of genetic maps and whole genome sequences obtained from meningcoccal and gonococcal isolates. Two gonococcal isolates (MS11 and FA1090), as well as two meningococcal isolates (B1940 [serogroup B, uncommon ET] and Z2491 [serogroup A, subgroup IV-1]), have been mapped by restriction mapping (BAUTSCH 1998; BIHLMAIER et al. 1991; DEMPSEY and CANNON 1994; GAHER et al. 1996). Furthermore, the genomes of strain Z2491, of which a restriction map is available, and of the strain MC58 (serogroup B, ET-5 complex) have been published (PARKHILL et al. 2000; TETTELIN et al. 2000). Restriction maps MS11, FA1090, B1940, and Z2491 revealed that the overall order of genes is rather conserved in *Neisseria*. However, it has been suggested that approximately 40% of the chromosomes have been subject to genome rearrangements, when gonococci and meningococci were compared (BAUTSCH 1998). The conserved gene order demonstrated by comparison of the maps obtained from the two meningococcal isolates (B1940, Z2491) is contrasted by the comparison of the genome sequences of Z2491 and MC58. A tremendous inversion of 955kb comprising almost half of the genome was revealed by comparison of the genome sequences (TETTELIN et al. 2000). The dimensions of this inversion are highly surprising, and there is need for confirmation of this result by independent methods because a restriction map of MC58 is not available. Nevertheless, it is not surprising per se that large inversions and genomic deletions occur in meningococci. The genome sequences revealed a large amount of repetitive DNA, theoretically giving rise to intra-chromosomal recombination. MC58 contains 1,980 DUS, of which almost 50% are organised as inverted repeats. Twenty-two intact insertion sequences have been found in this strain. The report of the Z2491 sequence (PARKHILL et al. 2000) focused especially on repeated DNA. Fourteen copies of IS*1016* were found, 22 of IS*1106*, and 7 of IS*1655*. Besides 1,892 DUS, there were hundreds of other repeat elements (Correia elements, AT-rich elements, RS-elements). It was suggested that the abundance of repeats contributes to the genome fluidity of the meningococcal genome, and theoretical evidence was provided that antigenic variation of many genes is driven in part by repeat mediated genomic rearrangements.

5 Evolution of Pathogenicity

Two distinct neisserial diseases developed during evolution of humans and *Neisseriae*. Gonococci cause urogenital inflammation and purulent infection, which might lead to severe pelvic inflammatory disease. Serogroup A, B, C, W135 and Y meningococci cause sepsis and meningitis. Furthermore, serogroup Y meningococci have been observed in broncho-pulmonary infections (ROSENSTEIN et al. 1999). The isolation of gonococci from the human urogenital tract is a pathological finding, whereas colonisation by meningococci only under certain circumstances results in meningococcal disease. A major difference between meningococci and gonococci is that virulence in gonococci does not disrupt transmission; however, this is the case in meningococci, where untreated infection is frequently lethal and terminates transmission. This view on meningococcal infection has been described by the term *evolutionary dead-end* (LEVIN and BULL 1994). Nevertheless, infections by both pathogenic *Neisseriae* depend on quite similar properties of the infectious agents. One of those is the ability of the organisms to adhere to and invade epithelial cells. Another is serum resistance, which is indispensable for both pathogenic *Neisseriae* to cause severe infections (VOGEL and FROSCH 1999). A variety of factors are involved in the biology of neisserial infections, some of which are present in both meningococci and gonococci; others are specific to a species. The interaction of meningococci and gonococci with epithelial cells is mediated by a protein called Opa, by pili, the IgA protease and porins, whereas a variety of hypervirulent meningococci (for example of the ET-5 complex, but not of the ET-37 complex), also rely on the membrane protein OpcA. Serum resistance in gonococci is mediated by porins and LPS structures, whereas the predominant factor of serum resistance in meningococci is the polysaccharide capsule, and porins and LPS seem to have adjuvant effects only. It is unclear which factors besides pili are relied on in meningococcal interaction with the meninges and brain endothelial cells, respectively. In the following sections, we will discuss the evolution of some of the virulence associated determinants described previously, i.e. OpcA, IgA protease, porins, and the capsule.

5.1 OpcA

Adherence to epithelial cells is a major step in neisserial infection. A meningococcal adhesin besides pili and Opa proteins is the protein OpcA (MERKER et al. 1997; OLYHOEK et al. 1991). This adhesin has been shown to contribute to adhesion of meningococci, an effect, which under experimental conditions is best seen with unpiliated and unencapsulated strains (DE VRIES et al. 1998; HARDY et al. 2000; VIRJI et al. 1992, 1993). OpcA is a transmembrane protein with five surface exposed loops (MERKER et al. 1997). It binds to heparan sulfate proteoglycans on epithelial surfaces (DE VRIES et al. 1998). The expression of the *opcA* gene exhibits phase variation due to slipped strand mispairing in the 5'-untranslated region of the gene

(SAKARI et al. 1994). As pointed out previously, the *opcA* gene is differentially distributed among pathogenic *Neisseriae* (WANG et al. 1993). Although it is widely distributed among meningococci, strains of the ET-37 complex and most strains of the cluster A4 are devoid of this marker. Sequence analysis of isolates possessing *opcA* revealed a rather low level of sequence variability and an unexpectedly low linkage of clonal groupings and *opcA* alleles (SEILER et al. 1996). It was assumed that *opcA* was acquired recently and spread rapidly within the species, probably due to some selective advantage resulting from improved colonisation of the human nasopharynx. A carefully performed consecutive analysis of the *opcA* region in ET-37 complex meningococci, serogroup A meningococci and gonococci, however, revealed that the hypothesis of a recent import of *opcA* into many, but not all clonal groupings of meningococci, does not explain the current distribution of the gene (ZHU et al. 1999). The sequence data suggest that the *opcA* region should be viewed as an island, which was imported into meningococci and gonococci, and which was deleted from some lineages later on. Loss of the *opcA* from this region is not an unlikely event because the region is characterised by a high level of genome plasticity giving rise to deletions and insertion-sequence integration. Furthermore, a paralogue ΨopcB pseudogene generated by an ancient duplication event was shown to be carried by gonococci, serogroup A meningococci, and also by ET-37 complex meningococci, which suggests that the latter lost the *opcA* gene after the ancient duplication. It is still an unresolved issue why the *opcA* genes of gonococci and meningococci are rather unrelated (55% homology) whereas only a few polymorphisms are found among the alleles of a single species. One explanation could be that both species acquired orthologous genes from an unrelated species. From a pathogenicity point of view, it will be interesting to rule out whether the deletion of *opcA* accounts for characteristics of the ET-37 complex, i.e. its potential to cause severe cases of systemic disease, and the different age distribution of ET-37 complex meningococci compared with other lineages such as the ET-5 complex (ERICKSON and DE WALS 1998; ROSENSTEIN et al. 1999).

5.2 IgA Protease

Neisserial IgA proteases represent one of the few traits clearly correlated to the capability of a species to cause both forms of neisserial disease (HALTER et al. 1984; HALTER et al. 1989; KOOMEY et al. 1982, 1984; POHLNER et al. 1987; REINHOLDT and KILIAN 1997). Pathogenic *Neisseriae* as well as e.g. *Haemophilus influenzae* express proteases capable of cleaving human IgA1; apathogenic neisserial species do not (MÜLLER 1983; REINHOLDT and KILIAN 1997; WOLFF and STERN 1995). The in vivo importance of IgA1 cleavage could not be confirmed by the human challenge model of urethral infection (JOHANNSEN et al. 1999), and in vivo cleavage of IgA by IgA proteases is still a matter of debate (HEDGES et al. 1998). However, IgA protease has been shown to exhibit interesting features with respect to cellular microbiology. IgA1 protease cleaves LAMP-1, thus interfering with phagosome maturation (AYALA et al. 1998; HAUCK and MEYER 1997; LIN et al. 1997).

Accordingly, IgA1 mutants have a defect in their capacity to transmigrate T84 epithelial cells (HOPPER et al. 2000). It has been shown that IgA1 protease induces pro-inflammatory cytokines in blood mononuclear cells (LORENZEN et al. 1999). Furthermore, cleavage of the TNF receptor II by IgA1 protease was associated with an inhibition of TNF-α induced apoptosis of human monocytic cells (BECK et al. 2000). There are two types of IgA proteases in *Neisseriae* with different cleavage specificity (type 1 and type 2) (LOMHOLT et al. 1995). Gonococcal and meningococcal *iga* genes are quite closely related (about 85% identity). Evidence for horizontal gene transfer came from the discovery of a mosaic-like structure of *iga* genes (HALTER et al. 1989). The identities of the *Haemophilus* and the neisserial *iga* genes are about 55%, when the genome sequences were compared (FLEISCH-MANN et al. 1995; TETTELIN et al. 2000). Furthermore, in the meningococcal genome sequences *iga* is found adjacent to the *trpB* gene (tryptophan synthase β-chain), whereas in *H. influenzae*, it is not (http://www.tigr.org/tdb/CMR/ghi/htmls/SplashPage.html). The orthologue genes in *Haemophilus influenzae* and pathogenic *Neisseriae* also exhibit rather different A + T contents (gonococci 55%, meningococci 53%, *H. influenzae* 62%), which make it unlikely that the gene was acquired by *Haemophilus* and *Neisseriae* from the same source. Taken together, the *iga* genes exemplify genetic material that entered pathogenic but not apathogenic neisserial species. Furthermore, pathogenic haemophili developed a comparable trait, which suggests that increase of fitness of pathogens by *iga* genes is a general phenomenon.

5.3 Porins

Porins are major outer membrane proteins in pathogenic and apathogenic *Neisseriae*. There are complex genetic relationships between different porin classes of pathogenic *Neisseriae*, which will be discussed below. PorA (the meningococcal class I porin) is only expressed in meningococci. Gonococci harbour a *porA* pseudogene, which is closely related to the meningococcal *porA* gene (FEAVERS and MAIDEN 1998). Besides the *porA* genes, both meningococci and gonococci express a *porB* gene, of which three types have been described (CARBONETTI et al. 1987; DERRICK et al. 1999; GOTSCHLICH et al. 1987; MURAKAMI et al. 1989):

a. The meningococcal class 3 *porB* (*porB3*), which is related to the gonococcal *porB1a* gene encoding P.IA
b. Class 2 *porB* (*porB2*) of meningococci
c. The gonococcal *porB1b* gene encoding P.IB, which is related to the *N. lactamica* porin.

Porins are underlying strong selective pressure resulting in rapid antigenic variation (SMITH et al. 1995). Horizontal gene transfer has been described for porin genes (DERRICK et al. 1999; VAZQUEZ et al. 1995). The trimeric porins function as voltage gated channels maintaining bacterial metabolism (JUDD 1989; MAURO et al. 1988; MINETTI et al. 1997, 1998; RUDEL et al. 1996; VAN PUTTEN et al. 1998) and contribute to the surface charge of the bacteria (SWANSON et al. 1997). Interesting impacts of porins on pathogenicity have been elucidated. In a GTP-controlled process, porins contribute to epithelial cell invasion, a property not conferred by porins of *N. lactamica*, although the *N. lactamica* porin increases phagocytosis and respiratory burst in HL60 phagocytic cells (BAUER et al. 1999). Interestingly, the interaction of gonococcal PorB with epithelial cells is modified by protein translocation from the bacterial to the host cell membrane, where the proteins cause rapid calcium influx and, thus, induce apoptosis (MÜLLER et al. 1999). Meningococcal porins have been shown to translocate into mitochondrial membranes of lymphoid cells, protecting target cells from apoptosis induced by apoptotic signals (MASSARI et al. 2000). The different effects on apoptosis seen in the two studies may be the result of the use of different porins and different cell types. Translocation of porin molecules might also result in cytoskeleton rearrangements due to association of porin with actin filaments (WEN et al. 2000). Porins act as second signals in induction of T cell independent antibodies against polysaccharides (SNAPPER et al. 1997). They have been shown to induce porin-specific T cells of the Th2 subset (SIMPSON et al. 1999). Finally, P.IA and probably class 3 PorB enhance serum resistance of pathogenic *Neisseriae* by binding the inhibitory complement factor H, whereas P.IB gonococci rely on factor H binding to sialylated LPS (RAM et al. 1998, 1998b, 1999).

Derrick et al. recently reported a refined phylogenetic analysis of the neisserial porins, which was performed on structurally conserved regions of the *porA* and *porB* genes (DERRICK et al. 1999). Split graph analysis illustrated that meningococcal and gonococcal *porA* (the latter a pseudogene) represent closely related genes forming an outgroup relative to other porins. Meningococcal class 3 *porB* (*porB3*), the gonococcal P.IA gene (*porB1a*), and *N. lactamica* porin gene cluster together, whereas the phylogenetic origin of the meningococcal *porB2* remains obscure because it is positioned between *porB3* genes and the *N. flavescens por* gene. The phylogenetic data on *porB* imply that all *porB* genes of meningococci, gonococci, and *N. lactamica*, except *porB2*, emerged in early interspecies genetic exchange during the emergence of the species. *PorB2* entered meningococci by horizontal gene transfer. Therefore, it is assumed that ET-37 complex and cluster A4 meningococci acquired a commensal *porB* gene, which, however, was lacking the GTP binding site found in *porB* of pathogenic *Neisseria* (and few non-pathogenic species). Since *porB2* exhibits the GTP-binding site, it was suggested that *porB2* entered meningococci by recombination of ancestral *porB* genes from a commensal and a pathogenic species. The fact that the GTP binding site was maintained during evolution demonstrates that it exhibits a selective advantage, most likely for interaction with host cells.

Gonococcal P.1 A (PorB1 A) gives rise to a more virulent phenotype when compared to P.1B (PorB1B) as a result of a more efficient complement degradation in P.1 A strains via factor H binding (RAM et al. 1998). Furthermore, GTP is more efficiently bound by P.1 A than by P.1B, which might contribute to enhanced cell invasion (VAN PUTTEN et al. 1998). This is probably why P.1 A strains are more frequently associated with disseminated gonococcal disease than P.1B strains (MORELLO and BOHNHOFF 1989). In meningococci, the contribution of porins is more complex because meningococci express two porin types at the same time. In light of the evolutionary findings discussed above, it will be most challenging to analyse the role of PorB2 for the altered pathogenicity profile of ET-37 complex strains, as has been discussed previously in the context of the *opcA* gene.

5.4 The Meningococcal Capsule

The polysaccharide capsule is the major pathogenicity factor of meningococci (KAHLER et al. 1998; MACKINNON et al. 1993; MASSON and HOLBEIN 1985; MASSON et al. 1981; VOGEL et al. 1996). Serogroup B, C, W135 and Y meningococci express capsules containing sialic acid either as hetero- or as homo-polymers (BHATTACHARJEE et al. 1976; CLAUS et al. 1997; FROSCH et al. 1989; LIU et al. 1971; SWARTLEY et al. 1997). The fifth serogroup associated with meningococcal disease, the serogroup A, does not synthesise polysialic acid, but a polysaccharide composed of *N*-acetyl-D-mannosamine-phosphate (LIU et al 1971b; SWARTLEY et al. 1998). All other serogroups, e.g. Z, 29 E, are not associated with disease, and the molecular biology of capsule synthesis has not been investigated to date. The genes necessary for capsule synthesis, transport, and modification are clustered on a large chromosomal region called the *cps*, which comprises more than 20kb (FROSCH et al. 1989). The following regions have been defined:

a. Region A: harbours the capsule synthesis operon (*sia* [sometimes also called *syn* (SWARTLEY et al. 1997)] genes in the case of the serogroups B, C, W135, Y; *myn* genes in the case of the serogroup A) (CLAUS et al. 1997; EDWARDS et al. 1994; FROSCH et al. 1989)
b. Region B: harbours the *lip* genes, whose gene products modify the polysaccharide by phospholipid substitution (FROSCH and MÜLLER 1993)
c. Region C: harbours the genes necessary for polysaccharide transport (*ctr* genes) (FROSCH et al. 1991, 1992)
d. Region D: harbours genes necessary for lipopolysaccharide synthesis, i.e. the *galE* gene and three *rfb* genes (HAMMERSCHMIDT et al. 1994; JENNINGS et al. 1993; PETERING et al. 1996; ROBERTSON et al. 1993)
e. Region D': this region evolved from duplication of region D in meningococci, with a 5'-truncation of the *galE* gene (PETERING et al. 1996)
f. Region E: comprises one large open reading frame encoding a protein with putative DNA binding properties (E. Wintermeyer and M. Frosch, unpublished)
g. Region MT (VOGEL and CLAUS 2000): this region carries methyltransferase genes and is truncated in meningococci

Region E, region D and the region MT seem to represent the ancient core, which is also present in gonococci (VOGEL and CLAUS 2000). The capsule specific regions A, C, and B most likely were incorporated into the meningococcal ancestor, an event that resulted in duplication of the region D. Certainly, it cannot be ruled out that the gonococcus lost the capsule specific regions of the *cps* (see Fig. 2). Furthermore, unpublished PCR analysis from our laboratory revealed that *galE*

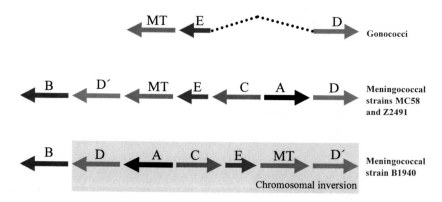

Fig. 2. Schematic depiction of the *cps* locus of the serogroup B strain B1940 in comparison to the strains Z2491 and MC58. The *capital letters* represent the regions of the *cps*. The regions present also in the gonococcus were included in the figure

and region E are present in *N. lactamica* and in some other commensal species as well, which supports the hypothesis that the regions A, C, and B entered the meningococcal ancestor, whereas the regions D and E represent the ancient core (D. Alber and U. Vogel, unpublished).

We have recently reviewed our current understanding of the evolution of the capsule locus deduced from the genome sequence data (VOGEL and CLAUS 2000). Therefore, in this paper, we focus on aspects of genome plasticity, i.e. chromosomal rearrangements within the *cps* locus and insertion sequences.

5.4.1 Chromosomal Rearrangements within the cps Locus

Figure 2 shows the order of regions of the *cps* in serogroup A meningococci (deduced from the genome sequence of the serogroup A strain Z2491 (PARKHILL et al. 2000), in serogroup B meningococci (deduced from the genome sequence of the strain MC58, which belongs to the ET-5 complex (TETTELIN et al. 2000), and from several publications cited previously on the strain B1940, which was the type of strain first used for the study of the *cps*), and gonococci (deduced from several publications cited previously and the preliminary genome sequence; http://www.genome.ou.edu/gono.html). The figure demonstrates that in strain B1940, the region B is found downstream of the region D, but not of region D' as in the strains Z2491 and MC58. This altered order of regions is caused by rearrangements within the *cps*, probably mediated by intrachromosomal recombination between homologous sequences of the regions D and D'. A systematic analysis of this inversion of the *cps* in a wide spectrum of sequence types of meningococci is under way in our laboratory. This study will elucidate the frequency of chromosomal rearrangements within the *cps* locus. Taken together, the finding of rearrangements within *cps* illustrates the genomic plasticity within this important virulence gene cluster of meningococci.

5.4.2 Insertion Sequence IS*1301*

Capsule expression in meningococci is subject to phase variation (HAMMERSCHMIDT et al. 1996, 1996b). We recently analysed 830 meningococcal carrier strains for capsular genotypes and phenotypes (U. Vogel and M. Frosch, unpublished data). Interestingly, 33% of all strains identified as serogroup B, C, W135, and Y by hybridisation with serogroup specific *siaD* gene probes (derived from the region A) did not express a polysaccharide as determined by ELISA using serogroup specific monoclonal antibodies. The molecular mechanisms of phase variation of capsule expression have been elucidated previously using the strain B1940 (HAMMERSCH-MIDT et al. 1996, 1996b). This strain either switched off capsule expression by a slipped strand mispairing mechanism within the *siaD* gene or by insertion of the insertion sequence IS*1301* into the *siaA* gene, the first gene of the operon in region A. IS*1301* is a mobile insertion sequence with a specific insertion site, which can be present in meningococci in as many as 17 copies per chromosome (HILSE et al. 1996, 2000). In consecutive studies, we have frequently found copies of the IS*1301* in the *cps* locus of a variety of meningococcal strains; however, other locations like the *porA* gene have also been reported (NEWCOMBE et al. 1998). It is likely that IS*1301* accounts for much of the phase variation in serogroup Y and W135 strains within our carrier collection because in a previous survey, we found that 84% of the serogroup Y strains and 46% of the serogroup W135 strains obtained from worldwide strain collections harboured IS*1301* (HILSE et al. 1996, 2000). In contrast, IS*1301* is rare in serogroup C strains of the hypervirulent ET-37 complex and the cluster A4; less than 3% of these strains harboured IS*1301* (HILSE et al. 2000). Furthermore, only 4% of the serogroup B strains of the ET-5 complex harboured IS*1301*. These data indicate that IS*1301* is underrepresented in hypervirulent lineages. Interestingly, the proportion of IS*1301* positive serogroup B and C strains not belonging to hypervirulent lineages was much higher with 26% and 29%, respectively. This might explain, why serogroup B strains of the ET-37 complex (usually serogroup C), and serogroup C strains of the ET-5 complex (usually serogroup B), which evolved by horizontal gene transfer of *siaD* genes, more frequently carried IS*1301* than their parent strains with the original serogroup: the IS*1301* was probably co-imported with the *siaD* gene.

The epidemiological data described above allow two scenarios:

a. Hypervirulent lineages exclude IS*1301* positive strains because IS*1301* affects the fitness of hypervirulent strains. This can be due to reduced transmission caused by IS*1301* mediated generation of unencapsulated variants, which might be impaired in aerosol transmission. However, this scenario would imply that the capsule is more important for the aerosol transmission of hypervirulent strains than for commensal strains.

b. IS*1301* positive descendents of hypervirulent strains are less virulent than their parents because capsule switch variants do not cause disease. Therefore, they are not found very often in strain collections because there is a sampling bias towards disease isolates in strain collections.

It will be very difficult to rule out whether IS*1301* indeed affects virulence or transmission. Epidemiological analysis is hampered by the very low frequency of hypervirulent strains even in large carrier strain collections. The comparative analysis of virulence of strains derived from hypervirulent lineages carrying IS*1301* or not is made difficult due to a lack of appropriate animal models and because of antigenic and genetic variability found even in strains derived from the same clonal grouping.

6 Conclusion

We described the population structure of neisserial species and discussed the evolution of pathogenicty within this genus. Retrospective analysis of historical evolutionary events will forever be a speculative issue. Nevertheless, the expanding knowledge about neisserial macro- and micro-evolution raises new questions regarding clone-specific traits and refines earlier analyses of pathogenicity, which often depended on random selection of isolates. Putting together the results from population biology and pathogenicity research, therefore, inspires comparative experimentation elucidating lineage specific characteristics. It would be impossible to date evolutionary events resulting in speciation of *Neisseriae* as has been done for Enterobacteriaceae. However, the understanding of macro-evolution and micro-evolution will allow the development of a more precise species concept of the genus *Neisseria*, which has been difficult to accomplish by most classical methods assuming clonality for their interpretation.

Acknowledgements. The authors' work on meningococcal population structure and epidemiology is supported by the Deutsche Forschungsgemeinschaft (grant no. Vo 718/3). We thank Martin Maiden, Oxford, and Mark Achtman, Berlin, for helpful discussions and fruitful cooperation. We acknowledge the Gonococcal Genome Sequencing Project supported by USPHS/NIH grant no. AI38399, and B.A. Roe, L. Song, S. P. Lin, X. Yuan, S. Clifton, Tom Ducey, Lisa Lewis and D.W. Dyer at the University of Oklahoma. The GenBank accession number for the completed *Neisseria gonorrhoeae* genome is AE004969.

References

Achtman M (1995) Global epidemiology of meningococcal disease. In: Cartwright K (ed.) Meningococcal disease. Wiley, Chichester, pp 159–175
Achtman M (1997) Microevolution and epidemic spread of serogroup A *Neisseria meningitidis* – a review. Gene 192:135–140
Achtman M, Azuma T, Berg DE, Ito Y, Morelli G, Pan ZJ, Suerbaum S, Thompson SA, van Der Ende A, van Doorn LJ (1999a) Recombination and clonal groupings within *Helicobacter pylori* from different geographical regions. Mol Microbiol 32:459–470

Achtman M, Zurth K, Morelli G, Torrea G, Guiyoule A, Carniel E (1999b) *Yersinia pestis*, the cause of plague, is a recently emerged clone of *Yersinia pseudotuberculosis*. Proc Natl Acad Sci USA 96:14043–14048

Ayala P, Lin L, Hopper S, Fukuda M, So M (1998) Infection of epithelial cells by pathogenic *Neisseriae* reduces the levels of multiple lysosomal constituents. Infect Immun 66:5001–5007

Bart A, Dankert J, van der Ende A (2000) Representational difference analysis of *Neisseria meningitidis* identifies sequences that are specific for the hyper-virulent lineage III clone. FEMS Microbiol Lett 188:111–114

Bauer FJ, Rudel T, Stein M, Meyer TF (1999) Mutagenesis of the *Neisseria gonorrhoeae* porin reduces invasion in epithelial cells and enhances phagocyte responsiveness. Mol Microbiol 31:903–913

Bautsch W (1998) Comparison of the genome organization of pathogenic neisseriae. Electrophoresis 19:577–581

Beck SC, Meyer TF (2000) IgA1 protease from *Neisseria gonorrhoeae* inhibits TNFalpha-mediated apoptosis of human monocytic cells. FEBS Lett 472:287–292

Bhattacharjee AK, Jennings HJ, Kenny CP, Martin A, Smith IC (1976) Structural determination of the polysaccharide antigens of *Neisseria meningitidis* serogroups Y, W-135, and BO1. Can J Biochem 54:1–8

Bihlmaier A, Römling U, Meyer TF, Tümmler B, Gibbs CP (1991) Physical and genetic map of the *Neisseria gonorrhoeae* strain MS11-N198 chromosome. Mol Microbiol 5:2529–2539

Biswas GD, Sparling PF (1981) Entry of double-stranded deoxyribonucleic acid during transformation of *Neisseria gonorrhoeae*. J Bacteriol 145:638–640

Blakebrough IS, Greenwood BM, Whittle HC, Bradley AK, Gilles HM (1982) The epidemiology of infections due to *Neisseria meningitidis* and *Neisseria lactamica* in a northern Nigerian community. J Infect Dis 146:626–637

Bowler LD, Zhang QY, Riou JY, Spratt BG (1994) Interspecies recombination between the *penA* genes of *Neisseria meningitidis* and commensal *Neisseria* species during the emergence of penicillin resistance in *N. meningitidis*: natural events and laboratory simulation. J Bacteriol 176:333–337

Bygraves JA, Urwin R, Fox AJ, Gray SJ, Russell JE, Feavers IM, Maiden MC (1999) Population genetic and evolutionary approaches to analysis of *Neisseria meningitidis* isolates belonging to the ET-5 complex. J Bacteriol 181:5551–5556

Carbonetti NH, Sparling PF (1987) Molecular cloning and characterization of the structural gene for protein I, the major outer membrane protein of *Neisseria gonorrhoeae*. Proc Natl Acad Sci USA 84:9084–9088

Cartwright K (1995) Meningococcal carriage and disease. In: Cartwright K (ed.) Meningococcal disease. John Wiley and Sons, Chichester, England, pp 115–146

Cartwright KA, Stuart JM, Jones DM, Noah ND (1987) The Stonehouse survey: nasopharyngeal carriage of meningococci and *Neisseria lactamica*. Epidemiol Infect 99:591–601

Caugant DA, Froholm LO, Bovre K, Holten E, Frasch CE, Mocca LF, Zollinger WD, Selander RK (1986) Intercontinental spread of a genetically distinctive complex of clones of *Neisseria meningitidis* causing epidemic disease. Proc Natl Acad Sci USA 83:4927–4931

Caugant DA, Mocca LF, Frasch CE, Froholm LO, Zollinger WD, Selander RK (1987) Genetic structure of *Neisseria meningitidis* populations in relation to serogroup, serotype, and outer membrane protein pattern. J Bacteriol 169:2781–2792

Caugant DA, Kristiansen BE, Froholm LO, Bovre K, Selander RK (1988) Clonal diversity of *Neisseria meningitidis* from a population of asymptomatic carriers. Infect Immun 56:2060–2068

Chaussee MS, Hill SA (1998) Formation of single-stranded DNA during DNA transformation of *Neisseria gonorrhoeae*. J Bacteriol 180:5117–5122

Claus H, Vogel U, Mühlenhoff M, Gerardy-Schahn R, Frosch M (1997) Molecular divergence of the *sia* locus in different serogroups of *Neisseria meningitidis* expressing polysialic acid capsules. Mol Gen Genet 257:28–34

Claus H, Frosch M, Vogel U (1998) Identification of a hotspot for transformation of *Neisseria meningitidis* by shuttle mutagenesis using signature-tagged transposons. Mol Gen Genet 259:363–371

Claus H, Friedrich A, Frosch M, Vogel U (2000) Differential distribution of two novel restriction-modification systems in clonal lineages of *Neisseria meningitidis*. J Bacteriol 182:1296–1303

Coen PG, Cartwright K, Stuart J (2000) Mathematical modelling of infection and disease due to *Neisseria meningitidis* and *Neisseria lactamica*. Int J Epidemiol 29:180–188

de Vries FP, Cole R, Dankert J, Frosch M, van Putten JP (1998) *Neisseria meningitidis* producing the Opc adhesin binds epithelial cell proteoglycan receptors. Mol Microbiol 27:1203–1212

Dempsey JA, Cannon JG (1994) Locations of genetic markers on the physical map of the chromosome of *Neisseria gonorrhoeae* FA1090. J Bacteriol 176:2055–2060

Denning DW, Gill SS (1991) *Neisseria lactamica* meningitis following skull trauma. Rev Infect Dis 13:216–218

Derrick JP, Urwin R, Suker J, Feavers IM, Maiden MC (1999) Structural and evolutionary inference from molecular variation in *Neisseria* porins. Infect Immun 67:2406–2413

Edwards U, Müller A, Hammerschmidt S, Gerardy-Schahn R, Frosch M (1994) Molecular analysis of the biosynthesis pathway of the alpha-2, 8 polysialic acid capsule by *Neisseria meningitidis* serogroup B. Mol Microbiol 14:141–149

Elkins C, Thomas CE, Seifert HS, Sparling PF (1991) Species-specific uptake of DNA by gonococci is mediated by a 10-base-pair sequence. J Bacteriol 173:3911–3913

Enright MC, Spratt BG (1999) Multilocus sequence typing. Trends Microbiol 7:482–487

Erickson L, de Wals P (1998) Complications and sequelae of meningococcal disease in Quebec, Canada, 1990–1994. Clin Infect Dis 26:1159–1164

Feavers IM, Maiden MC (1998) A gonococcal porA pseudogene: implications for understanding the evolution and pathogenicity of *Neisseria gonorrhoeae*. Mol Microbiol 30:647–656

Feil E, Zhou J, Maynard Smith J, Spratt BG (1996) A comparison of the nucleotide sequences of the *adk* and *recA* genes of pathogenic and commensal Neisseria species: evidence for extensive interspecies recombination within *adk*. J Mol Evol 43:631–640

Feil EJ, Maiden MC, Achtman M, Spratt BG (1999) The relative contributions of recombination and mutation to the divergence of clones of *Neisseria meningitidis*. Mol Biol Evol 16:1496–1502

Fleischmann RD, Adams MD, White O, Clayton RA, Kirkness EF, Kerlavage AR, Bult CJ, Tomb JF, Dougherty BA, Merrick JM, et al. (1995) Whole-genome random sequencing and assembly of *Haemophilus influenzae* Rd. Science 269:496–512

Frosch M, Müller A (1993) Phospholipid substitution of capsular polysaccharides and mechanisms of capsule formation in *Neisseria meningitidis*. Mol Microbiol 8:483–493

Frosch M, Weisgerber C, Meyer TF (1989) Molecular characterization and expression in *Escherichia coli* of the gene complex encoding the polysaccharide capsule of *Neisseria meningitidis* group B. Proc Natl Acad Sci USA 86:1669–1673

Frosch M, Edwards U, Bousset K, Krauße B, Weisgerber C (1991) Evidence for a common molecular origin of the capsule gene loci in gram-negative bacteria expressing group II capsular polysaccharides. Mol Microbiol 5:1251–1263

Frosch M, Müller D, Bousset K, Müller A (1992) Conserved outer membrane protein of *Neisseria meningitidis* involved in capsule expression. Infect Immun 60:798–803

Gaher M, Einsiedler K, Crass T, Bautsch W (1996) A physical and genetic map of *Neisseria meningitidis* B1940. Mol Microbiol 19:249–259

Gold R, Goldschneider I, Lepow ML, Draper TF, Randolph M (1978) Carriage of *Neisseria meningitidis* and *Neisseria lactamica* in infants and children. J Infect Dis 137:112–121

Goodman SD, Scocca JJ (1988) Identification and arrangement of the DNA sequence recognized in specific transformation of *Neisseria gonorrhoeae*. Proc Natl Acad Sci USA 85:6982–6986

Gordts F, Halewyck S, Pierard D, Kaufman L, Clement PA (2000) Microbiology of the middle meatus: a comparison between normal adults and children. J Laryngol Otol 114:184–188

Gotschlich EC, Seiff ME, Blake MS, Koomey M (1987) Porin protein of *Neisseria gonorrhoeae*: cloning and gene structure. Proc Natl Acad Sci USA 84:8135–8139

Gutjahr TS, O'Rourke M, Ison CA, Spratt BG (1997) Arginine-, hypoxanthine-, uracil-requiring isolates of *Neisseria gonorrhoeae* are a clonal lineage with a non-clonal population. Microbiology 143:633–640

Halter R, Pohlner J, Meyer TF (1984) IgA protease of *Neisseria gonorrhoeae*: isolation and characterization of the gene and its extracellular product. EMBO J 3:1595–1601

Halter R, Pohlner J, Meyer TF (1989) Mosaic-like organization of IgA protease genes in *Neisseria gonorrhoeae* generated by horizontal genetic exchange in vivo. EMBO J 8:2737–2744

Hammerschmidt S, Birkholz C, Zähringer U, Robertson BD, van Putten J, Ebeling O, Frosch M (1994) Contribution of genes from the capsule gene complex (*cps*) to lipooligosaccharide biosynthesis and serum resistance in *Neisseria meningitidis*. Mol Microbiol 11:885–896

Hammerschmidt S, Hilse R, van Putten JP, Gerardy-Schahn R, Unkmeir A, Frosch M (1996) Modulation of cell surface sialic acid expression in *Neisseria meningitidis* via a transposable genetic element. EMBO J 15:192–198

Hammerschmidt S, Müller A, Sillmann H, Mühlenhoff M, Borrow R, Fox A, van Putten J, Zollinger WD, Gerardy-Schahn R, Frosch M (1996b) Capsule phase variation in *Neisseria meningitidis* serogroup B by slipped strand mispairing in the polysialyltransferase gene (*siaD*): correlation with bacterial invasion and the outbreak of meningococcal disease. Mol Microbiol 20:1211–1220

Hardy SJ, Christodoulides M, Weller RO, Heckels JE (2000) Interactions of *Neisseria meningitidis* with cells of the human meninges. Mol Microbiol 36:817–829

Hauck CR, Meyer TF (1997) The lysosomal/phagosomal membrane protein h-lamp-1 is a target of the IgA1 protease of *Neisseria gonorrhoeae*. FEBS Lett 405:86–90

Hedges SR, Mayo MS, Kallman L, Mestecky J, Hook EW, Russell MW (1998) Evaluation of immunoglobulin A1 (IgA1) protease and IgA1 protease-inhibitory activity in human female genital infection with *Neisseria gonorrhoeae*. Infect Immun 66:5826–5832

Hilse R, Hammerschmidt S, Bautsch W, Frosch M (1996) Site-specific insertion of IS*1301* and distribution in *Neisseria meningitidis* strains. J Bacteriol 178:2527–2532

Hilse R, Stoevesandt J, Caugant DA, Claus H, Frosch M, Vogel U (2000) Distribution of the meningococcal insertion sequence IS1301 in clonal lineages of *Neisseria meningitidis*. Epidemiol Infect 124:337–340

Hoke C, Vedros NA (1982) Taxonomy of the Neisseriae: Deoxyribonucleic acid base composition, interspecific transformation, and deoxyribonucleic acid hybridization. Int J Syst Bacteriol 32:57–66

Holmes EC, Urwin R, Maiden MC (1999) The influence of recombination on the population structure and evolution of the human pathogen *Neisseria meningitidis*. Mol Biol Evol 16:741–749

Hopper S, Vasquez B, Merz A, Clary S, Wilbur JS, So M (2000) Effects of the immunoglobulin A1 protease on *Neisseria gonorrhoeae* trafficking across polarized T84 epithelial monolayers. Infect Immun 68:906–911

Jennings MP, van der Ley P, Wilks KE, Maskell DJ, Poolman JT, Moxon ER (1993) Cloning and molecular analysis of the *galE* gene of *Neisseria meningitidis* and its role in lipopolysaccharide biosynthesis. Mol Microbiol 10:361–369

Johannsen DB, Johnston DM, Koymen HO, Cohen MS, Cannon JG (1999) A *Neisseria gonorrhoeae* immunoglobulin A1 protease mutant is infectious in the human challenge model of urethral infection. Infect Immun 67:3009–3013

Jones D (1995) Epidemiology of meningococcal disease in Europe and the USA. In: Cartwright K (ed.) Meningococcal disease. Wiley, Chichester, pp 147–158

Judd RC (1989) Protein I: structure, function, and genetics. Clin Microbiol Rev 2 [Suppl]:S41–8

Kahler CM, Martin LE, Shih GC, Rahman MM, Carlson RW, Stephens DS (1998) The (alpha 2 → 8)-linked polysialic acid capsule and lipooligosaccharide structure both contribute to the ability of serogroup B *Neisseria meningitidis* to resist the bactericidal activity of normal human serum. Infect Immun 66:5939–5947

Kertesz DA, Coulthart MB, Ryan JA, Johnson WM, Ashton FE (1998) Serogroup B, electrophoretic type 15 *Neisseria meningitidis* in Canada. J Infect Dis 177:1754–1757

Kim JJ, Mandrell RE, Griffiss JM (1989) *Neisseria lactamica* and *Neisseria meningitidis* share lipooligosaccharide epitopes but lack common capsular and class 1, 2, and 3 protein epitopes. Infect Immun 57:602–608

Klee SR, Nassif X, Kusecek B, Merker P, Beretti JL, Achtman M, Tinsley CR (2000) Molecular and biological analysis of eight genetic islands that distinguish *Neisseria meningitidis* from the closely related pathogen *Neisseria gonorrhoeae*. Infect Immun 68:2082–2095

Koomey JM, Falkow S (1984) Nucleotide sequence homology between the immunoglobulin A1 protease genes of *Neisseria gonorrhoeae*, *Neisseria meningitidis*, and *Haemophilus influenzae*. Infect Immun 43:101–107

Koomey JM, Gill RE, Falkow S (1982) Genetic and biochemical analysis of gonococcal IgA1 protease: cloning in *Escherichia coli* and construction of mutants of gonococci that fail to produce the activity. Proc Natl Acad Sci USA 79:7881–7885

Kremastinou J, Tzanakaki G, Pagalis A, Theodondou M, Weir DM, Blackwell CC (1999) Detection of IgG and IgM to meningococcal outer membrane proteins in relation to carriage of *Neisseria meningitidis* or *Neisseria lactamica*. FEMS Immunol Med Microbiol 24:73–78

Kriz P, Musilek M, Skoczynska A, Hryniewicz W (2000) Genetic and antigenetic characteristics of *Neisseria meningitidis* strains isolated in the Czech Republic in 1997–1998. Eur J Clin Microbiol Infect Dis 19:452–459

Lacks SA, Springhorn SS (1984) Transfer of recombinant plasmids containing the gene for *Dpn*II DNA methylase into strains of *Streptococcus pneumoniae* that produce *Dpn*I or *Dpn*II restriction endonucleases. J Bacteriol 158:905–909

Lavitola A, Bucci C, Salvatore P, Maresca G, Bruni CB, Alifano P (1999) Intracistronic transcription termination in polysialyltransferase gene (*siaD*) affects phase variation in *Neisseria meningitidis*. Mol Microbiol 33:119–127

Levin BR, Bull JJ (1994) Short-sighted evolution and the virulence of pathogenic microorganisms. Trends Microbiol 2:76–81

Lin L, Ayala P, Larson J, Mulks M, Fukuda M, Carlsson SR, Enns C, So M (1997) The *Neisseria* type 2 IgA1 protease cleaves LAMP1 and promotes survival of bacteria within epithelial cells. Mol Microbiol 24:1083–1094

Linz B, Schenker M, Zhu P, Achtman M (2000) Frequent interspecific genetic exchange between commensal *Neisseriae* and *Neisseria meningitidis*. Mol Microbiol 36:1049–1058

Liu TY, Gotschlich EC, Dunne FT, Jonssen EK (1971) Studies on the meningococcal polysaccharides. II. Composition and chemical properties of the group B and group C polysaccharide. J Biol Chem 246:4703–4712

Liu TY, Gotschlich EC, Jonssen EK, Wysocki JR (1971b) Studies on the meningococcal polysaccharides. I. Composition and chemical properties of the group A polysaccharide. J Biol Chem 246:2849–2850

Lloyd-Still JD, Shwachman H (1975) Duodenal microflora: a prospective study in pediatric gastrointestinal disorders. Am J Dig Dis 20:708–715

Lomholt H, Poulsen K, Kilian M (1995) Comparative characterization of the iga gene encoding IgA1 protease in *Neisseria meningitidis*, *Neisseria gonorrhoeae* and *Haemophilus influenzae*. Mol Microbiol 15:495–506

Lorenz MG, Wackernagel W (1994) Bacterial gene transfer by natural genetic transformation in the environment. Microbiol Rev 58:563–602

Lorenzen DR, Dux F, Wolk U, Tsirpouchtsidis A, Haas G, Meyer TF (1999) Immunoglobulin A1 protease, an exoenzyme of pathogenic *Neisseriae*, is a potent inducer of proinflammatory cytokines. J Exp Med 190:1049–1058

Lujan R, Zhang QY, Saez Nieto JA, Jones DM, Spratt BG (1991) Penicillin-resistant isolates of *Neisseria lactamica* produce altered forms of penicillin-binding protein 2 that arose by interspecies horizontal gene transfer. Antimicrob Agents Chemother 35:300–304

Mackinnon FG, Borrow R, Gorringe AR, Fox AJ, Jones DM, Robinson A (1993) Demonstration of lipooligosaccharide immunotype and capsule as virulence factors for *Neisseria meningitidis* using an infant mouse intranasal infection model. Microb Pathog 15:359–366

Maiden MC, Bygraves JA, Feil E, Morelli G, Russell JE, Urwin R, Zhang Q, Zhou J, Zurth K, Caugant DA, Feavers DA, Achtman M, Spratt BG (1998) Multilocus sequence typing: a portable approach to the identification of clones within populations of pathogenic microorganisms. Proc Natl Acad Sci USA 95:3140–3145

Maiden MC, Malorny B, Achtman M (1996) A global gene pool in the neisseriae [letter]. Mol Microbiol 21:1297–1298

Majewski J, Cohan FM (1998) The effect of mismatch repair and heteroduplex formation on sexual isolation in *Bacillus*. Genetics 148:13–18

Majewski J, Zawadzki P, Pickerill P, Cohan FM, Dowson CG (2000) Barriers to genetic exchange between bacterial species: *Streptococcus pneumoniae* transformation. J Bacteriol 182:1016–1023

Massari P, Ho Y, Wetzler LM (2000) *Neisseria meningitidis* porin PorB interacts with mitochondria and protects cells from apoptosis. Proc Natl Acad Sci USA 97:9070–9075

Masson L, Holbein BE (1985) Influence of nutrient limitation and low pH on serogroup B *Neisseria meningitidis* capsular polysaccharide levels: correlation with virulence for mice. Infect Immun 47:465–471

Masson L, Holbein BE, Ashton F (1981) Virulence linked to polysaccharide production in serogroup B *Neisseria meningitidis*. FEMS Microbiol Lett 13:187–190

Mauro A, Blake M, Labarca P (1988) Voltage gating of conductance in lipid bilayers induced by porin from outer membrane of *Neisseria gonorrhoeae*. Proc Natl Acad Sci USA 85:1071–1075

Merker P, Tommassen J, Kusecek B, Virji M, Sesardic D, Achtman M (1997) Two-dimensional structure of the Opc invasin from *Neisseria meningitidis*. Mol Microbiol 23:281–293

Minetti CA, Tai JY, Blake MS, Pullen JK, Liang SM, Remeta DP (1997) Structural and functional characterization of a recombinant PorB class 2 protein from *Neisseria meningitidis*. Conformational stability and porin activity. J Biol Chem 272:10710–10720

Minetti CA, Blake MS, Remeta DP (1998) Characterization of the structure, function, and conformational stability of PorB class 3 protein from *Neisseria meningitidis*. A porin with unusual physicochemical properties. J Biol Chem 273:25329–25338

Morello JA, Bohnhoff M (1989) Serovars and serum resistance of *Neisseria gonorrhoeae* from disseminated and uncomplicated infections. J Infect Dis 160:1012–1017

Morschhäuser J, Köhler G, Ziehbur W, Blum-Oehler G, Dobrindt U, Hacker J (2000) Evolution of microbial pathogens. Philos Trans R Soc Lond B Biol Sci 355:695–704

Müller A, Gunther D, Dux F, Naumann M, Meyer TF, Rudel T (1999) Neisserial porin (PorB) causes rapid calcium influx in target cells and induces apoptosis by the activation of cysteine proteases. EMBO J 18:339–352

Müller HE (1983) Lack of immunoglobulin A protease in *Neisseria lactamica* [letter]. Eur J Clin Microbiol 2:153–154

Murakami K, Gotschlich EC, Seiff ME (1989) Cloning and characterization of the structural gene for the class 2 protein of *Neisseria meningitidis*. Infect Immun 57:2318–2323

Newcombe J, Cartwright K, Dyer S, McFadden J (1998) Naturally occurring insertional inactivation of the porA gene of *Neisseria meningitidis* by integration of IS1301 [letter]. Mol Microbiol 30:453–454

O'Rourke M, Spratt BG (1994) Further evidence for the non-clonal population structure of *Neisseria gonorrhoeae*: extensive genetic diversity within isolates of the same electrophoretic type. Microbiology 140:1285–1290

O'Rourke M, Stevens E (1993) Genetic structure of *Neisseria gonorrhoeae* populations: a non-clonal pathogen. J Gen Microbiol 139:2603–2611

Olsen SF, Djurhuus B, Rasmussen K, Joensen HD, Larsen SO, Zoffman H, Lind I (1991) Pharyngeal carriage of *Neisseria meningitidis* and *Neisseria lactamica* in households with infants within areas with high and low incidences of meningococcal disease. Epidemiol Infect 106:445–457

Olyhoek AJ, Sarkari J, Bopp M, Morelli G, Achtman M (1991) Cloning and expression in *Escherichia coli* of opc, the gene for an unusual class 5 outer membrane protein from *Neisseria meningitidis*. Microb Pathog 11:249–257

Parkhill J, Achtman M, James KD, et al. (2000) Complete DNA sequence of a serogroup A strain of *Neisseria meningitidis* Z2491. Nature 404:502–506

Pedersen LM, Madsen OR, Gutschik E (1993) Septicaemia caused by an unusual *Neisseria meningitidis* species following dental extraction. Scand J Infect Dis 25:137–139

Perrin A, Nassif X, Tinsley C (1999) Identification of regions of the chromosome of *Neisseria meningitidis* and *Neisseria gonorrhoeae*, which are specific to the pathogenic *Neisseria* species. Infect Immun 67:6119–6129

Petering H, Hammerschmidt S, Frosch M, van Putten JP, Ison CA, Robertson BD (1996) Genes associated with meningococcal capsule complex are also found in *Neisseria gonorrhoeae*. J Bacteriol 178:3342–3345

Pohlner J, Halter R, Beyreuther K, Meyer TF (1987) Gene structure and extracellular secretion of *Neisseria gonorrhoeae* IgA protease. Nature 325:458–462

Ram S, Mackinnon FG, Gulati S, McQuillen DP, Vogel U, Frosch M, Elkins C, Guttormsen HK, Wetzler LM, Oppermann M, Pangburn MK, Rice PA (1999) The contrasting mechanisms of serum resistance of *Neisseria gonorrhoeae* and group B *Neisseria meningitidis*. Mol Immunol 36:915–928

Ram S, McQuillen DP, Gulati S, Elkins C, Pangburn MK, Rice PA (1998) Binding of complement factor H to loop 5 of porin protein 1 A: a molecular mechanism of serum resistance of nonsialylated *Neisseria gonorrhoeae*. J Exp Med 188:671–680

Ram S, Sharma AK, Simpson SD, Gulati S, McQuillen DP, Pangburn MK, Rice PA (1998b) A novel sialic acid binding site on factor H mediates serum resistance of sialylated *Neisseria gonorrhoeae*. J Exp Med 187:743–752

Reinholdt J, Kilian M (1997) Comparative analysis of immunoglobulin A1 protease activity among bacteria representing different genera, species, and strains. Infect Immun 65:4452–4459

Robertson BD, Frosch M, van Putten JP (1993) The role of galE in the biosynthesis and function of gonococcal lipopolysaccharide. Mol Microbiol 8:891–901

Rokbi B, Renauld-Mongenie G, Mignon M, Danve B, Poncet D, Chabanel C, Caugant DA, Quentin-Millet M-J (2000) Allelic diversity of the two transferrin binding protein B gene isotypes among a collection of *Neisseria meningitidis* strains representative of serogroup B disease: implication for the composition of a recombinant TbpB-based vaccine. Infect Immun 68:4938–4947

Rosenstein NE, Perkins BA, Stephens DS, Lefkowitz L, Cartter ML, Danila R, Cieslak P, Shutt KA, Popovic T, Schuchat A, Harrison LH, Reingold AL (1999) The changing epidemiology of meningococcal disease in the United States, 1992–1996. J Infect Dis 180:1894–1901

Rotimi VO, Duerden BI (1981) The development of the bacterial flora in normal neonates. J Med Microbiol 14:51–62

Rudel T, Schmid A, Benz R, Kolb HA, Lang F, Meyer TF (1996) Modulation of Neisseria porin (PorB) by cytosolic ATP/GTP of target cells: parallels between pathogen accommodation and mitochondrial endosymbiosis. Cell 85:391–402

Saez-Nieto JA, Lujan R, Martinez-Suarez JV, Berron S, Vazquez JA, Vinas M, Campos J (1990) *Neisseria lactamica* and *Neisseria polysaccharea* as possible sources of meningococcal beta-lactam resistance by genetic transformation. Antimicrob Agents Chemother 34:2269–2272

Sarkari J, Pandit N, Moxon ER, Achtman M (1994) Variable expression of the Opc outer membrane protein in *Neisseria meningitidis* is caused by size variation of a promoter containing poly-cytidine. Mol Microbiol 13:207–217

Seiler A, Reinhardt R, Sarkari J, Caugant DA, Achtman M (1996) Allelic polymorphism and site-specific recombination in the opc locus of *Neisseria meningitidis*. Mol Microbiol 19:841–856

Simpson SD, Ho Y, Rice PA, Wetzler LM (1999) T lymphocyte response to *Neisseria gonorrhoeae* porin in individuals with mucosal gonococcal infections. J Infect Dis 180:762–773

Smith HO, Gwinn ML, Salzberg SL (1999) DNA uptake signal sequences in naturally transformable bacteria. Res Microbiol 150:603–616

Smith NH, Holmes EC, Donovan GM, Carpenter GA, Spratt BG (1999b) Networks and groups within the genus Neisseria: analysis of *argF, recA, rho,* and 16S rRNA sequences from human *Neisseria* species. Mol Biol Evol 16:773–783

Smith NH, Maynard Smith J, Spratt BG (1995) Sequence evolution of the porB gene of *Neisseria gonorrhoeae* and *Neisseria meningitidis*: evidence of positive Darwinian selection. Mol Biol Evol 12:363–370

Snapper CM, Rosas FR, Kehry MR, Mond JJ, Wetzler LM (1997) Neisserial porins may provide critical second signals to polysaccharide-activated murine B cells for induction of immunoglobulin secretion. Infect Immun 65:3203–3208

Spratt BG, Maiden MC (1999) Bacterial population genetics, evolution and epidemiology. Philos Trans R Soc Lond B Biol Sci 354:701–710

Stein DC (1991) Transformation of *Neisseria gonorrhoeae*: physical requirements of the transforming DNA. Can J Microbiol 37:345–349

Suerbaum S (2000) Genetic variability within *Helicobacter pylori*. Int J Med Microbiol 290:175–181

Suerbaum S, Achtman M (1999) Evolution of *Helicobacter pylori*: the role of recombination. Trends Microbiol 7:182–184

Suerbaum S, Smith JM, Bapumia K, Morelli G, Smith NH, Kunstmann E, Dyrek I, Achtman M (1998) Free recombination within *Helicobacter pylori*. Proc Natl Acad Sci USA 95:12619–12624

Swanson J, Dorward D, Lubke L, Kao D (1997) Porin polypeptide contributes to surface charge of gonococci. J Bacteriol 179:3541–3548

Swartley JS, Marfin AA, Edupuganti S, Liu LJ, Cieslak P, Perkins B, Wenger JD, Stephens DS (1997) Capsule switching of *Neisseria meningitidis*. Proc Natl Acad Sci USA 94:271–276

Swartley JS, Liu LJ, Miller YK, Martin LE, Edupuganti S, Stephens DS (1998) Characterization of the gene cassette required for biosynthesis of the (alpha 1→6)-linked N-acetyl-D-mannosamine-1-phosphate capsule of serogroup A *Neisseria meningitidis*. J Bacteriol 180:1533–1539

Tettelin H, Saunders NJ, Heidelberg J, et al. (2000) Complete genome sequence of *Neisseria meningitidis* serogroup B strain MC58. Science 287:1809–1815

Tinsley CR, Nassif X (1996) Analysis of the genetic differences between *Neisseria meningitidis* and *Neisseria gonorrhoeae*: two closely related bacteria expressing two different pathogenicities. Proc Natl Acad Sci USA 93:11109–11114

Troncoso G, Sanchez S, Moreda M, Criado MT, Ferreiros CM (2000) Antigenic cross-reactivity between outer membrane proteins of *Neisseria meningitidis* and commensal Neisseria species. FEMS Immunol Med Microbiol 27:103–109

van Der Ende A, Hopman CT, Zaat S, Essink BB, Berkhout B, Dankert J (1995) Variable expression of class 1 outer membrane protein in *Neisseria meningitidis* is caused by variation in the spacing between the -10 and -35 regions of the promoter. J Bacteriol 177:2475–2480

van Putten JP, Duensing TD, Carlson J (1998) Gonococcal invasion of epithelial cells driven by P.IA, a bacterial ion channel with GTP binding properties. J Exp Med 188:941–952

Vazquez JA, Berron S, O'Rourke M, Carpenter G, Feil E, Smith NH, Spratt BG (1995) Interspecies recombination in nature: a meningococcus that has acquired a gonococcal PIB porin. Mol Microbiol 15:1001–1007

Virji M, Makepeace K, Ferguson DJ, Achtman M, Sarkari J, Moxon ER (1992) Expression of the Opc protein correlates with invasion of epithelial and endothelial cells by *Neisseria meningitidis*. Mol Microbiol 6:2785–2795

Virji M, Makepeace K, Ferguson DJ, Achtman M, Moxon ER (1993) Meningococcal Opa and Opc proteins: their role in colonization and invasion of human epithelial and endothelial cells. Mol Microbiol 10:499–510

Vogel U, Claus H (2000) The evolution of human pathogens: examples and clinical implications. Int J Med Microbiol 290:511–518

Vogel U, Frosch M (1999) Mechanisms of neisserial serum resistance. Mol Microbiol 32:1133–1139

Vogel U, Hammerschmidt S, Frosch M (1996) Sialic acids of both the capsule and the sialylated lipooligosaccharide of *Neisseria meningitidis* serogroup B are prerequisites for virulence of meningococci in the infant rat. Med Microbiol Immunol (Berl) 185:81–87

Vogel U, Morelli G, Zurth K, Claus H, Kriener E, Achtman M, Frosch M (1998) Necessity of molecular techniques to distinguish between *Neisseria meningitidis* strains isolated from patients with meningococcal disease and from their healthy contacts. J Clin Microbiol 36:2465–2470

Wang JF, Caugant DA, Morelli G, Koumare B, Achtman M (1993) Antigenic and epidemiologic properties of the ET-37 complex of *Neisseria meningitidis*. J Infect Dis 167:1320–1329

Wen KK, Giardina PC, Blake MS, Edwards J, Apicella MA, Rubenstein PA (2000) Interaction of the gonococcal porin P.IB with G- and F-actin. Biochemistry 39:8638–8647

Wolff K, Stern A (1995) Identification and characterization of specific sequences encoding pathogenicity associated proteins in the genome of commensal *Neisseria* species. FEMS Microbiol Lett 125:255–263

Zawadzki P, Roberts MS, Cohan FM (1995) The log-linear relationship between sexual isolation and sequence divergence in Bacillus transformation is robust. Genetics 140:917–932

Zhou J, Spratt BG (1992) Sequence diversity within the *argF*, *fbp* and *recA* genes of natural isolates of *Neisseria meningitidis*: interspecies recombination within the *argF* gene. Mol Microbiol 6:2135–2146

Zhou J, Bowler LD, Spratt BG (1997) Interspecies recombination, and phylogenetic distortions, within the glutamine synthetase and shikimate dehydrogenase genes of *Neisseria meningitidis* and commensal *Neisseria* species. Mol Microbiol 23:799–812

Zhu P, Morelli G, Achtman M (1999) The *opcA* and Ψ*opcB* regions in *Neisseria*: genes, pseudogenes, deletions, insertion elements and DNA islands. Mol Microbiol 33:635–650

Genomic Islands of *Dichelobacter nodosus*

J.I. ROOD

1 Introduction

Dichelobacter nodosus is an anaerobic bacterium that is the causative agent of footrot in sheep and other ruminants. The organism is a slow-growing gram negative rod that is almost exclusively found on the ruminant hoof (STEWART 1989) and is a member of the family *Cardiobacteriaceae*, which belongs in the gamma division of the *Proteobacteria* (DEWHIRST et al. 1990). The organism has a relatively small genome of 1.54Mb that only has three rRNA operons (LA FONTAINE and ROOD 1996, 1997).

Ovine footrot is a mixed bacterial infection, but *D. nodosus* must be present for disease to occur. Under appropriate climatic conditions, the organism infects the interdigital skin and then progressively underruns the junction between the horn of the hoof and the soft tissue. The end result is the separation of the hard tissue of the horn, resulting in lameness, inability to feed and loss of body condition and wool quality (EGERTON et al. 1969; STEWART 1989). The disease is of considerable economic significance in almost all wool- and sheep meat-producing countries.

The virulence of the *D. nodosus* strain infecting the hoof is one of the major factors in the pathogenesis of the disease. Clinical *D. nodosus* isolates are described as virulent if they cause highly infectious disease outbreaks that lead to a significant separation of the horn of the hoof. By contrast, benign isolates only cause an

Bacterial Pathogenesis Research Group, Department of Microbiology, Monash University, Victoria 3800, Australia

interdigital dermatitis, even under optimal climatic conditions for the transmission of the disease. There are also many strains of intermediate virulence (STEWART 1989).

The major *D. nodosus*-encoded virulence factors believed to be involved in the disease are polar type IV fimbriae and extracellular proteases (BILLINGTON et al. 1996a). The type IV fimbriae are the major protective antigens on the surface of *D. nodosus* cells (CLAXTON 1989) and, like type IV fimbriae from other bacterial species, impart twitching motility upon their host cells (STROM and LORY 1993). It is thought that the fimbriae are involved in the translocation of the organism through the lesion, but, until recently, there have been no genetic methods of analysis available in *D. nodosus*. However, recent studies that involved the insertional inactivation of the fimbrial subunit gene, *fimA*, and virulence testing of the resultant mutants, have shown that this gene is essential for virulence (KENNAN et al. 2001).

Several of the genes involved in fimbrial biogenesis in *D. nodosus* have been cloned and sequenced and shown to be closely related to similar genes from other bacteria that produce type IV fimbriae (HOBBS et al. 1991; JOHNSTON et al. 1995, 1998; MATTICK et al. 1993). These genes are not localized to one area of the *D. nodosus* chromosome and, therefore, do not appear to be located in pathogenicity islands (LA FONTAINE and ROOD 1997).

Virulent isolates of *D. nodosus* produce several extracellular serine protease isoenzymes, which are encoded by the *aprV2*, *aprV5*, and *bprV* genes (LILLEY et al. 1992; RIFFKIN et al. 1993, 1995). Closely related protease genes, *aprB2*, *aprB5*, and *bprB*, are found in benign isolates (LILLEY et al. 1995; RIFFKIN et al. 1993, 1995). The enzymes encoded by the benign genes have different biochemical properties to the virulent proteases, forming the basis for tests that are used for the differential diagnosis of *D. nodosus* isolates (DEPIAZZI et al. 1991; PALMER 1993; SKERMAN 1989). Once more, the precise role of these genes in the disease process remains to be determined. The *apr5* and *bprV* genes are located 1kb apart on the *D. nodosus* genome (BILLINGTON et al. 1996a), but the location of the *aprV2* gene has not been determined.

2 Genomic Islands in *D. nodosus*

To develop gene probes that could be used for the differential diagnosis of ovine footrot, a comparative hybridization approach was used to isolate gene regions that were present in virulent isolates of *D. nodosus* but were not found in benign strains (KATZ et al. 1991). Three distinct recombinant plasmids were isolated and sequenced. One of these plasmids was subsequently found to be present in three copies on the chromosome of the reference *D. nodosus* strain A198 and was designated as part of the *vap* locus (KATZ et al. 1992, 1994). The other plasmids were subsequently shown to be part of a 27-kb locus known as the *vrl* region

(BILLINGTON et al. 1999; HARING et al. 1995). Both the *vap* and *vrl* loci have similarities to pathogenicity islands.

Screening of 101 virulent, intermediate and benign isolates of *D. nodosus* revealed that although all of the virulent isolates hybridized to both *vap* and *vrl* specific gene probes, 33% of the benign isolates also hybridized to the *vap* probe. By contrast, only 6% of the benign isolates were homologous to the *vrl* probes. These results indicated that the *vap* locus was more commonly found in virulent isolates but was also present in benign strains and strains of intermediate virulence. The *vrl* region appeared to be a better indicator of the virulence of an unknown *D. nodosus* isolate (KATZ et al. 1991).

Subsequently, a more comprehensive survey of 771 *D. nodosus* isolates was carried out, using both gene probe and PCR methods (ROOD et al. 1996). The results showed that 87% of the virulent isolates carried the *vrl* region, compared to only 6% of the benign isolates. These data correlated well with conventional laboratory tests for virulence, such as elastase and protease thermostability tests. Once more, the presence of the *vap* locus did not correlate as well with virulence. Although these studies examined 872 isolates (KATZ et al. 1991; ROOD et al. 1996), they did not identify a single isolate that had only the *vrl* region. All 311 *vrl* positive strains also carried the *vap* locus. By contrast, 289 strains that had *vap* but not *vrl* were detected (ROOD et al. 1996). Based on these data, it appears that the *vap* locus is essential for the acquisition or maintenance of the *vrl* region.

3 The *vrl* Locus

The elucidation of a physical and genetic map of the strain A198 genome revealed that it contained a single copy of the *vrl* region, which was located between the 260-kb and 650-kb *Stu*I fragments (LA FONTAINE and ROOD 1997). The *vrl* region from strain A198 has been cloned and completely sequenced (BILLINGTON et al. 1999; HARING et al. 1995; ROOD et al. 1993). It consists of a contiguous 27.1kb DNA segment that has a G + C content of 59.7% (BILLINGTON et al. 1999), which is much higher than the value of 45% reported for the overall genome (HOLDEMAN et al. 1984) and explains why it contains 22 *Eag*I and *Stu*I sites, compared to only 11 such sites in the rest of the 1.54-Mb genome (BILLINGTON et al. 1999; LA FONTAINE and ROOD 1997). The locus contains 22 potential genes, all of which are located on the same strand and appear to be organized in operon-like structures with overlapping or closely juxtaposed genes and ribosome binding sites (Fig. 1) (BILLINGTON et al. 1999). There is a potential promoter located in the 126-bp gap between *vrlH* and *vrlI*. The only other significant non-coding region is 245-bp of sequence located between *vrlD* and *vrlE*.

Comparison of the deduced amino acid sequences of the *vrl* gene products revealed several regions of similarity to plasmid or bacteriophage encoded proteins but did not identify any homologues of known virulence genes (BILLINGTON et al.

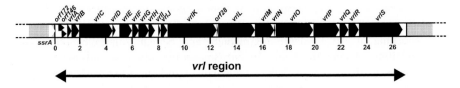

Fig. 1. Genetic organization of the *vrl* region. *vrl* genes are indicated by the *black arrows*, *ssrA* by the *white arrow*. The region outside the *vrl* locus is shown in *gray*. Size markers are in kb

1999). The VrlC protein has some similarity to extracellular glycosidases, such as chitinase, amylase, cellulase and pullulanase but does not appear to be secreted. It also has two Asp boxes, four of which are commonly found in sialidase enzymes. The possibility that VrlC may have endoglycosidase activity does have potential relevance to virulence. However, the level of sequence similarity is not high, and any designation of this protein as a virulence factor would have to be regarded as highly speculative.

VrlD has limited C-terminal similarity to the NorQ protein from *Bradyrhizobium japonicum*, which is a putative chaperone protein involved in nitric oxide reductase activity (GenBank Accession No. AJ132911), and VrlG has 24% identity to the glutaminase subunit of glutamine amidotransferases (BILLINGTON et al. 1999). Neither of these proteins is likely to be involved in virulence.

Several of the Vrl proteins have similarity to bacteriophage or plasmid encoded proteins. VrlJ, VrlO and VrlS each have ATP-binding domains (BILLINGTON et al. 1999), with the latter proteins each having the seven signature motifs of the DEAH family of ATP-dependent helicases. Similarly, VrlL appears to belong to the adenine-specific methyltransferase family. VrlK and VrlP have similarity to the *Streptomyces coelicolor* PglY and PglZ proteins, which are involved in bacteriophage φ31 resistance. The genes encoding the latter proteins are juxtaposed in *S. coelicolor*, unlike *vrlK* and *vrlP*, which are 7kb apart. However, the five intervening ORFs have a much lower percentage G + C content, suggesting that this region was of a different genetic origin and had been inserted into the *vrl* locus. Finally, VrlI shares a helix-turn-helix motif with the 37.3 protein from the *Bacillus subtilis* bacteriophage SPP1 and may be a DNA-binding transcriptional activator. Although not necessarily significant on an individual protein basis, taken together, these comparisons suggest that the *vrl* region is likely to have had an extrachromosomal origin. However, the *vrl* region does not appear to carry any genes that encode a site-specific recombinase, such as an integrase. Therefore, it appears that if the *vrl* region has evolved by the site-specific insertion of an extrachromosomal element into the *D. nodosus* chromosome, then either the site-specific recombinase gene has been subsequently deleted or the recombination process involved a host-encoded enzyme. The fact that the *vrl* region is only present in strains that also carry one or more copies of the *vap* region (ROOD et al. 1996) suggests that this recombinase may be *vap*-encoded (BILLINGTON et al. 1999).

There is evidence that the *vrl* region has inserted by a site-specific recombination event typical of bacterial pathogenicity islands. Most pathogenicity islands carry integrase genes that mediate site-specific recombination in or near tRNA genes, such as *selC* or *leuX* or other small RNA genes, such as *ssrA* (HACKER et al. 1997; HACKER and KAPER 1999). The *ssrA* gene encodes the 10Sa RNA molecule known as tmRNA (FELDEN et al. 1997), which can act as both a tRNA and an mRNA molecule (MUTO et al. 1998). tmRNA is important in the process of *trans*-translation, whereby the release of mRNA molecules from stalled or arrested ribosomes is mediated by the provision of a sequence encoding a peptide tag that contains a protease recognition site (KEILER et al. 1996; WILLIAMS et al. 1999). The resultant truncated protein is then degraded, primarily by the ClpP proteases (GOTTESMAN et al. 1998). tmRNA also has a role in gene regulation, which although initially thought to be mediated by a different mechanism (RETALLACK and FRIEDMAN 1995), is now also considered to involve *trans*-translation (ABO et al. 2000; WITHEY and FRIEDMAN 1999).

The VPI pathogenicity island of *Vibrio cholerae* (KARAOLIS et al. 1998; KOVACH et al. 1996) and the *iviXXII* virulence region of *Salmonella enterica* serovar Typhimurium (JULIO et al. 2000) have both inserted near the end of an *ssrA* gene. In *S.* Typhimurium, *ssrA* has been shown to be required for virulence in BALB/c mice (JULIO et al. 2000). The *D. nodosus vrl* region has also inserted into the end of an *ssrA* gene (HARING et al. 1995) (Fig. 1). The *vrl* sequence has inserted six nucleotides after the site at which the precursor is processed to form the mature tmRNA molecule (Fig. 2). The insertion site is preceded by a bacteriophage *att*-like sequence, and a potential transcriptional terminator is located immediately within the left end of the *vrl* locus. Since the site of *vrl* insertion is before the end of the precursor gene, insertion is likely to affect the processing of the *ssrA* transcript. It

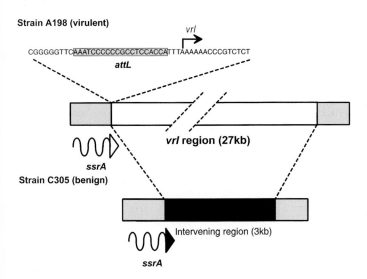

Fig. 2. The insertion site of the *vrl* region. Regions on either side of the *vrl* locus are shown in *grey*. The *vrl* region is in *white*, with the sequence located at the equivalent site in strain C305 shown in *black*. The *attL* site located at the junction between *vrl* and the chromosome is shown by the insert. Modified from Fig. 4 of BILLINGTON et al. (1996a)

was postulated that the *vrl* region may affect virulence as a result of its effects on the structure of the tmRNA precursor rather than as a result of carrying specific virulence genes (HARING et al. 1995). The implication is that, as in other bacteria, tmRNA has a global regulatory role and that insertion of *vrl* into the end of *ssrA* gene has affected the production of a functional processed tmRNA molecule such that there is an altered level of expression of one or more unknown virulence genes. Further experiments are required to verify this hypothesis. These experiments are now feasible because genetic methods for the construction of chromosomal mutants of *D. nodosus* have recently been developed (KENNAN et al. 1998).

Analysis of the benign strain C305 has revealed that a 3kb intervening region is present at the same site at which the *vrl* region is inserted in the virulent strain A198 (HARING et al. 1995) (Fig. 2). This region has no sequence similarity to the *vrl* locus. Any model that is developed to describe the potential role in virulence of the *vrl* locus must take into account this insertion. In addition, we have identified (BILLINGTON et al. 1999) a small group of strains that have large deletions within the *vrl* locus, from *vrlC* to *vrlP* (17.4kb) or from within the *att* site in *ssrA* to *vrlO* (17.0kb). Several of these strains are still virulent, suggesting that the region of the *vrl* locus that has been deleted is not essential for virulence. In addition, the *vrl* region does not appear to encode any gene products that are recognized in either experimental infections or vaccination experiments (BILLINGTON et al. 1999). Therefore, it is possible that the *vrl* region is not directly involved in virulence but is merely associated with virulent strains in a clonal manner.

4 The *vap* Loci

The reference virulent strain of *D. nodosus*, A198 or VCS1001, has three copies of the *vap* region (KATZ et al. 1991, 1994). There is extensive variation among these copies, indicating that there has been a significant level of genetic recombination and rearrangement since these regions were introduced into *D. nodosus*. The *vap* region is present in virtually all virulent strains of *D. nodosus* and in 32% of benign strains; therefore, it is not an absolute indicator of virulence in this species, although almost all virulent strains appear to have from one to three copies (KATZ et al. 1991). The three copies originally detected in strain A198 were designated as *vap* regions 1, 2 and 3 (KATZ et al. 1994), but subsequent studies (CHEETHAM et al. 1995) have shown that regions 1 and 3 are juxtaposed on the chromosome and form a discrete genomic island known as the *intA* element (WHITTLE et al. 1999).

The 11.5kb *intA* element consists of at least 16 genes, several of which (*vapADEG*) appear to have been duplicated (Fig. 3). The products of many of these genes have sequence similarity to proteins encoded by bacterial plasmids or other mobile genetic elements (CHEETHAM et al. 1999). The VapE protein is related to Orf11, which is found on a mobile 15.2kb toxic shock toxin pathogenicity island, SaPI1 from *Staphylococcus aureus* (LINDSAY et al. 1998) and VapE from the plant

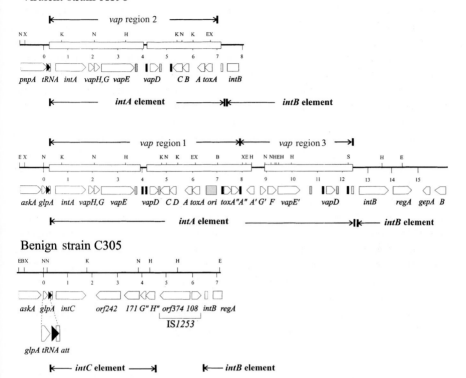

Fig. 3. Genetic organization of the *vap* regions. Both the original *vap* regions 1, 2 and 3 and the recently designated *intA*, *intB* and *intC* elements are shown. Genes are indicated by the *open arrows*. Size markers are in kb. Modified from Fig. 1 of Whittle et al. (1999)

pathogen *Xylella fastidiosa* (Simpson et al. 2000). However, there is no evidence that these homologues are involved in virulence. Comparative analysis of VapD reveals that there are related proteins encoded on various plasmids, including ORF5 from the *Neisseria gonorrhoeae* cryptic plasmid and plasmids from *Actinobacillus actinomycetemcomitans* and *Treponema denticola* (Billington et al. 1996a). There are also VapD-like proteins encoded on the chromosomes of *Helicobacter pylori*, *Riemerella anatipestifer*, *Haemophilus influenzae*, *Neisseria meningitidis* and *X. fastidiosa*. Unfortunately, none of these proteins has any known function.

The *vapBC* gene region is similar to the *trbH* region of the F plasmid and the *vagCD* region of the *Salmonella dublin* virulence plasmid. These genes appear to encode proteins involved in plasmid maintenance (Pullinger and Lax 1992). The putative 135 amino acid VapC protein has the conserved PIN or PilT N-terminal domain. This 100 amino acid domain is of unknown function but has been postulated to be involved in signaling because it is found in a plasmid-encoded transcriptional regulator and other regulatory proteins (Makarova et al.

1999). VapB is a homologue of VagC. In addition, there are homologues of VapB, VapC and VapD encoded on the *H. influenzae* genome (FLEISCHMANN et al. 1995).

Functions have been assigned to *toxA* and *vapA*, the next genes in the *vap* loci (Fig. 3). The ToxA and VapA proteins have sequence similarity to the HigB and HigA proteins of the Rts1 plasmid killer system (BILLINGTON et al. 1996b; TIAN et al. 1996b). The latter proteins act as a host cell toxic protein and its cognate antidote protein, respectively, with the HigA antidote protein also acting to repress the expression of the *higBA* operon (TIAN et al. 1996a). It appears that the VapA and ToxA proteins act in a similar manner (BLOOMFIELD et al. 1997). The VapA protein also has a helix-turn-helix motif typically found in repressor proteins. It has been postulated that the ToxA/VapA system serves to maintain the *vap* locus in the host cell (BLOOMFIELD et al. 1997).

Unlike the *vrl* locus, a recombinase has been identified in the *vap* regions. At the left end of *vap* regions 1/3 and 2 there is a gene, *intA* (Fig. 3), whose product has sequence similarity to the lambda integrase family of site-specific recombinases, including the conserved residues known to be essential for integrase function (BLOOMFIELD et al. 1997; CHEETHAM et al. 1995). Examination of the sites at which the *vap* loci appear to have inserted suggests that insertion of *vap* region 1/3 and *vap* region 2 has occurred at typical bacteriophage-like *att* sites located downstream of either a tRNA-ser_{GCU} gene, *serV*, or a tRNA-ser_{GGA} gene, respectively (BLOOMFIELD et al. 1997). Based on these results, it was concluded that in strain A198, *vap* region 1 and *vap* region 2 were derived by separate insertion events that involved different tRNA-*ser* genes. It is uncertain whether *vap* region 3 arose by partial duplication of *vap* region 1 or by a separate insertion event. Both *vap* regions 1/3 and *vap* region 2 have now been designated as variants of the *intA* genetic element (WHITTLE et al. 1999).

The presence in the *vap* region of genes with functional or sequence similarity to several plasmid encoded genes suggests that the *vap* loci were originally extra-chromosomal. A 10-kb plasmid, pJIR896, has been identified in *D. nodosus* strain AC3577 (BILLINGTON et al. 1996b). This plasmid consists of *vap* region 1, part of *vap* region 3, a single *att* site, and a copy of IS*1253*, an insertion sequence that is also found on the *D. nodosus* chromosome. The analysis of this plasmid supports the hypothesis that the chromosomal *vap* regions were derived from the insertion of an extrachromosomal element by integrase-mediated site-specific recombination events.

Other genetic elements that carry integrase genes have been identified in *D. nodosus* (BLOOMFIELD et al. 1997; WHITTLE et al. 1999). Next to the right end of the *vap* 3 region of the *intA* element in strain A198 (Fig. 3), there is a second integrase gene, *intB*, whose complete product has 31% sequence identity to IntA, although it is unlikely to be functional since *intB* carries an internal stop codon (BLOOMFIELD et al. 1997). Downstream of *intB* there is a gene, *regA*, that appears to encode a regulatory protein that has a helix-turn-helix motif, followed by several genes, including *gepA*, whose product has similarity to a protein encoded by a conjugative transposon from *Bacteroides thetaiotamicron*. The *intB* element appears to have inserted into the *att* site located at the right end of the *intA* element. There is another *intB* gene located at the right end of the *intA* element previously designated as *vap* region 2. Although the previous internal *intB* stop codon is not present, the gene still appears to be truncated (BLOOMFIELD et al. 1997). Analysis of four additional *D. nodosus* strains revealed that they all had *intB* genes at the same position relative to the *intA* element, although two of these strains had additional *intB* sequences that were not associated with *vap* sequences (BLOOMFIELD et al. 1997). Based on these data, the regions downstream of the *intA* elements were subsequently designated as *intB* genetic elements, and it was postulated that they were derived from separate integrase-mediated recombination events (WHITTLE et al. 1999).

A third genetic element, the *intC* element, has been identified in the benign *D. nodosus* strain C305. This 6.6kb element carries a third integrase gene, *intC*, a copy of IS*1253*, variants of the *vapG* and *vapH* genes, and is inserted at the same tRNA-*ser*$_{GCU}$ site that has the *intA* element in strain A198 (WHITTLE et al. 1999). There is a truncated *intB* element located immediately downstream, as it would be if the inserted region were an *intA* element. Therefore, it appears that the tRNA-*ser*$_{GCU}$ gene can act as the site of insertion for either *intA* or *intC* elements. A survey of other *D. nodosus* isolates revealed that 10/15 strains carried *intC* elements, all at the same site as in strain C305. The virulent strain 1311 also carries the 5.1kb broad host range plasmid pDN1 (WHITTLE et al. 2000). In a derivative that had lost pDN1, strain 1311 A, the much larger (>14kb) *intC* element was also deleted, although the tRNA-*ser*$_{GCU}$ gene was not affected by the deletion (WHITTLE et al. 1999). Comparison of the thermostabilities of protease preparations from strains 1311 and 1311 A revealed that loss of pDN1 and the *intC* element was associated with a loss of thermostability, a well-known virulence-related property of clinical *D. nodosus* isolates. In addition, strain 1311 A produced less protease on solid media. These effects on protease production were not due to the loss of pDN1. Unfortunately, since only one *intC* deletion derivative has been isolated and analyzed, the precise relationship between the *intC* element and protease production remains to be determined.

To the left of the tRNA-*ser*$_{GCU}$ gene in strains A198, C305 and 1311, there are two genes, *glpA* and *askA* (WHITTLE et al. 1999). The *askA* gene encodes the enzyme aspartokinase, a housekeeping gene unlikely to be involved in virulence. The *glpA* gene encodes a putative 64 amino acid protein that has 74% identity to the first 50 amino acids of the RsmA protein from the plant pathogen *Erwinia carotovora* and the *Escherichia coli* CsrA protein (ROMEO 1998). The *csrA* gene is located next to *serV* in *E. coli*, at the same position as *glpA* in *D. nodosus*. RsmA is an RNA-binding protein that is a global post-transcriptional repressor of virulence factors and other gene products in *E. carotovora* (CUI et al. 1996; CUI et al. 1999; MUKHERJEE et al. 1996). CsrA acts in the same way to activate exponential phase metabolic pathways (ROMEO 1998). To the left of the tRNA-*ser*$_{GGA}$ gene in strain A198, which is the site of insertion of the *vap* region 2 *intA* element, there is a gene that encodes the PnpA protein, which is a polynucleotide phosphorylase and, like CsrA, has the KH domain found in several RNA binding proteins (LIU et al. 1995; WHITTLE et al. 1999).

It has been postulated that the effect of the *vap* elements on virulence is mediated by their ability to modulate the functional expression of the *pnpA* and *glpA* genes (WHITTLE et al. 1999). Specifically, it is proposed that in virulent isolates the *intA* element is inserted next to *pnpA* and that *intA* or *intC* is inserted next to *glpA*. Termination of the *pnpA*-tRNA or *glpA*-tRNA transcripts is postulated to vary, depending on which element is integrated at each site, affecting the functional expression of the PnpA and GlpA proteins. Variation in the levels of these putative RNA binding proteins, or the respective tRNA molecules, is proposed to have global regulatory effects, including effects on virulence gene expression. Additional experiments are required to verify this hypothesis. RNA studies are needed to confirm that the nature of the various transcripts is dependent upon the element inserted downstream of each respective gene. In addition, it will be necessary to insertionally inactivate these genes and study the resultant effects on virulence gene expression and virulence in sheep. These experiments are feasible now that methods for the genetic manipulation of *D. nodosus* are available (KENNAN et al. 1998).

5 Are the *vrl* and *vap* Elements Pathogenicity Islands?

Pathogenicity islands have been defined as discrete, relatively large, genetic elements that have several common features (HACKER et al. 1997; HACKER and KAPER 1999, 2000). These properties include the presence of one or more virulence genes, often genes encoding adhesins, invasins or type III or type IV secretion systems. They also have a different percentage G + C content compared to the host chromosome, reflecting their acquisition by horizontal gene transfer. They insert in or near tRNA genes or IS sequences, carry IS elements, transposases or integrases, and exhibit genetic instability. Pathogenicity islands are found primarily in virulent strains, although they may be present in a sporadic manner in less virulent isolates. The site at which they are inserted is often an important factor in determining whether the genes encoded on a pathogenicity island are expressed.

The *vrl* element has many properties in common with pathogenicity islands (BILLINGTON et al. 1999; CHEETHAM et al. 1999). It consists of a large discrete genetic unit that has a different percentage G + C content to that of the *D. nodosus* chromosome; it is primarily, but not exclusively, found in virulent isolates, and it is associated with an *ssrA* gene, which has similarity to tRNA genes and has been shown to act as a pathogenicity island insertion site in other bacteria (JULIO et al. 2000; KARAOLIS et al. 1998). However, the *vrl* locus does not carry any known virulence genes and has not been shown to confer virulence. In addition, *vrl* does not carry any integrase or resolvase genes, although its absolute association with the *vap* loci and presumed dependence upon the *vap* integrase for insertion, provides an explanation for this observation.

A similar situation exists with the *intA* or *vap* elements (CHEETHAM et al. 1999; WHITTLE et al. 1999). These elements are smaller, have a percentage G + C content that is similar to that of the chromosome, have an integrase gene, and are inserted into tRNA genes. Like the *vrl* region, the *intA* elements do not carry any known virulence genes and have not been shown to confer virulence. For both the *vrl* and *intA* elements, it has been proposed that they modulate virulence as a result of the effect of their insertion on the functional expression of genes transcribed at the insertion sites. However, these hypotheses have not been experimentally verified, primarily because genetic methods of analysis have only recently become available for *D. nodosus*. The *intB* and *intC* elements have also been identified in some strains of this organism. These elements are yet to be completely defined but have been shown to carry integrase genes and to insert into typical pathogenicity island insertion sites. There is preliminary evidence that in one strain deletion of the *intC* element may alter extracellular protease production (WHITTLE et al. 1999).

In summary, the *vrl* and *intA* elements appear to meet almost all of the criteria normally used to define pathogenicity islands, except that they have not been positively shown to carry virulence genes or to confer virulence on their hosts. Therefore, they technically should be referred to as genomic islands rather than pathogenicity islands. However, such a distinction is really a matter of semantics, as there is little evolutionary point in distinguishing between pathogenicity islands, genomic islands or metabolic fitness islands (HACKER and KAPER 1999). The important feature of the *D. nodosus* elements is that they clearly represent either mobile genetic elements, or derivatives of mobile genetic elements, that have been acquired by horizontal gene transfer and potentially have the ability to modulate the genetic potential of their host. With genetic studies on *D. nodosus* in their infancy but now technically quite straightforward, the author looks forward to exciting developments in this field as these methods are applied with skill and rigor to the analysis of this important pathogenic bacterium.

Acknowledgements. The author thanks the Australian Research Council for supporting the research carried out in his laboratory and Dr Brian Cheetham for providing an electronic copy of Fig. 1 from WHITTLE et al. (1999).

References

Abo T, Inada T, Ogawa K, Aiba H (2000) SsrA-mediated tagging and proteolysis of LacI and its role in the regulation of *lac* operon. EMBO J 19:3762–3769

Billington SJ, Johnston JL, Rood JI (1996a) Virulence regions and virulence factors of the ovine footrot pathogen, *Dichelobacter nodosus*. FEMS Microbiol Lett 145:147–156

Billington SJ, Sinistaj M, Cheetham BF, Ayres A, Moses EK, Katz ME, Rood JI (1996b) Identification of a native *Dichelobacter nodosus* plasmid and implications for the evolution of the *vap* regions. Gene 172:111–116

Billington SJ, Huggins AS, Johanesen P, Crellin PK, Cheung J, Katz ME, Wright CL, Haring V, Rood JI (1999) Complete nucleotide sequence of the 27-kb virulence related locus (*vrl*) of *Dichelobacter nodosus*: evidence for an extrachromosomal origin. Infect Immun 67:1277–1286

Bloomfield GA, Whittle G, McDonagh MB, Katz ME, Cheetham BF (1997) Analysis of sequences flanking the *vap* regions of *Dichelobacter nodosus*: evidence for multiple integration events and a new genetic element. Microbiology 143:553–562

Cheetham BF, Tattersall DB, Bloomfield GA, Rood JI, Katz ME (1995) Identification of a bacterio-phage-related integrase gene in a *vap* region of the genome of *D. nodosus*. Gene 162:53–58

Cheetham B, Whittle G, Katz ME (1999) Are the *vap* regions of *Dichelobacter nodosus* pathogenicity islands? In: Kaper J, Hacker J (eds) Pathogenicity islands and other mobile virulence elements. ASM Press, Washington, DC, pp 203–218

Claxton PD (1989) Antigenic classification of *Bacteroides nodosus*. In: Egerton JR, Yong WK, Riffkin GG (eds) Footrot and foot abscess of ruminants. CRC Press, Inc., Boca Raton, pp 155–166

Cui Y, Madi L, Mukherjee A, Dumenyo CK, Chatterjee AK (1996) The RsmA- mutants of *Erwinia carotovora* subsp. *carotovora* strain Ecc71 overexpress hrpNEcc and elicit a hypersensitive reaction-like response in tobacco leaves. Mol Plant Microbe Interact 9:565–573

Cui Y, Mukherjee A, Dumenyo CK, Liu Y, Chatterjee AK (1999) *rsmC* of the soft-rotting bacterium *Erwinia carotovora* subsp. *carotovora* negatively controls extracellular enzyme and harpin(Ecc) production and virulence by modulating levels of regulatory RNA (rsmB) and RNA-binding protein (RsmA). J Bacteriol 181:6042–6052

Depiazzi LJ, Richards RB, Henderson J, Rood JI, Palmer M, Penhale WJ (1991) Characterisation of virulent and benign strains of *Bacteroides nodosus*. Vet Microbiol 26:151–160

Dewhirst FE, Paster BJ, La Fontaine S, Rood JI (1990) Transfer of *Kingella indologenes* (Snell and Lapage 1976) to the genus *Suttonella* gen. nov. as *Suttonella indologenes* comb. nov.; Transfer of *Bacteroides nodosus* (Beveridge 1941) to the genus *Dichelobacter* gen. nov. as *Dichelobacter nodosus* comb. nov.; and assignment of the genera *Cardiobacterium*, *Dichelobacter*, and *Suttonella* to *Cardiobacteriaceae* fam. nov. in the gamma division of *Proteobacteria* based on 16 S Ribosomal Ribonucleic Acid Sequence Comparisons. Int J Syst Bacteriol 40:426–433

Egerton JR, Roberts DS, Parsonson IM (1969) The aetiology and pathogenesis of ovine footrot. I. A histological study of the bacterial invasion. J Comp Pathol 81:179–185

Felden B, Himeno H, Muto A, McCutcheon JP, Atkins JF, Gesteland RF (1997) Probing the structure of the Escherichia coli 10Sa RNA (tmRNA). RNA 3:89–103

Fleischmann RD, Adams MD, White O, Clayton RA, Kirkness EF, Kerlavage AR, Bult CJ, Tomb J-F, Dougherty BA, Merrick JM, McKenney K, Sutton G, FitzHugh W, Fields C, Gocayne JD, Scott J, Shirley R, Liu L-I, Glodek A, Kelley JM, Weidman JF, Phillips CA, Spriggs T, Hedblom E, Cotton MD, Utterback TR, Hanna MC, Nguyen DT, Saudek DM, Brandon RC, Fine LD, Fritchman JL, Fuhrmann JL, Geoghagen NSM, Gnehm CL, McDonald LA, Small KV, Fraser CM, Smith HO, Venter JC (1995) Whole-genome random sequencing and assembly of *Haemophilus influenzae* Rd. Science 269:496–512

Gottesman S, Roche E, Zhou Y, Sauer RT (1998) The ClpXP and ClpAP proteases degrade proteins with carboxy-terminal peptide tails added by the SsrA-tagging system. Genes Dev 12:1338–1347

Hacker J, Kaper J (1999) The concept of pathogenicity islands. In: Kaper J, Hacker J (eds) Pathogenicity islands and other mobile virulence elements. ASM Press, Washington, DC, pp 1–11

Hacker J, Kaper JB (2000) Pathogenicity islands and the evolution of microbes. Annu Rev Microbiol 54:641–679

Hacker J, Blum-Oehler G, Mühldorfer I, Tschäpe H (1997) Pathogenicity islands of virulent bacteria: structure, function and impact on microbial evolution. Mol Microbiol 23:1089–1097

Haring V, Billington SJ, Wright CL, Huggins AS, Katz ME, Rood JI (1995) Delineation of the virulence related locus *vrl* of *Dichelobacter nodosus*. Microbiology 141:2081–2091

Hobbs M, Dalrymple BP, Cox PT, Livingstone SP, Delaney SF, Mattick JS (1991) Organization of the fimbrial gene region of *Bacteroides nodosus*: class I and class II strains. Mol Microbiol 5: 543–560

Holdeman LV, Kelley RW, Moore WEC (1984) Genus I. *Bacteroides* Castellani and Chalmers 1919, 959[AL]. In: Krieg NR, Holt JG (eds) Bergey's manual of systematic bacteriology. The Williams and Wilkins Co., Baltimore, pp 604–631

Johnston JL, Billington SJ, Haring V, Rood JI (1995) Identification of fimbrial assembly genes from *Dichelobacter nodosus*: evidence that *fimP* encodes the typeIV prepilin peptidase. Gene 161:21–26

Johnston JL, Billington SJ, Haring V, Rood JI (1998) Complementation analysis of the *Dichelobacter nodosus fimN*, *fimO*, and *fimP* genes in *Pseudomonas aeruginosa* and transcriptional analysis of the *fimNOP* gene region. Infect Immun 66:297–304

Julio SM, Heithoff DM, Mahan MJ (2000) *ssrA* (tmRNA) plays a role in *Salmonella enterica* serovar Typhimurium pathogenesis. J Bacteriol 182:1558–1563

Karaolis DK, Johnson JA, Bailey CC, Boedeker EC, Kaper JB, Reeves PR (1998) A *Vibrio cholerae* pathogenicity island associated with epidemic and pandemic strains. Proc Natl Acad Sci USA 95:3134–3139

Katz ME, Howarth PM, Yong WK, Riffkin GG, Depiazzi LJ, Rood JI (1991) Identification of three gene
regions associated with virulence in *Dichelobacter nodosus*, the causative agent of ovine footrot. J Gen
Microbiol 137:2117–2124

Katz ME, Strugnell RA, Rood JI (1992) Molecular characterization of a genomic region associated with
virulence in *Dichelobacter nodosus*. Infect Immun 60:4586–4592

Katz ME, Wright CL, Gartside TS, Cheetham BF, Doidge CV, Moses EK, Rood JI (1994) Genetic
organization of the duplicated *vap* region of the *Dichelobacter nodosus* genome. J Bacteriol 176:2663–
2669

Keiler KC, Waller PRH, Sauer RT (1996) Role of a peptide tagging system in degradation of proteins
synthesized from damaged messenger RNA. Science 271:990–993

Kennan RM, Billington SJ, Rood JI (1998) Electroporation-mediated transformation of the ovine footrot
pathogen *Dichelobacter nodosus*. FEMS Microbiol Lett 169:383–389

Kennan RM, Dhungyel OP, Whittington RJ, Egerton JR, Rood JI (2001) The type IV fimbrial subunit
gene (*fimA*) of *Dichelobacter nodosus* is essential for virulence, protease secretion and natural competence. J Bacteriol 183:4451–4458

Kovach ME, Shaffer MD, Peterson KM (1996) A putative integrase gene defines the distal end of a large
cluster of ToxR-regulated colonization genes in *Vibrio cholerae*. Microbiology 142:2165–2174

La Fontaine S, Rood JI (1996) Organization of ribosomal RNA genes from the footrot pathogen
Dichelobacter nodosus. Microbiology 142:889–899

La Fontaine S, Rood JI (1997) Physical and genetic map of the chromosome of *Dichelobacter nodosus*
strain A198. Gene 184:291–298

Lilley GG, Riffkin MC, Stewart DJ, Kortt AA (1995) Nucleotide and deduced protein sequence of the
extracellular, serine basic protease gene (*bprB*) from *Dichelobacter nodosus* strain 305: comparison
with the basic protease gene (*bprV*) from virulent strain 198. Biochem Mol Biol Int 36:101–111

Lilley GG, Stewart DJ, Kortt AA (1992) Amino acid and DNA sequences of an extracellular basic
protease of *Dichelobacter nodosus* show that it is a member of the subtilisin family of proteases. Eur J
Biochem 210:13–21

Lindsay JA, Ruzin A, Ross HF, Kurepina N, Novick RP (1998) The gene for toxic shock toxin is carried
by a family of mobile pathogenicity islands in *Staphylococcus aureus*. Mol Microbiol 29:527–543

Liu M, Yang H, Romeo T (1995) The product of the pleiotropic *Escherichia coli* gene *csrA* modulates
glycogen biosynthesis via effects on mRNA stability. J Bacteriol 177:2663–2672

Makarova KS, Aravind L, Galperin MY, Grishin NV, Tatusov RL, Wolf YI, Koonin EV (1999)
Comparative genomics of the *Archaea* (*Euryarchaeota*): evolution of conserved protein families, the
stable core, and the variable shell. Genome Res 9:608–628

Mattick JM, Hobbs M, Cox PT, Dalrymple BP (1993) Molecular biology of the fimbriae of *Dichelobacter*
(previously *Bacteroides*) *nodosus*. In: Sebald M (eds) Genetics and molecular biology of anaerobic
bacteria. Springer, Berlin Heidelberg New York, pp 517–545

Mukherjee A, Cui Y, Liu Y, Dumenyo CK, Chatterjee AK (1996) Global regulation in *Erwinia* species by
Erwinia carotovora rsmA, a homologue of *Escherichia coli csrA*: repression of secondary metabolites,
pathogenicity and hypersensitive reaction. Microbiology 142:427–434

Muto A, Ushida C, Himeno H (1998) A bacterial RNA that functions as both a tRNA and an mRNA.
Trends Biochem Sci 23:25–29

Palmer MA (1993) A gelatin test to detect activity and stability of proteases produced by *Dichelobacter
nodosus*. Vet Microbiol 36:113–122

Pullinger GD, Lax AJ (1992) A *Salmonella dublin* virulence plasmid locus that affects bacterial growth
under nutrient-limited conditions. Mol Microbiol 6:1631–1643

Retallack DM, Friedman DI (1995) A role for a small stable RNA in modulating the activity of
DNA-binding proteins. Cell 83:227–235

Riffkin MC, Focareta A, Edwards RD, Stewart DJ, Kortt AA (1993) Cloning, sequence and expression
of the gene (*aprV5*) encoding extracellular serine acidic protease V5 from *Dichelobacter nodosus*. Gene
137:259–264

Riffkin MC, Wang LF, Kortt AA, Stewart DJ (1995) A single amino-acid change between the
antigenically different extracellular serine proteases V2 and B2 from *Dichelobacter nodosus*. Gene
167:279–283

Romeo T (1998) Global regulation by the small RNA-binding protein CsrA and the non-coding RNA
molecule CsrB. Mol Microbiol 29:1321–1330

Rood JI, Wright CL, Haring V, Katz ME (1993) Molecular analysis of the virulence associated gene
regions from the ovine footrot pathogen, *Dichelobacter nodosus*. In: Kado CI, Crosa J II, (eds)
Molecular mechanism of Bacterial Virulence. Kluwer Academic Publishers, Netherlands

Rood JI, Howarth PA, Haring V, Billington SJ, Yong WK, Liu D, Palmer MA, Pitman DA, Links I, Stewart DA, Vaughan JA (1996) Comparison of gene probe and conventional methods for the differentiation of ovine footrot isolates of *Dichelobacter nodosus*. Vet Microbiol 52:127–141

Simpson AJ, Reinach FC, Arruda P, Abreu FA, Acencio M, Alvarenga R, Alves LM, Araya JE, Baia GS, Baptista CS, Barros MH, Bonaccorsi ED, Bordin S, Bove JM, Briones MR, Bueno MR, Camargo AA, Camargo LE, Carraro DM, Carrer H, Colauto NB, Colombo C, Costa FF, Costa MC, Costa-Neto CM, Coutinho LL, Cristofani M, Dias-Neto E, Docena C, El-Dorry H, Facincani AP, Ferreira AJ, Ferreira VC, Ferro JA, Fraga JS, Franca SC, Franco MC, Frohme M, Furlan LR, Garnier M, Goldman GH, Goldman MH, Gomes SL, Gruber A, Ho PL, Hoheisel JD, Junqueira ML, Kemper EL, Kitajima JP, Krieger JE, Kuramae EE, Laigret F, Lambais MR, Leite LC, Lemos EG, Lemos MV, Lopes SA, Lopes CR, Machado JA, Machado MA, Madeira AM, Madeira HM, Marino CL (2000) The genome sequence of the plant pathogen *Xylella fastidiosa*. The *Xylella fastidiosa* consortium of the organization for nucleotide sequencing and analysis. Nature 406:151–157

Skerman TM (1989) Isolation and identification of *Bacteroides nodosus*. In: Egerton JR, Yong WK, Riffkin GG (eds) Footrot and foot abscess of ruminants. CRC Press, Inc., Boca Raton, pp 85–104

Stewart DJ (1989) Footrot of sheep. In: Egerton JR, Yong WK, Riffkin GG (eds) Footrot and foot abscess of ruminants. CRC Press, Boca Raton, pp 5–45

Strom MS, Lory S (1993) Structure-function and biogenesis of the type IV pili. Annu Rev Microbiol 47:565–596

Tian QB, Hayashi T, Murata T, Terawaki Y (1996a) Gene product identification and promoter analysis of *hig* locus of plasmid Rts1. Biochem Biophys Res Commun 225:679–684

Tian QB, Ohnishi M, Tabushi A, Terawaki Y (1996b) A new plasmid-encoded proteic killer gene system: cloning, sequencing and analyzing locus of plasmid Rts1. Biochem Biophys Res Commun 220: 280–284

Whittle G, Bloomfield G, Katz M, Cheetham B (1999) The site-specific integration of genetic elements may modulate thermostable protease production, a virulence factor in *Dichelobacter nodosus*, the causative agent of ovine footrot. Microbiology 145:2845–2855

Whittle G, Katz ME, Clayton EH, Cheetham BF (2000) Identification and characterization of a native *Dichelobacter nodosus* plasmid, pDN1. Plasmid 43:230–234

Williams KP, Martindale KA, Bartel DP (1999) Resuming translation on tmRNA: a unique mode of determining a reading frame. EMBO J 18:5423–5433

Withey J, Friedman D (1999) Analysis of the role of *trans*-translation in the requirement of tmRNA for λimm^{P22} growth in *Escherichia coli*. J Bacteriol 181:2148–2157

Genomic Structure and Evolution of *Legionella* Species

K. Heuner[1], M. Steinert[1], R. Marre[2], and J. Hacker[1]

1 Introduction

Legionella pneumophila is the causative agent of legionnaires' disease. This atypical pneumonia was first described after a big outbreak in Philadelphia, Pa., during the 56th annual American Legion convention (Fraser et al. 1977; McDade et al. 1977). In humans *Legionella* also causes Pontiac fever, which is a nonpneumonic illness with fever and headache. Pontiac fever is self-limiting, and the mortality rate is zero. *L. pneumophila* is a classic opportunistic pathogen, which mainly infects immunocompromised humans.

Legionella is commonly found in aquatic habitats. High concentrations of *Legionella* can regularly be detected in man-made hot-water systems (Fields et al. 1989; Wadowsky et al. 1988). *L. pneumophila* is able to replicate intracellularly in many different host cells (Fields 1996). In the environment, *Legionella* replicates in

[1] Institut für Molekulare Infektionsbiologie, Julius-Maximilians Universität Würzburg, Röntgenring 11, 97070 Würzburg, Germany
[2] Institut für medizinische Mikrobiologie und Hygiene, Universität Ulm, Robert-Koch-Strasse 8, 89081 Ulm, Germany

protozoa and during infection in human alveolar macrophages. Macrophages, monocytes and also alveolar epithelial cells support intracellular replication of *L. pneumophila* (CIANCIOTTO et al. 1995; HORWITZ and SILVERSTEIN 1980; ROWBOTHAM 1980). The introduction of man-made hot-water systems created the conditions for successful transmission of *L. pneumophila* to humans (FIELDS 1996). Therefore, it was speculated that the capability to multiply in protozoa is the evolutionary prerequisite for *Legionella* to become a human pathogen.

2 Taxonomy and Evolution of *Legionellaceae*

Legionella organisms are non-spore-forming gram negative bacilli. *Legionella* is a member of the gamma-subgroup of proteobacteria, and so far, 42 species and 65 serogroups of Legionellae have been described (FREY et al. 1991; WINN 1999). Nutritionally, they are fastidious, and it is thought that intracellular replication within selected host cells is the primary and perhaps sole means of proliferation in the environment (FIELDS 1993). There are approximately 19 human pathogenic species, but *L. pneumophila* is the most frequently isolated species associated with disease (BENSON and FIELDS 1998; MARSTON et al. 1994; WINN 1988). In cold-water systems, only low concentrations of legionellae (10 bacteria/l) are found, whereas man-made hot-water systems may harbour up to 10^6 bacteria/l (GROOTHUIS et al. 1985). A large number of *Legionella*-like amoebal pathogens (LLAPs) have been described, which are clustered in 12 phylogenetic groups belonging to five species (ADELEKE et al. 1996, 2001) (Fig. 1). Although the ecology and genetic composition of LLAPs are similar to *Legionella*, these isolates are difficult to grow on artificial media, and they rarely cause disease.

The chromosome of *L. pneumophila* is approximately 3.9Mb in size (BENDER et al. 1990). In the near future, the whole genome of *L. pneumophila* Philadelphia 1 will be sequenced, and the DNA fragments will be assembled by the group of H.A. Shuman and J.J. Russo (QU et al. 2001). The G + C content of *L. pneumophila* is 38% over most of its length. Information about the *Legionella* genome is available at the homepage (*http://genome3.cpmc.columbia.edu/~legion/*). Genome analysis of *Legionella* isolates by pulsed-field gel electrophoresis (PFGE) was shown to be useful for identification of individual strains. More recently, sequence-based phylogenetic schemes that utilize the variation in the 16S rRNA sequence have been used to classify and identify *Legionella*. Based on this knowledge, specific fluorescence labelled oligonucleotides, which hybridise with the complementary rRNA region of the target organism, have been designed. This powerful tool allows the analysis of the structure and dynamics in complex microbial biocenosis. Ratcliff et al. phylogenetically compared most *Legionella* species, using the species variation between the 16S rRNA and *mip* genes (RATCLIFF et al. 1997). In their study, they found over twice the variation in the *mip* gene at the DNA level (56% of base sites) when compared to the 16S rRNA (23% of base sites). In addition, the *mip*

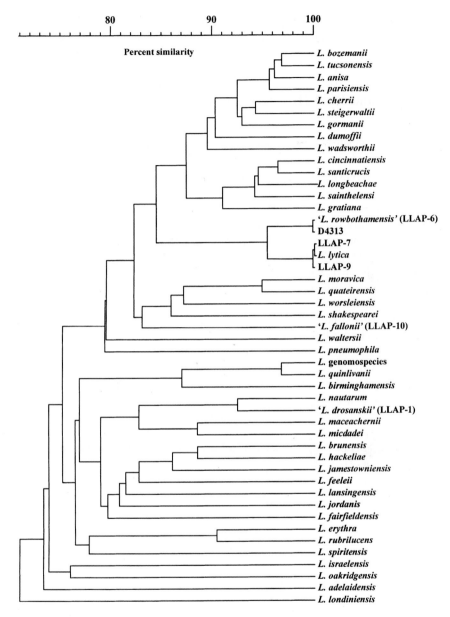

Fig. 1. UPGMA phylogenetic dendrogram of *mip* sequence similarities found among *Legionella* species and LLAP strains. The *vertical bar* joining two species or clusters indicates the level of similarity. The phylogenetic dendrogram was kindly provided by M.A. Halablab (ADELEKE et al. 2001)

sequence results were in complete agreement with serological, DNA/DNA hybridisation and fatty acid and ubiquinone results. Until now, there has been no evidence of horizontally genetic recombination across *Legionella* species. This sequence similarity among *Legionella* strains provides evidence that global migration of legionellae, probably within protozoan cysts, may occur.

3 Survival and Dual Host System of *Legionella*

Legionellae are widely distributed in natural aquatic environments and also in manmade aquatic habitats. It is still unclear whether *L. pneumophila* is able to multiply extracellularly (KEEVIL 2000; SURMAN et al. 2001). However, recently it was demonstrated that *L. pneumophila* is not capable of growing extracellularly in a biofilm model with five pre-selected organisms (FIELDS 2001). Up to now, it has been assumed that intracellular replication in protozoa is central for the survival of *L. pneumophila*. In addition, amoebae may reactivate viable but nonculturable (VBNC) *L. pneumophila*. This dormancy state often represents the majority of a population in the environment. The virulence of these resuscitated bacteria seemed not to be reduced. Interestingly, no resuscitation was observed in guinea pigs (STEINERT et al. 1997).

In 1980, Rowbotham described the ability of *L. pneumophila* to infect protozoa and to replicate intracellularly in *Acanthamoeba* and *Naegleria* (ROWBOTHAM 1980). Since then, it was shown that *L. pneumophila* is able to multiply in 16 species of amoebae and two species of ciliated protozoa (Table 1) (reviewed in FIELDS 1996). *Acanthamoeba* and *Hartmannella* were used in most of the studies investigating the pathogenic mechanisms of *L. pneumophila*. Intracellular growth of *L. pneumophila* in amoebae was shown to change the bacterial surface properties (BARKER et al. 1993) to increase the resistance of *Legionella* to antibiotics as well as to chemical biocides (BARKER et al. 1992, 1995) and to enhance invasion into human monocytes (CIRILLO et al. 1994, 1999; NEUMEISTER et al. 2000). Mice co-infected with *Legionella* and amoebae exhibited more severe symptoms than those infected with amoebae or *L. pneumophila* alone (BRIELAND et al. 1996; CIRILLO et al. 1999).

Table 1. Organisms supporting intracellular growth of *L. pneumophila*

Protozoan	Organism	References
Amoebae[a]	*Acanthamoebae castellanii*	ROWBOTHAM 1986
	A. polyphage	ROWBOTHAM 1986
	Echinamoeba exundans	FIELDS et al. 1990
	Hartmannella vermiformis	ROWBOTHAM 1986
	Naegleria fowleri	NEWSOME et al. 1985
	Saccamoeba spp.	ROHR et al. 1998
	Vahlkampfia jugosa	ROWBOTHAM 1986
Myxamoebae	*Dictyostelium discoideum*	HÄGELE et al. 2000; SOLOMON et al. 2000
Ciliata	*Cyclidium* spp.	BARBAREE et al. 1986
	Tetrahymena pyriformis	FIELDS et al. 1984

[a] *L. pneumophila* is able to replicate in 16 species of amoebae.

Person-to-person spread was never documented. Therefore, the human host seems to be a "dead end" for *L. pneumophila* transmission. Aerosols, which contain respirable vesicles of *A. castellanii* with viable *L. pneumophila*, were suggested to be an effective way of entering the human host (BERK et al. 1998). This illustrates that the ability of *L. pneumophila* to multiply intracellularly in amoebae could be the prerequisite to cause disease in humans. The ability to infect the human lung may be the consequence of the evolutionary capacity of *L. pneumophila* to survive in the environment by intracellular multiplication in protozoan hosts. This idea is supported by the fact that most of the genes required for intracellular replication of *L. pneumophila* are required for both hosts, human and protozoan (SEGAL and SHUMAN 1999b; GAO et al. 1997). However, certain genes (*rpoS*, *ligA*, *lsp*) are only required for multiplication in amoebae (HALES and SHUMAN 1999a,b; FETTES et al. 2000). The generation of genes that are especially required for the survival in macrophages, for example, the macrophage specific infectivity loci (*mil*) described by GAO et al. (1998a), still lack an evolutionary explanation. It might be speculated that these genes evolved during the interaction with yet unidentified hosts.

4 Virulence and Fitness Factors of *Legionella*

Most of the genes required for intracellular replication of *L. pneumophila* are required in both human and protozoan host cells (Table 2). Good examples in this respect are the macrophage infectivity potentiator gene (*mip*), and the pilus biogenesis (*pil*), protozoan and macrophage infectivity (*pmi*), *prp* and most of the intracellular multiplication/defect in organelle trafficking (*icm/dot*) loci (ANDREWS et al. 1998; CIANCIOTTO and FIELDS 1992; GAO et al. 1998b; LILES et al. 1999; SEGAL and SHUMAN 1999b; STONE et al. 1999; for recent reviews see ABU KWAIK 1998, BRAND and HACKER 1997, SWANSON and HAMMER 2000 and VOGEL and ISBERG 1999).

4.1 Factors Needed for Replication in Protozoa and Human Macrophages

The homodimeric Mip protein has been shown to contribute to intracellular survival of *L. pneumophila* within human macrophages, human monocytes and protozoa (CIANCIOTTO et al. 1990b; CIANCIOTTO and FIELDS 1992; WINTERMEYER et al. 1995). The 24-kDa surface protein is expressed constitutively during intracellular replication and belongs to the enzyme family of FK-506-binding proteins, which exhibit peptidyl-prolyl *cis/trans* isomerase (PPIase) activity (FISCHER et al. 1992; KÖHLER et al. 2000a). Although the PPIase activity is not required in monocellular amoeba hosts, it significantly influences the infection process in guinea pigs (KÖHLER et al. 2000b).

Table 2. Factors involved in intracellular replication and fitness of *L. pneumophila*

Gene or locus	Name or function	Affected property	References
Factors relevant for macrophages and protozoa:			
dot/icm	Defect in organelle trafficking/ intracellular multiplication; Type IVB secretion system	Required for macrophage killing, intracellular multiplication and RSF1010 conjugation	ANDREWS et al. 1998; BERGER and ISBERG 1993; BRAND et al. 1994; CHRISTIE and VOGEL 2000; SEGAL and SHUMAN 1997; SEGAL et al. 1998; VOGEL et al. 1998
eml	Early stage macrophage induced locus	Survival during early stage of infection	ABU KWAIK and PEDERSON 1996
flaA	Flagellin; core protein of the flagellum	Reduced entry into macrophages	DIETRICH et al. 2000; HEUNER et al. 1995
mip	Macrophage infectivity potentiator peptidyl-prolyl *cis/trans* isomerase	Intracellular replication and PPIase activity	CIANCIOTTO et al. 1990b; ENGELBERG et al. 1989; FISCHER et al. 1992; WINTERMEYER et al. 1995
pilBCD	Type IV pilus biogeneseis and Type II protein secretion	Intracellular multiplication in *A. castellanii*, survival in animal model of infection	ARAGON et al 2000; LILES et al. 1998, 1999
pmi	Protozoan and macrophage infectivity loci	Intracellular replication	GAO et al. 1997, 1998b
prp	Putative biosynthetic pathway	Intracellular replication	STONE et al. 1999
Macrophage specific factors:			
mil loci	Macrophage-specific infectivity loci, putative transport protein	Replication in human macrophages	GAO et al. 1998b; HARB and ABU KWAIK 2000
milA	Macrophage-specific infectivity locus A, putative transport protein	Replication in human macrophages	HARB and ABU KWAIK 2000
Protozoa specific factors:			
ligA	*L. pneumophila* infectivity gene	Replication in *A. castellanii*	FETTES et al. 2000
lsp	Type II protein secretion system	Replication in *A. castellanii*	HALES and SHUMAN 1999b
rpoS	Alternative sigma factor	Intracellular replication in *A. castellanii*	HALES and SHUMAN 1999a

Recently, a locus of 4kb was identified, which encodes homologues of *P. aeruginosa* PilB, PilC and PilD, proteins essential for type II protein secretion and type IV pilus production (LILES et al. 1998). The type II secretion system associated with the *pilD* gene seems to be required for the release of virulence factors. A *pilD* mutant strain was greatly impaired in its ability to grow within *Hartmannella vermiformis* and U937 cells, suggesting that proteins (for example the acid phosphatase, monoacylglycerol lipase and others) secreted by the type II secretion system promote the ability of *L. pneumophila* to replicate intracellularly (ARAGON et al. 2000; LILES et al. 1999). At the same time, the PilE homologue encoding gene, responsible for the existence of long pili of *L. pneumophila*, was cloned by another group (STONE and ABU KWAIK 1998). While the *pilE* mutant strain showed wild-type phenotype for intracellular replication in human epithelial cells, human macrophage-like U937 cells and *A. castellanii*, it exhibited a 50% decreased adherence to these cells (STONE and ABU KWAIK 1998).

The type IV secretion system encoded by the *icm/dot* loci seemed to be required for replication of *Legionella* in both host systems (SEGAL and SHUMAN 1999b), whereas the second type IV secretion system (*lvh* operon) was found to be dispensable for intracellular growth (SEGAL et al. 1999). These secretion systems will be discussed in another context in the next paragraph.

4.2 Factors Relevant for Replication in Protozoa or Human Macrophages

Recently, genes specifically required for multiplication in amoebae were identified, for example the *rpoS*, *ligA* and *lsp* genes (FETTES et al. 2000; HALES and SHUMAN 1999a, b). On the other hand, macrophage specific infectivity loci (*mil*) were described by GAO et al. (1998a,b), which are specifically required for the replication of *L. pneumophila* in macrophages (Table 2).

The *rpoS* gene codes for the stationary-phase sigma factor RpoS, which may regulate genes in *L. pneumophila* that are required for growth in amoebae. RpoS is not needed for the stationary growth dependent resistance to stress (HALES and SHUMAN 1999a). The *L. pneumophila* infectivity gene A (*ligA*) encodes for a structure, which could be part of a regulatory system, which is, similar to RpoS, involved in the survival of *L. pneumophila* in the environment (FETTES et al. 2000). The *lspFGHIJK* genes encode proteins of the general secretion pathway (type II secretion) of *L. pneumophila*. The *lspGH* mutant strain was unable to secrete the Msp protease and did not multiply within *A. castellanii*. But this strain was still able to kill HL-60 derived macrophages (HALES and SHUMAN 1999b).

The *mil* mutant strains of *L. pneumophila* are impaired from surviving in macrophages (GAO et al. 1998a,b). The identified *milA* gene encodes a putative transport protein. The growth defect of the *milA* mutant strain could be linked with the presence of the endosomal/lysosomal markers LAMP-2 and BiP on the phagosome. It has been speculated that the MilA protein is involved in the phagosome maturation process (HARB and ABU KWAIK 2000). The other mutant strains are still under investigation, and the results will be helpful to learn more about macrophage specific infectivity loci.

5 Determinants Encoding Type IV Secretion Systems – Parts of Pathogenicity Islands?

Pathogenicity islands (PAIs) are characterized as large genomic regions, with a different DNA composition compared to the overall DNA composition of the rest of the chromosome, which encodes essential virulence factors (HACKER et al. 1997). They were first described in uropathogenic *Escherichia coli* (BLUM et al. 1994), then in ETEC, EPEC (ELLIOTT et al. 1998), EHEC (KAPER et al. 1999), *Salmonella* spp. (OCHMAN et al. 1996), *Yersinia enterocolitica* (CARNIEL et al. 1996), *Helicobacter pylori* (CENSINI et al. 1996) and many other bacteria.

So far, very little is known about PAIs in the genus *Legionella*. However, there are three putative candidates of PAIs, the *lvh* region encoding a type IV secretion system (SEGAL et al. 1999) and the two *icm/dot* regions (region I and II, Fig. 2) encoding another type IV secretion system of *L. pneumophila* (ANDREWS et al. 1998; SEGAL and SHUMAN 1997; SEGAL et al. 1998).

SEGAL et al. (1999) described a type IV-like secretion system in *Legionella* containing 11 genes homologous to genes of other type IV secretion systems (Fig. 2). The *lvh* genes seem to be located on a genomic island with a higher G + C content compared to the overall G + C content of the chromosome. The G + C content of *L. pneumophila* chromosome is 38% (BRENNER et al. 1978), but the *lvh* genes were found to have a G + C content of 44% (SEGAL et al. 1999). A region containing lower G + C content (37%) was found upstream of the putative PAI. However, no other features of a typical PAI were described. The *lvh* genes were shown to be not required for intracellular replication in HL-60 cells or in *A. castellanii*, but they are partially required for RSF1010 conjugation and were able to substitute for some components of the *icm/dot* secretion system (SEGAL et al. 1999). Allowing better classification of type IV secretion systems, CHRISTIE and VOGEL (2000) propose the Lvh system, which is able to transfer an IncQ plasmid as a type IVA system (VirB-based). Other type IV systems, derived from IncI Tra homologues, were proposed as type IVB.

The second type IV secretion system of *L. pneumophila* (*icm/dot* encoded), classified as type IVB (CHRISTIE and VOGEL 2000), is required for RSF1010 conjugation but also for intracellular multiplication in both host systems (SEGAL et al. 1998; SEGAL and SHUMAN 1999b; VOGEL et al. 1998). It was speculated, that *L. pneumophila* may have acquired the *dot* secretion system by integrating the conjugation system of a plasmid (VOGEL and ISBERG 1999) (Fig. 2). This was also hypothesized by SEGAL and SHUMAN (1999a). They showed that in *Coxiella burnetii*, which is evolutionarily closely related to *L. pneumophila*, homologues of the *icm/dot* genes are more similar than the *icm/dot* and the *tra/trb* genes (Tra region of the IncI ColIb-P9 plasmid of *Shigella flexneri*) (SEGAL and SHUMAN 1999a; CHRISTIE and VOGEL 2000). The authors suggest that *L. pneumophila* and *C. burnetii* might have incorporated an IncI-plasmid conjugation system to export effector molecules into host cells.

The *icm/dot* loci are found on two genomic islands of approximately 20kb each (SEGAL and SHUMAN 1999b; VOGEL et al. 1998). The G + C content of the icm locus was found to be 39%, and the authors suggested that this may indicate that the icm locus is not a typical pathogenicity island (SEGAL et al. 1998). Sixteen of the 18 *icm* genes were found to be required for macrophage killing (SEGAL et al. 1998), and these genes are also required for intracellular growth in *A. castellanii* (SEGAL and SHUMAN 1999b).

As the genome of *L. pneumophila* is sequenced and will be assembled in the near future, it will be possible to analyse the genome for the existence of putative pathogenicity islands or other foreign genomic islands of *L. pneumophila*.

6 Plasmids in *Legionella*

The first report of a plasmid in *Legionella* was a 30MDa cryptic plasmid found in *L. pneumophila* (KNUDSON and MIKESELL 1980). Meanwhile, cryptic plasmids have also been identified in other *Legionella* species, like *L. micdadei*, *L. longbeachae*, *L. gormanii*, *L. dumoffii* and some others (BROWN et al. 1982, JOHNSON and SCHALLA 1982, MAHER et al. 1983). *L. pneumophila* strains with plasmids seem to persist longer in the environment than strains lacking plasmids (BROWN et al. 1982). It was shown that a 36-MDa plasmid of *L. pneumophila* conferred resistance to short wave UV light, and, therefore, it may be important for survival of the bacteria in its natural environment (TULLY et al. 1991). The plasmids of *Legionella* seem to be generally stable upon passage on laboratory media or in animals (BROWN et al. 1982, EDELSTEIN et al. 1986), and they are mostly self-transmissible by conjugation (JOHNSON and SCHALLA 1982; MINTZ et al. 1992).

There are reports about the existence of a 30-kb instable genetic element in *L. pneumophila*, which is responsible for (LPS) phase variation. In the virulent wild-type strain, the genetic element is integrated in the chromosome, whereas in the avirulent phase variation strain, the genetic element is excised and replicates as a high copy plasmid (LÜNEBERG 2000, LÜNEBERG et al. 2000). It remains to be shown which virulence factors or regulators of virulence are encoded by this mobile genetic element. Recently, another plasmid encoding a putative regulator was described (DOYLE et al. 2000). The plasmid of *L. longbeachae* encodes a putative transcriptional regulator (LrpR) with homology to OmpR and a protein with homology to a two-component system sensor kinase. The *lrpR* mutant strain was attenuated for intracellular multiplication within *Acanthamoeba* and was also attenuated in an animal model of infection, suggesting that this plasmid (pA5H5) is involved in the pathogenicity of *L. longbeachae* SG1.

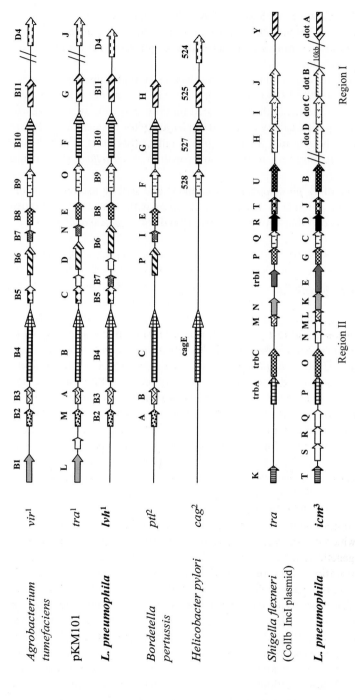

Fig. 2. *L. pneumophila lvh* and *dot/icm* genes in comparison to other type IV secretion systems. Homologous genes are *shaded in the same pattern*. Genes *not shaded* are not type IV related. *1*, representative conjugation systems; *2*, transfer systems thought to function as exporters of effector proteins during infection; *3*, *L. pneumophila icm/dot* system is also thought to export effector molecules during infection but is related with the transfer region of the *Shigella flexneri* CollB IncI plasmid. The *trbI* homologue is from the IncP plasmid RK2. (Figure from Christie and Vogel 2000; modified)

DAAKA et al. (1994) first showed a putative correlation between strains containing a plasmid and virulence of these strains in a mouse A-J macrophage cell line model. However, the role of plasmids for the pathogenicity of *Legionella* has yet to be determined.

7 *L. pneumophila* Specific Genes – an Indication of Horizontal Gene Transfer or Gene Deletion?

Many cloned genes of *L. pneumophila* possess homologues in other *Legionella* species, as shown for the *fur*, *mip*, *flaA*, *pilB*, *htpB*, *ompS* and *sodB* gene (AMEMURA-MAEKAWA et al. 1996; CIANCIOTTO 1990a; HEUNER et al. 1995; HICKEY and CIANCIOTTO, 1994; HOFFMAN et al. 1990, 1992; LILES et al. 1998; RATCLIFF et al. 1997; WEERATNA et al. 1994). As discussed above, *L. pneumophila* utilizes the same genes to grow in protozoa and human alveolar macrophages with only a few exceptions. Nevertheless, differences in the entry mechanisms of *L. pneumophila* are observed between human and protozoan cells and within the spectrum of host amoebae (HARB et al. 1998). A comparative analysis of *L. pneumophila* and *L. micdadei* virulence traits revealed dramatic differences in the mechanisms of infection between both species (GAO et al. 1999; JOSHI and SWANSON 1999).

Recently, some *L. pneumophila*-specific genes were identified (Table 3). There was a report about the cloning of an *L. pneumophila*-specific putative adhesin, the 16kDa *pneumophila*-specific outer membrane protein (Pom). A Pom negative mutant strain possesses a reduced initial uptake compared to the wild-type strain (STEUDEL et al. 2000).

Our group recently described the flagellum as a factor involved in the early stages of the invasion process of macrophages by *L. pneumophila* (DIETRICH et al. 2000). The expression of the flagellum of *L. pneumophila* is modulated by different environmental factors (HEUNER et al. 1999). The promoter of the *flaA* gene is recognized by the alternative sigma-28 factor (*fliA*) of *L. pneumophila* (HEUNER et al. 1995), and the *fliA* gene is able to complement an *E. coli fliA* mutant strain (HEUNER et al. 1997). By screening a genomic library of *L. pneumophila* for factors that negatively regulate *flaA* promoter dependent reporter gene expression, we identified a *L. pneumophila*-specific transcriptional factor, belonging to the LysR type of transcriptional regulators (HEUNER et al. 2000). Yet it is unclear what role this regulator plays in flagellum expression or on general gene expression events in *L. pneumophila*.

The *L. pneumophila*-specific infectivity gene A (*ligA*) encodes a structure that is necessary for *L. pneumophila* to replicate within *A. castellanii* (FETTES et al. 2000). The *L. pneumophila*-specific *frgA* gene encodes a protein that has homology with the aerobactin synthetases IucA and IucC of *E. coli*. The authors speculated that *L. pneumophila* encodes a siderophore, which is required for optimal intracellular growth, since an *frgA* mutant strain was reduced 80-fold in intracellular growth in

Table 3. *Legionella pneumophila* specific genes

Gene	Name or function	References
frgA	*fur* regulated gene, putative siderophore	HICKEY and CIANCIOTTO 1997
flaR	Transcription factor; member of the LysR family of transcriptional regulators	HEUNER et al. 2000
hpb[a]	Hemin binding protein	O'CONNELL et al. 1996
iraAB[a]	Putative methyltransferase and a putative peptide transporter	VISWANATHAN et al. 2000
ligA	*L. pneumophila* infectivity gene	FETTES et al. 2000
LPS gene locus[a]	LPS (O-chain) biosynthesis	LÜNEBERG et al. 2000
pom	putative adhesin, outer membrane protein	STEUDEL et al. 2000
sodC	copper-zinc superoxide dismutase	AMEMURA-MAEKAWA et al. 1996

[a] Largely limited to strains of *L. pneumophila*.

U937 cells (HICKEY and CIANCIOTTO 1997). The *iraAB* locus is largely limited to *L. pneumophila* strains (except two other species) and is required for iron assimilation. While the gene product of *iraA*, a methyltransferase, is critical for virulence, the gene product of *iraB*, a homologue of di- and tri-peptide transporters, is not. The *iraB* gene seems to have a role in iron acquisition (VISWANATHAN et al. 2000).

It is possible that in the group of *L. pneumophila*-specific genes factors or regulators will be identified, which may help to explain why *L. pneumophila* is such a potent pathogen compared with the non-*L. pneumophila* strains. For example, the *L. pneumophila*-specific gene *ligA* is found near to the very conserved Mip encoding gene (FETTES et al. 2000), and the authors hypothesized the possibility of incorporation of foreign genes, which contribute to pathogenicity. However, they also mentioned the possibility that species other than *L. pneumophila* may have lost *ligA* during evolution. The loss of genes might have been the reason for the reduction in the ability to replicate in many different host cells, as seen in some non-*L. pneumophila* species.

Comparative analysis of *Legionella* genus conserved regions flanking *L. pneumophila*-specific ones with the sequenced genome of *L. pneumophila* will help to elucidate the question if there is horizontal gene transfer of virulence factors in *L. pneumophila* strains. But it is also possible that non-*L. pneumophila* species may have lost genes during the evolutionary process, optimizing replication in only one specific host.

8 Conclusions

L. pneumophila is a human pathogen that is ubiquitous in the environment. The ability of *L. pneumophila* to replicate intracellularly in a wide range of protozoa in its environment is thought to be the prerequisite to become a human pathogen. It is not clear why *L. pneumophila* is predominantly isolated from humans with legionnaires' disease, although it is not more frequently found in the environment. The ability of *L. pneumophila* to survive and to replicate in man-made hot-water systems might be the prerequisite for successful transmission of *L. pneumophila* to humans. Nevertheless, *L. pneumohila* is not really adapted to the human host. No human-to-human spread has been ever documented, and, therefore, the human host appears to be a dead end for the distribution of *L. pneumophila*.

It is suggested that *L. pneumophila*-specific genes may be responsible for the virulence of *L. pneumophila*, and further research on *L. pneumophila*-specific genes might reveal the role of these genes. Probably *L. pneumophila* has acquired some foreign genetic elements that make *L. pneumophila* more virulent or alternatively, certain non-*L. pneumophila* species may have lost some genes during evolution. Since *L. pneumophila* is able to conjugate plasmids via the type IV secretion system, horizontal gene transfer in *Legionella* is conceivable. One PAI-like island, the *lvh* region encoding a type IV secretion system, has been identified in *Legionella*. Furthermore, it is proposed that *Legionella* has acquired the *icm/dot* genes, encoding another type IV secretion system, by horizontal gene transfer and integrating the conjugation system of a plasmid. The complete genome of *L. pneumophila* is sequenced now, and the subsequent analysis may reveal the presence of foreign DNA elements in *L. pneumophila*. This will contribute to more detailed knowledge about the evolution of *Legionellaceae*.

References

Abu Kwaik Y, Pederson LL (1996) The use of differential display-PCR to isolate and characterize a *Legionella pneumophila* locus induced during the intracellular infection of macrophages. Mol Microbiol 21:543–556

Abu Kwaik Y, Gao LY, Stone BJ, Venkataraman C, Harb OS (1998) Invasion of protozoa by *Legionella pneumophila* and its role in bacterial ecology and pathogenesis. Appl Environ Microbiol 64:3127–3133

Adeleke AA, Pruckler JM, Benson RF, Rowbotham T, Halablab MA, Fields BS (1996) *Legionella*-like amoebal pathogens – phylogenetic status and possible role in respiratory disease. Emerg Infect Dis 2:225–230

Adeleke AA, Fields BS, Benson RF, Daneshvar MJ, Pruckler JM, Ratcliff RM, Harrison TG, Weyant RS, Birtles RJ, Raoult D, Halablab MA (2001) *Legionella drosanskii* sp. nov., *Legionella rowbothamii* sp. nov. and *Legionella fallonii* sp. nov.: three unusual new *Legionella* species. Int J Syst Evol Microbiol 51:1151–1160

Amemura-Maekawa J, Kura F, Watanabe H (1996) Cloning and nucleotide sequences of iron and copper-zinc superoxide dismutase genes of *Legionella pneumophila* and their distribution among *Legionella* species. Jpn J Med Sci Biol 49:167–186

Andrews HL, Vogel JP, Isberg RR (1998) Identification of linked *Legionella pneumophila* genes essential for intracellular growth and evasion of the endocytic pathway. Infect Immun 66:950–958

Aragon V, Kurtz S, Flieger A, Neumeister B, Cianciotto NP (2000) Secreted enzymatic activities of wild-type and *pilD*-deficient *Legionella pneumophila*. Infect Immun 68:1855–1863

Barbaree JM, Fields BS, Feeley JC, Gorman GW, Martin WT (1986) Isolation of protozoa from water associated with a legionellosis outbreak and demonstration of intracellular multiplication of *Legionella pneumophila*. Appl Environ Microbiol 51:422–424

Barker J, Brown MR, Collier PJ, Farrell I, Gilbert P (1992) Relationship between *Legionella pneumophila* and *Acanthamoeba polyphaga*: physiological status and susceptibility to chemical inactivation. Appl Environ Microbiol 58:2420–2425

Barker J, Lambert PA, Brown MR (1993) Influence of intra-amoebic and other growth conditions on the surface properties of *Legionella pneumophila*. Infect Immun 61:3503–3510

Barker J, Scaife H, Brown MR (1995) Intraphagocytic growth induces an antibiotic-resistant phenotype of *Legionella pneumophila*. Antimicrob Agents Chemother 39:2684–2688

Bender L, Ott M, Marre R, Hacker J (1990) Genome analysis of *Legionella* ssp. by orthogonal field alternation gel electrophoresis (OFAGE). FEMS Microbiol Lett 60:253–257

Benson RF, Fields BS (1998) Classification of the genus *Legionella*. Semin Respir Infect 13:90–99

Berger KH, Isberg RR (1993) Two distinct defects in intracellular growth complemented by a single genetic locus in *Legionella pneumophila*. Mol Microbiol 7:7–19

Berk SG, Ting RS, Turner GW, Ashburn RJ (1998) Production of respirable vesicles containing live *Legionella pneumophila* cells by two *Acanthamoeba* spp. Appl Environ Microbiol 64:279–286

Blum G, Ott M, Lischewski A, Ritter A, Imrich H, Tschape H, Hacker J (1994) Excision of large DNA regions termed pathogenicity islands from tRNA-specific loci in the chromosome of an *Escherichia coli* wild-type pathogen. Infect Immun 62:606–614

Brand BC, Sadosky AB, Shuman HA (1994) The *Legionella pneumophila icm* locus: a set of genes required for intracellular multiplication in human macrophages. Mol Microbiol 14:797–808

Brand BC, Hacker J (1997) The biology of *Legionella* infection. In: Kaufmann SHE (ed) Host response to intracellular pathogens. Chapman and Hall, pp 291–312

Brenner DJ, Steigerwalt AG, Weaver RE, McDade JE, Feeley JC, Mandel M (1978) Classification of the legionnaires' disease bacterium: an interim report. Curr Microbiol 1:71–75

Brieland J, McClain M, Heath L, Chrisp C, Huffnagle G, LeGendre M, Hurley M, Fantone J, Engleberg C (1996) Coinoculation with *Hartmannella vermiformis* enhances replicative *Legionella pneumophila* lung infection in a murine model of legionnaires' disease. Infect Immun 64:2449–2456

Brown A, Vickers RM, Elder EM, Lema M, Garrity GM (1982) Plasmids and surface antigen markers of endemic and epidemic *Legionella pneumophila* strains. J Clin Microbiol 16:230–235

Carniel E, Guilvout I, Prentice (1996) Characterization of a large chromosomal "high-pathogenicity island" in biotype 1B *Yersinia enterocolitica*. J Bacteriol 178:6743–6751

Censini S, Lange C, Xiang Z, Crabtree JE, Ghiara P, Borodovsky M, Rappuoli R, Covacci A (1996) Cag, a pathogenicity island of *Helicobacter pylori*, encodes type I-specific and disease-associated virulence factors. Proc Natl Acad Sci USA 93:14648–14653

Christie PJ, Vogel JP (2000) Bacterial type IV secretion: conjugation systems adapted to deliver effector molecules to host cells. Trends Microbiol 8:354–360

Cianciotto NP, Fields BS (1992) *Legionella pneumophila mip* gene potentiates intracellular infection of protozoa and human macrophages. Proc Natl Acad Sci USA 89:5188–5191

Cianciotto NP, Bangsborg JM, Eisenstein BI, Engleberg NC (1990a) Identification of *mip*-like genes in the genus *Legionella*. Infect Immun 58:2912–2918

Cianciotto NP, Eisenstein BI, Mody CH, Engleberg NC (1990b) A mutation in the *mip* gene results in an attenuation of *Legionella pneumophila* virulence. J Infect Dis 162:121–126

Cianciotto NP, Stamos JK, Kamp DW (1995) Infectivity of *Legionella pneumophila mip* mutant for alveolar epithelial cells. Curr Microbiol 30:247–250

Cirillo JD, Falkow S, Tompkins LS (1994) Growth of *Legionella pneumophila* in *Acanthamoeba castellanii* enhances invasion. Infect Immun 62:3254–3261

Cirillo JD, Cirillo SL, Yan L, Bermudez LE, Falkow S, Tompkins LS (1999) Intracellular growth in *Acanthamoeba castellanii* affects monocyte entry mechanisms and enhances virulence of *Legionella pneumophila*. Infect Immun 67:4427–4434

Daaka Y, Yamamoto Y, Klein TW, Newton C, Friedman H (1994) Correlation of *Legionella pneumophila* virulence with the presence of a plasmid. Curr Microbiol 28:217–223

Dietrich C, Heuner K, Brand BC, Steinert M, Hacker J (2000) The flagellum of *Legionella pneumophila* positively affects the early phase of infection of eukaryotic host cells. Infect Immun 64:2116–2122

Doyle RM, Heuzenroeder MW (2000) A mutation in an *ompR*-like gene on a *Legionella longbeacheae* serogroup 1 plasmid attenuates virulence. International Conference on Legionella, 5th, Ulm, Germany, (abstract book) p 34 (abstract) P11

Edelstein PH, Nakahama C, Tobin JO, Calarco K, Beer KB, Joly JR, Selander RK (1986) Paleoepidemiologic investigation of legionnaires' disease at Wadsworth Veterans Administration Hospital by using three typing methods for comparison of legionellae from clinical and environmental sources. J Clin Microbiol 23:1121–1126

Elliott SJ, Wainwright LA, McDaniel TK, Jarvis KG, Deng YK, Lai LC, McNamara BP, Donnenberg MS, Kaper JB (1998) The complete sequence of the locus of enterocyte effacement (LEE) from enteropathogenic *Escherichia coli* E2348/69. Mol Microbiol 28:1–4

Engleberg NC, Carter C, Weber DR, Cianciotto NP, Eisenstein BI (1989) DNA sequence of *mip*, a *Legionella pneumophila* gene associated with macrophage infectivity. Infect Immun 57:1263–1270

Fettes PS, Susa M, Hacker J, Marre R (2000) Characterization of the *Legionella pneumophila* gene *ligA*. Int J Med Microbiol 290:239–250

Fields BS (1993) *Legionella* and protozoa: interaction of a pathogen and its natural host. In: Barbaree JM, Breimann RF, Dufour AP (eds) *Legionella*: current status and emerging perspectives. ASM, Washington DC, pp 129–136

Fields BS (1996) The molecular ecology of legionellae. Trends Microbiol 4:286–290

Fields BS (2001) The social life of Legionellae. *Legionella* – Proceedings of the 5th International Symposium. Marre R, Abu Kwaik Y, Bartlett C, Cianciotto N, Fields BS, Frosch M, Hacker J, Lück PC. ASM press, Washington DC, (in press)

Fields BS, Shotts EB Jr, Feeley JC, Gorman GW, Martin WT (1984) Proliferation of *Legionella pneumophila* as an intracellular parasite of the ciliated protozoan *Tetrahymena pyriformis*. Appl Environ Microbiol 47:467–471

Fields BS, Sanden GN, Barbaree JM, Morrill WE, Wadowsky RM, White EW, Feeley JC (1989) Intracellular multiplication of *Legionella pneumophila* in amoebae isolated from hospital hot-water tanks. Curr Microbiol 18:131–137

Fields BS, Nerad TA, Sawyer TK, King CH, Barbaree JM, Martin WT, Morrill WE, Sanden GN (1990) Characterization of an axenic strain of *Hartmannella vermiformis* obtained from an investigation of nosocomial legionellosis. J Protozool 37:581–583

Fischer G, Bang H, Ludwig B, Mann K, Hacker J (1992) Mip protein of *Legionella pneumophila* exhibits peptidyl-prolyl-cis/trans isomerase (PPlase) activity. Mol Microbiol 6:1375–1383

Fraser DW, Tsai TR, Orenstein W, Parkin WE, Beecham HJ, Sharrar RG, Harris J, Mallison GF, Martin SM, McDade JE, Shepard CC, Brachman PS (1977) Legionnaires' disease: description of an epidemic of pneumonia. N Engl J Med 297:1189–1197

Frey NK, Warwick S, Saunders NA, Embley TM (1991) The use of 16S ribosomal RNA analysis to investigate the phylogeny of the family *Legionellaceae*. J Gen Microbiol 137:1215–1222

Gao LY, Harb OS, Kwaik YA (1997) Utilization of similar mechanisms by *Legionella pneumophila* to parasitize two evolutionary distant Host Cells, mammalian macrophages and protozoa. Infect Immun 65:4738–4746

Gao LY, Harb OS, Kwaik YA (1998a) Identification of macrophage specific infectivity loci (*mil*) of *Legionella pneumophila* that are not required for infectivity of protozoan. Infect Immun 66:883–892

Gao LY, Stone BJ, Brieland JK, Abu Kwaik Y (1998b) Different fates of *Legionella pneumophila pmi* and *mil* mutants within macrophages and alveolar epithelial cells. Microb Pathog 25:291–306

Gao LY, Susa M, Ticac B, Abu Kwaik Y (1999) Heterogeneity in intracellular replication and cytopathogenicity of *Legionella pneumophila* and *Legionella micdadei* in mammalian and protozoan cells. Microb Pathog 27:273–287

Groothuis DG, Veenendal HR, Dijkstra HL (1985) Influence of temperature on the number of *Legionella pneumophila* in hot-water systems. J Appl Bacteriol 59:529–536

Hacker J, Blum-Oehler G, Muhldorfer I, Tschape H (1997) Pathogenicity islands of virulent bacteria: structure, function and impact on microbial evolution. Mol Microbiol 23:1089–1097

Hägele S, Köhler R, Merkert H, Schleicher M, Hacker J, Steinert M (2000) *Dictyostelium discoideum*: a new host model system for intracellular pathogens of the genus *Legionella*. Cell Microbiol 2:165–171

Hales LM, Shuman HA (1999a) The *Legionella pneumophila rpo*S gene is required for growth within *Acanthamoeba castellanii*. J Bacteriol 181:4879–4989

Hales LM, Shuman HA (1999b) *Legionella pneumophila* contains a type II general secretion pathway required for growth in amoebae as well as for secretion of the Msp protease. Infect Immun 67: 3662–3666

Harb OS, Venkataraman C, Haack BJ, Gao LY, Kwaik YA (1998) Heterogeneity in the attachment and uptake mechanisms of the legionnaires' disease bacterium, *Legionella pneumophila*, by protozoan hosts. Appl Environ Microbiol 64:126–132

Harb OS, Abu Kwaik Y (2000) Characterization of a macrophage-specific infectivity locus (*milA*) of *Legionella pneumophila*. Infect Immun 68:368–376

Heuner K, Bender-Beck L, Brand BC, Lück PC, Mann KH, Marre R, Ott M, Hacker J (1995) Cloning and genetic characterization of the flagellum subunit gene (*flaA*) of *Legionella pneumophila* serogroup 1. Infect Immun 63:2499–2507

Heuner K, Hacker J, Brand BC (1997) The alternative sigma factor σ^{28} of *Legionella pneumophila* restores flagellation and motility to an *Escherichia coli fliA* mutant. J Bacteriol 179:17–23

Heuner K, Brand BC, Hacker J (1999) The expression of the flagellum of *Legionella pneumophila* is modulated by different environmental factors. FEMS Microbiol Lett 175:69–77

Heuner K, Dietrich C, Steinert M, Göbel UB, Hacker J (2000) Cloning and characterization of a *Legionella pneumophila*-specific gene encoding a member of the LysR family of transcriptional regulators. Mol Gen Genet 264:204–211

Hickey EK, Cianciotto NP (1994) Cloning and sequencing of the *Legionella pneumophila fur* gene. Gene 143:117–121

Hickey EK, Cianciotto NP (1997) An iron- and fur-repressed *Legionella pneumophila* gene that promotes intracellular infection and encodes a protein with similarity to the *Escherichia coli* aerobactin synthetases. Infect Immun 65:133–143

Hoffman PS, Houston L, Butler CA (1990) *Legionella pneumophila htpAB* heat shock operon: nucleotide sequence and expression of the 60-kilodalton antigen in *L. pneumophila*-infected HeLa cells. Infect Immun 58:3380–3387

Hoffman PS, Ripley M, Weeratna R (1992) Cloning and nucleotide sequence of a gene (*ompS*) encoding the major outer membrane protein of *Legionella pneumophila*. J Bacteriol 174:914–920

Horwitz MA, Silverstein SC (1980) Legionnaires' disease bacterium (*Legionella pneumophila*) multiples intracellulary in human monocytes. J Exp Med 66:441–450

Johnson SR, Schalla WO (1982) Plasmids of serogroup 1 strains of *Legionella pneumophila*. Curr Microbiol 7:143–146

Joshi AD, Swanson MS (1999) Comparative analysis of *Legionella pneumophila* and *Legionella micdadei* virulence traits. Infect Immun 67:4134–4142

Kaper JB, Mellies JL, Nataro JP (1999) Pathogenicity islands and other mobile genetic elements of diarrheagenic *Escherichia coli*. In: Kaper JB, Hacker J (eds) Pathogenicity islands and other mobile virulence elements. ASM Press, Washington DC

Keevil CW (2000) Biofilms and *Legionella*. International Conference on *Legionella*, 5th, Ulm, Germany, (abstract book) p11 (abstract 017)

Knudson GB, Mikesell P (1980) A plasmid in *Legionella pneumophila*. Infect Immun 29:1092–1095

Köhler R, Bubert A, Goebel W, Steinert M, Hacker J, Bubert B (2000a) Expression and use of the green fluorescent protein as a reporter system in *Legionella pneumophila*. Mol Gen Genet 262:1060–1069

Köhler R, Fanghänel J, König B, Lüneberg E, Fischer G, Frosch M, Steinert M, Hacker J (2000b) Dimerization of the Mip protein is essential for the virulence of *Legionella*. International Conference on Legionella, 5th, Ulm, Germany, (abstract book) p 38 (abstract) p 19

Liles MR, Viswanathan VK, Cianciotto NP (1998) Identification and temperature regulation of *Legionella pneumophila* genes involved in type IV pilus biogenesis and type II protein secretion. Infect Immun 66:1776–1782

Liles MR, Edelstein PH, Cianciotto NP (1999) The prepilin peptidase is required for protein secretion by and the virulence of the intracellular pathogen *Legionella pneumophila*. Mol Microbiol 31: 959–970

Lüneberg E (2000) Phase variation of lipopolysaccharide and other virulence determinants in *Legionella pneumophila*. International Conference on *Legionella*, 5th, Ulm, Germany, (abstract book) p 11 (abstract 018)

Lüneberg E, Zetzmann N, Alber D, Knirel YA, Kooistra O, Zahringer U, Frosch M (2000) Cloning and functional characterization of a 30kb gene locus required for lipopolysaccharide biosynthesis in *Legionella pneumophila*. Int J Med Microbiol 290:37–49

Maher WE, Plouffe JF, Para MF (1983) Plasmid profiles of clinical and environmental isolates of *Legionella pneumophila* serogroup 1. J Clin Microbiol 18:1422–1423

Marston BJ, Lipman HB, Breiman RF (1994) Surveillance for legionnaires' disease. Risk factors for morbidity and mortality. Arch Intern Med 154:2417–2422

McDade JE, Shepard CC, Fraser DW, Tsai TR, Redus MA, Dowdle WR (1977) Legionnaires' disease: isolation of a bacterium and demonstration of its role in other respiratory disease. N Engl J Med 297:1197–1203

Mintz CS, Fields BS, Zou CH (1992) Isolation and characterization of a conjugative plasmid from *Legionella pneumophila*. J Gen Microbiol 138:1379–1386

Neumeister B, Reiff G, Faigle M, Dietz K, Northoff H, Lang F (2000) Influence of *Acanthamoeba castellanii* on intracellular growth of different *Legionella* species in human monocytes. Appl Environ Microbiol 66:914–919

Newsome AL, Baker RL, Miller RD, Arnold RR (1985) Interactions between *Naegleria fowleri* and *Legionella pneumophila*. Infect Immun 50:449–452

Ochman H, Groisman EA (1996) Distribution of pathogenicity islands in *Salmonella* spp. Infect Immun 64:5410–5412

O'Connell WA, Hickey EK, Cianciotto NP (1996) A *Legionella pneumophila* gene that promotes hemin binding. Infect Immun 64:842–848

Qu X, Morozova I, Chen M, Kalachikov S, Segal G, Chen J, Park H, Georghiou A, Asamani G, Feder M, Rineer J, Greenberg JP, Goldsberry C, Rzhetsky A, Fischer SG, DeJong P, Zhang P, Cayanis E, Shuman HA, Russo JJ (2001) The *Legionella pneumophila* sequencing project. *Legionella* – Proceedings of the 5th International Symposium. Marre R, Abu Kwaik Y, Bartlett C, Cianciotto N, Fields BS, Frosch M, Hacker J, Lück PC. ASM press, Washington DC, (in press)

Ratcliff RM, Donnellan SC, Lanser JA, Manning PA, Heuzenroeder MW (1997) Interspecies sequence differences in the Mip protein from the genus *Legionella*: implications for function and evolutionary relatedness. Mol Microbiol 25:1149–1158

Rohr U, Weber S, Michel R, Selenka F, Wilhelm M (1998) Comparison of free-living amoebae in hot water systems of hospitals with isolates from moist sanitary areas by identifying genera and determining temperature tolerance. Appl Environ Microbiol 64:1822–1824

Rowbotham TJ (1980) Preliminary report on the pathogenicity of *Legionella pneumophila* for freshwater and soil amoebae. J Clin Pathol 33:1179–1183

Rowbotham TJ (1986) Current view on the relationship between amoebae, legionellae and man. Isr J Med Sci 22:678–689

Segal G, Shuman H (1997) Characterization of a new region required for macrophage killing by *Legionella pneumophila*. Infect Immun 65:5057–5066

Segal G, Shuman HA (1999a) Possible origin of the *Legionella pneumophila* virulence genes and their relation to *Coxiella burnetii*. Mol Microbiol 33:669–670

Segal G, Shuman HA (1999b) *Legionella pneumophila* utilizes the same genes to multiply within *Acanthamoeba castellanii* and human macrophages. Infect Immun 67:2117–2124

Segal G, Purcell M, Shuman HA (1998) Host cell killing and bacterial conjugation require overlapping sets of genes within a 22-kb region of the *Legionella pneumophila* genome. Proc Natl Acad Sci USA 95:1669–1674

Segal G, Russo JJ, Shuman HA (1999) Relationships between a new type IV secretion system and the icm/dot virulence system of *Legionella pneumophila*. Mol Microbiol 1999 34:799–809

Solomon JM, Rupper A, Cardelli JA, Isberg RR (2000) Intracellular growth of *Legionella pneumophila* in *Dictyostelium discoideum*, a system for genetic analysis of host-pathogen interactions. Infect Immun 68:2939–2947

Steinert M, Emody L, Amann R, Hacker J (1997) Resuscitation of viable but nonculturable *Legionella pneumophila* Philadelphia JR32 by *Acanthamoeba castellanii*. Appl Environ Microbiol 63:2047–2053

Steudel C, Oettler W, Helbig JH, Lueck PC (2000) Characterization of a 16kDa species specific protein of *L. pneumophila* promoting uptake in amoebae. International Conference on *Legionella*, 5th, Ulm, Germany, (abstract book) P13 (abstract 021)

Stone BJ, Abu Kwaik Y (1998) Expression of multiple pili by *Legionella pneumophila*: identification and characterization of a type IV pilin gene and its role in adherence to mammalian and protozoan cells. Infect Immun 66:1768–1775

Stone BJ, Brier A, Kwaik YA (1999) The *Legionella pneumophila* prp locus; required during infection of macrophages and amoebae. Microb Pathog 27:369–376

Surman SB, Morton LHG, Keevil CW, Fitzgeorge, RB, Skinner A (2001) *Legionella pneumophila* proliferation is not dependent on intracellular replication. *Legionella* – Proceedings of the 5th International Symposium. Marre R, Abu Kwaik, Bartlett C, Cianciotto N, Fields BS, Frosch M, Hacker J, Lück PC. ASM press, Washington DC, (in press)

Swanson MS, Hammer BK (2000) *Legionella pneumophila* pathogenesis: a fateful journey from amoebae to macrophages. Annu Rev Microbiol 54:567–613

Tully M (1991) A plasmid from a virulent strain of *Legionella pneumophila* is conjugative and confers resistance to ultraviolet light. FEMS Microbiol Lett 90:43–48

Viswanathan VK, Edelstein PH, Pope CD, Cianciotto NP (2000) The *Legionella pneumophila* iraAB locus is required for iron assimilation, intracellular infection, and virulence. Infect Immun 68:1069–1079

Vogel JP, Andrews HL, Wong SK, Isberg RR (1998) Conjugative transfer by the virulence system of *Legionella pneumophila*. Science 279:873–876

Vogel JP, Isberg RR (1999) Cell biology of *Legionella pneumophila*. Curr Opin Microbiol 2:30–34

Wadowsky RM, Butler LJ, Cook MK, Verma SM, Paul MA, Fields BS, Keleti G, Sykora JL, Yee RB (1988) Growth-supporting activity for *Legionella pneumophila* in tap-water cultures and implication of *Hartmannelli* amoebae as growth factors. Appl Environ Microbiol 54:2677–2682

Weeratna R, Stamler DA, Edelstein PH, Ripley M, Marrie T, Hoskin D, Hoffman PS (1994) Human and guinea pig immune responses to *Legionella pneumophila* protein antigens OmpS and Hsp60. Infect Immun 62:3454–3462

Winn WC (1988) Legionnaires' disease: historical perspective. Clin Microbiol Rev 1:60–81

Winn WC (1999) *Legionella*. In: Murray PR, Baron EJ, Pfaller MA, Tenover FC, Yolken RH (eds) Manual of Clinical Microbiology. ASM, Washington DC, pp 572–585

Wintermeyer E, Ludwig B, Steinert M, Schmidt B, Fischer G, Hacker J (1995) Influence of site specifically altered Mip proteins on intracellular survival of *Legionella pneumophila* in eukaryotic cells. Infect Immun 63:4576–4583

Phages and Other Mobile Virulence Elements in Gram-Positive Pathogens

C. Gentry-Weeks[1], P.S. Coburn[2], and M.S. Gilmore[2,3]

1 Introduction

Over the past 30 years, gram-positive bacteria have re-emerged as leading agents of nosocomial and community-acquired infection. This resurgence correlates with the expansion of populations harboring virulence and multiple antibiotic resistance traits. Recent bacterial genome nucleotide sequence determinations show the heretofore unappreciated extent to which mobile genetic elements, including bacteriophages, conjugative plasmids, and transposons, have contributed to the horizontal dissemination of virulence factors and antibiotic resistance determinants. This chapter examines the role that phages, plasmids, and transposons have played in enhancing the ability of highly adapted gram-positive bacteria to cause human disease.

[1] Department of Microbiology, College of Veterinary Medicine and Biomedical Sciences, Colorado State University, Fort Collins, CO 80823, USA
[2] Department of Microbiology and Immunology, The University of Oklahoma Health Sciences Center, P.O. Box 26901, Oklahoma City, OK 73190, USA
[3] Department of Ophthalmology, Department of Microbiology and Immunology, The University of Oklahoma Health Sciences Center, P.O. Box 26901, Oklahoma City, OK 73190, USA

2 Bacteriophage Lysogenic Conversion to Virulence in Gram-Positive Pathogens: Historical Aspects and Possible Evolutionary Significance

Bacteriophages are capable of persisting in a bacterial population through integration into the bacterial chromosome (lysogeny) or through low-level replication in a subgroup of the population (BARKSDALE and ARDEN 1974). Both processes may result in significant phenotypic change of the infected cell, a process termed phage conversion (BARKSDALE and ARDEN 1974). Phage conversion benefits the phage if the newly expressed traits enhance the fitness of the host bacterial population, for example, by enabling it to expand into, or transiently inhabit, an otherwise excluded environmental niche (for instance by evading host defenses [MIAO and MILLER 1999]). Because phages can endure conditions not conducive to bacterial survival, maintenance within a phage population ensures the survival of these traits should the bacterial population encounter adverse environmental conditions (MIAO and MILLER 1999).

A number of bacterial virulence factors have been shown to be phage-encoded, including diphtheria toxin of *Corynebacterium diphtheriae* (FREEMAN 1951; GROMAN 1953; GROMAN 1984; LAIRD and GROMAN 1976b); erythrogenic exotoxins A and C of *Streptococcus pyogenes* (JOHNSON et al. 1986; NIDA and FERRETTI 1982; WEEKS and FERRETTI 1986); leukocidin (VIJVER et al. 1972), staphylokinase, exfoliative toxin A (YOSHIZAWA et al. 2000), and enterotoxin A of *Staphylococcus aureus* (COLEMAN et al. 1989; KONDO and FUJISE 1977), and neurotoxins C1 and D of *Clostridium botulinum* (EKLUND and POYSKY 1969; EKLUND et al. 1969; EKLUND et al. 1971; INOUE and IIDA 1971).

2.1 *Corynebacterium diphtheriae* Diphtheria Toxin Conversion Paradigm

Expression of diphtheria toxin by *Corynebacterium diphtheriae* has been long known to be dependent on lysogenic conversion (FREEMAN 1951). Phage conversion was found to require lysogenization by corynephage strain β, and subsequent elimination of this phage rendered strains nontoxinogenic (BARKSDALE and ARDEN 1974; BARKSDALE and PAPPENHEIMER 1954; GROMAN 1953; GROMAN 1984; HOLMES 2000). Analysis of corynephage β from mutated cells expressing inactive forms of diphtheria toxin that retained immunological cross-reactivity, demonstrated that corynephage β carried the structural gene for diphtheria toxin (HOLMES 1976; HOLMES 2000; UCHIDA et al. 1971). The wild-type toxin gene, *tox*, was cloned and sequenced (GREENFIELD et al. 1983), and localized to one end of the integrated phage genome adjacent to the *attP* site (HOLMES 1976; LAIRD and GROMAN 1976a). Based on the location within the phage genome, it has been suggested that the *tox* gene was acquired by an ancestral form of phage β, through specialized transduction (HOLMES 2000). The nature of the ancestral host bacterium is unclear, however, since all characterized toxinogenic *C. diphtheriae* strains appear to possess diphtheria toxin converting phages (HOLMES 2000).

Corynephage β has been shown to integrate into a homologous sequence within an arginine-tRNA gene of the *C. diphtheriae* chromosome (RAPPUOLI and RATTI 1984; RATTI et al. 1997). Expression of the *tox* gene was shown to be independent of phage life cycle, i.e., toxin production was shown to occur during vegetative phage replication as well as when the phage is integrated into the bacterial genome (GILL et al. 1972; HOLMES 2000; MATSUDA and BARKSDALE 1966; MATSUDA and BARKSDALE 1967).

Although carried by corynephage β, the *tox* gene is under the regulatory control of the host. Toxin production is repressed under iron replete conditions, and a host genome-encoded iron-binding protein is responsible for binding to the *tox* operator and repressing transcription (FOUREL et al. 1989; SCHMITT and HOLMES 1993; TAO et al. 1992; TAO and MURPHY 1992). The involvement of host and phage functions in regulating toxin expression may be viewed as evidence for the hypothesis that the *tox* gene was acquired by a nontoxinogenic phage from an ancestral bacterium.

While toxin production may be transiently advantageous to the infecting bacterium, recent observations on the consequences of selective pressure from widespread DTP (diphtheria-pertussis-tetanus) vaccination suggest that maintenance of the *tox* gene on an independent genetic element may be important for the fitness of the *C. diphtheriae* population. The currently used vaccine may select for mutant forms of the diphtheria toxin that retain function but do not react with anti-toxin antibodies made in response to formalin-treated diphtheria toxin preparations. Thus, phages may allow for the rapid dissemination of these altered *tox* determinants to nontoxinogenic *C. diphtheriae*. This phenomenon has been hypothesized to account for the recent diphtheria epidemic in Russia. However, while heterogeneity in the *tox* sequence was observed at the DNA level among *C. diphtheriae* isolates from this epidemic, none of the mutations resulted in amino acid alteration and thus preserved the immunogenicity of the toxin (reviewed in POPOVIC et al. 2000).

2.2 *Streptococcus pyogenes*

DNA sequence analysis of the *S. pyogenes* SF370 genome has revealed that 10% of the open reading frames are associated with bacteriophage and transposon genes, emphasizing the importance of these elements in the plasticity of the *S. pyogenes* genome (J.J. Ferretti, personal communication). Streptococcal phages play an important role in disease by encoding superantigens (erythrogenic exotoxins A and C) and hyaluronidases. Lysogenic conversion of nontoxinogenic strains of group A streptococci was first demonstrated in 1926 (CANTACUZENE and BONCIEU 1926), and since that time temperate converting phages have been detected in a high percentage of *S. pyogenes* strains. One study detected the presence of phage-associated sequences in 97% of strains analyzed (HYNES et al. 1995). The genomic DNA sequence of *S. pyogenes* SF370 revealed the presence of three complete (phages 370.1, 370.2, 370.3) and one partial phage genome (phage 370.4) (J.J. Ferretti, personal communication).

Phage T12, the prototypical *S. pyogenes* phage, specifies erythrogenic exotoxin A (also called streptococcal pyrogenic exotoxin A; SpeA) (JOHNSON and SCHLIEVERT 1984; JOHNSON et al. 1986; WEEKS and FERRETTI 1984; ZABRISKIE 1964), a toxin associated with scarlet fever, toxic-shock-like syndrome, and a number of other streptococcal diseases (JOHNSON et al. 1986; STEVENS et al. 1989; MUSSER et al. 1991). Evidence for horizontal transfer of *speA* toxin genes by phages includes the distribution of one allele (of four identified *speA* alleles) among diverse streptococcal strains from different phylogenetic lineages (MUSSER et al. 1991; NELSON et al. 1991). Erythrogenic exotoxin C (SpeC), like A, is a superantigen encoded by temperate phage CS112 (GOSHORN and SCHLIEVERT 1989). Two alleles of *speC* occur in diverse clones of *S. pyogenes*, again supporting the hypothesis that bacteriophages contribute to horizontal gene transfer in streptococci (KAPUR et al. 1992). The genes for erythrogenic toxins A and C are adjacent to the respective phage attachment sites suggesting, as hypothesized for corynephage β, that transduction or illegitimate recombination resulted in the acquisition of these toxin genes from an ancestral bacterial genome (JOHNSON et al. 1986; GOSHORN and SCHLIEVERT 1989). Similarly, the virulence-implicated genes on the phage genomes in *S. pyogenes* SF370 are located at the site of integration into the bacterial genome (J.J. Ferretti, personal communication). In the genome of this strain, four virulence associated genes – *speC*; a gene with homology to a previously described streptococcal mitogenic factor, MF; a homolog of a competence-specific nuclease, EndA; and the Dnase, streptodornase – are tandemly encoded at one end of the bacteriophage 370.1 genome near the integration site. It has been noted that the GC content of the virulence-associated genes in bacteriophages 370.1, 370.2, 370.3, and 370.4 ranges from 26–30%, while adjacent phage genes have a GC content of approximately 38.5% (a value close to that of the *S. pyogenes* genome) (J.J. Ferretti, personal communication). This discrepancy in GC content strengthens the hypothesis that the virulence genes were acquired from a distantly related organism by phage transfer.

Phage T12, which specifies the SpeA superantigen, inserts into a serine-tRNA gene within the genome (MCSHAN et al. 1997). However, not all *speA*-carrying phages integrate at this site, although other T12-related phages that lack *speA* do (MCSHAN and FERRETTI 1997). A common theme of pathogenicity islands (PAIs) of gram-negative bacteria is that they are associated with tRNA genes at their boundaries (HACKER et al. 1997). A 6-kb region (previously called the "vir regulon") encoding a regulator (*mga*), M and M-like proteins (*emm*, *enn*, *mrp*), and a C5a peptidase (*scpA*), has been identified in *S. pyogenes* (PODBIELSKI et al. 1996). This "vir regulon" has been referred to as a pathogenicity island (HACKER et al. 1997), although the hallmarks of gram-negative pathogenicity islands (tRNA loci or direct repeats at the end of the region, mobility genes [integrases, IS elements, transposases, etc.], and instability) are absent. The lack of association of the "vir regulon" with integrases or bacteriophages, suggests that although phages contribute to horizontal gene transfer and diversity, they are probably not associated with mobilization of putative pathogenicity islands of *S. pyogenes*.

In addition to the virulence factors described above, two genes encoding hyaluronidase activity (*hylP* and *hylP2*) are also associated with streptococcal phages (HYNES et al. 1995). Hyaluronidase has been proposed to potentiate dispersion from initial sites of infection by degrading hyaluronic acid found in connective tissue (HYNES et al. 1995). However, hyaluronidase activity may be of primary importance to the bacteriophage, since degradation of the hyaluronic acid capsule of *S. pyogenes* and exposure of phage receptors may facilitate phage infection (HYNES et al. 1995). Thus, this factor may benefit both the bacterial host and phage. Nine bacteriophage-encoded *hyl* alleles have been identified among *S. pyogenes* strains, and these alleles display a mosaicism that has been attributed to horizontal transfer and intragenic recombination (MARCIEL et al. 1997). As with erythrogenic exotoxins A and C, the association of multiple alleles of hyaluronidase with bacteriophage may contribute to genetic diversity and concomitant diversity in *S. pyogenes* disease.

2.3 *Staphylococcus aureus*

Several virulence factors of *S. aureus* are encoded by temperate phages, including enterotoxin A (and possibly enterotoxin E), staphylokinase, leukocidin, and exfoliative toxin A. Lysogenization in *S. aureus* occurs as single or multiple, simultaneous conversions, with phages mediating positive (acquisition of a virulence factor) and/or negative conversion (loss of a virulence factor). Single conversion to leukocidin or exfoliative toxin A production was observed to result from lysogenization by members of phage serotype group A, and by phage phi-ZM-1, respectively (VIJVER et al. 1972; YOSHIZAWA et al. 2000). Genetic analysis of enterotoxin A, staphylokinase, leukocidin, and exfoliative toxin A genes from bacteriophages definitively established that these virulence factors are also located on bacteriophage genomes (BETLEY and MEKALANOS 1985; SAKO et al. 1983; KANEKO et al. 1997; YOSHIZAWA et al. 2000). Although conclusive evidence is not available, it is possible that enterotoxin E is encoded by defective phages, since an enterotoxin E probe hybridizes to phage DNA induced from these strains (COUCH et al. 1988). A UV-inducible staphylococcal phage (designated FRI1106-1) also has been found to contain a silent variant enterotoxin gene that appears to be related to enterotoxin A (SOLTIS et al. 1990).

In contrast to positive conversion, chromosomally encoded traits such as β-hemolysin or lipase are lost following phage integration into the structural genes for these traits (COLEMAN et al. 1991; COLEMAN et al. 1986; LEE and IANDOLO 1986; WINKLER et al. 1965). Staphylococcal phages belonging to the serotype F group have been characterized that mediate both double and triple conversions. Cases of simultaneous loss of β-hemolysin expression and positive conversion to staphylokinase production (double conversion) (WINKLER et al. 1965), and of the simultaneous positive conversion to staphylokinase and enterotoxin A production and the loss of β hemolysin (triple conversion) (COLEMAN et al. 1989) have been reported. In the latter case, the staphylokinase and enterotoxin A genes were found to be closely linked on the phage genome immediately adjacent to the phage attachment site, whereas the bacterial attachment site was localized within the β-hemolysin (*hlb*) gene, resulting in its insertional inactivation upon integration. Clearly, bacteriophages modulate the virulence of *S. aureus*. Negative conversion events may serve to lessen the impact of *S. aureus* infection, allowing more stable colonization to the benefit of both bacterium and phage.

Bacteriophages probably play a role in the dissemination of toxic shock syndrome toxin (TSST-1), a potent superantigen, among *S. aureus* strains. The TSST-1 gene (*tst*) was initially found on an accessory genetic element (KREISWIRTH et al. 1989), and further studies have demonstrated that *tst* is located on mobile pathogenicity islands, designated SaPI1 or SaPI2, depending on the chromosomal insertion site (LINDSAY et al. 1998). The prototypical pathogenicity island, SaPI1, is a 15.2-kb element flanked by 17 nucleotide direct repeats and contains genes for a putative integrase, a possible second superantigen, and a gene of unknown function homologous to the *vapE* gene that is located on the *vap* pathogenicity island of *Dichelobacter nodosus*. SaPI1 can be excised and circularized by two staphylococcal phages, φ13 and 80α, and SaPI1and can be replicated, encapsidated, and transduced at high frequency by φ13. Bacteriophage transduction of SaPI1 represents the first documented case of mobilization of a pathogenicity island in bacteria and illustrates that bacteriophage infection can lead to rapid alteration of the phenotype of an *S. aureus* strain and intensification of disease.

Recently, methicillin resistance has been shown to be conferred by a unique genetic element, designated staphylococcus cassette chromosome *mec* (SCC*mec*) (KATAYAMA et al. 2000). SCC*mec* is a 52-kb element that is flanked by inverted repeats and contains two novel recombinases, CcrA and CcrB, that allow precise excision from the chromosome and formation of an extrachromosomal circular DNA. This element also contains plasmid pUB110 (encoding kanamycin-tobramycin and bleomycin resistance) inserted between two insertion sequences, and Tn*554* (encoding erythromycin and spectinomycin resistance). SCC*mec* is unusual in that it lacks additional virulence factors associated with pathogenicity islands, structural genes of bacteriophages, and *tra* genes of conjugative transposons. Methicillin resistance can be experimentally transduced among *S. aureus* strains by phages (COHEN and SWEENEY 1970); however, a phage capable of transducing the SSC*mec* element between staphylococcal species has not been identified at this time. These observations, however, raise the possibility that in addition to virulence factors, bacteriophages may be involved in the dissemination of methicillin and/or multi-drug resistance among *S. aureus*.

3 Conversions in Other Gram-Positive Pathogens: *Bacillus cereus* and *Rhodococcus equi*

Studies of bacteriophages have shown that they can confer other traits that affect bacterial fitness and niche control, such as bacteriocin production and possibly antibiotic resistance. Bacteriocin production by lysogens of *Bacillus cereus* has been observed (IVANOVICS et al. 1974); however, a role has yet to be ascribed for this trait in the pathogenesis of infection. In *Rhodococcus equi*, the causative agent of equine pneumonia as well as pneumonia in immunocompromised humans, production of phage was associated with bacterial virulence in a nude mouse model (NORDMANN et al. 1994). Resistant lysogens were not killed by β-lactam antibiotics, whereas strains not producing phage were β-lactam sensitive, suggesting a phage-associated β-lactam resistance mechanism (NORDMANN et al. 1994). Bacteriophages, therefore, are capable of carrying a number of potentially advantageous traits not considered traditionally as virulence factors but, nevertheless, increasing the fitness of an organism and potentially enhancing its ability to colonize.

4 Influence of Nonconverting Bacteriophages on *Streptococcus pneumoniae* Capsule Production

Phages of the human respiratory tract pathogen, *Streptococcus pneumoniae*, appear to lysogenize clinical isolates at a high rate (GINDREAU et al. 2000; RAMIREZ et al. 1999). It has been demonstrated that the primary pneumococcal virulence factor, the capsular polysaccharide, provides resistance to infection by phages of group ω (BERNHEIMER and TIRABY 1976). As a result, it has been suggested that phages capable of lysing unencapsulated pneumococcal strains exert selective pressure for the maintenance and evolution of the polysaccharide capsule, impacting the structure of natural pneumococcal populations (GINDREAU et al. 2000; RAMIREZ et al. 1999).

5 Conjugative Plasmids Encoding Virulence Traits

The emergence in the 1980s and '90s of enterococci and staphylococci as leading causes of nosocomial infection, is due in part to the acquisition of virulence traits and antibiotic resistances on mobile elements via conjugation. In the enterococci, pheromone-responsive conjugative plasmids have been described that express transfer-related genes following exposure to hepta- or octa-peptides expressed by a recipient cell of the same or closely related species (DUNNY et al. 1979; HIRT et al. 1996; WIRTH 1994; WIRTH and MARCINEK 1995). Each pheromone-responsive plasmid responds to a specific pheromone, and receipt of a particular plasmid does not preclude secretion of other pheromones and receipt of other pheromone-responsive plasmids (EHRENFELD et al. 1986).

One plasmid function induced by exposure to pheromones is a cell-surface protein, termed aggregation substance (AS). AS mediates the binding of donor with recipient (Galli et al. 1989) by interacting in part with lipoteichoic acid on the recipient surface (Bensing and Dunny 1993; Ehrenfeld et al. 1986). Aggregation substance expressed on the donor cell surface mediates the "clumping" reaction typical of the mating response. Additionally, aggregation substance can function as an adhesin that can facilitate bacterial attachment and colonization of host tissue. Aggregation substance can promote binding to cultured renal tubular cells (Kreft et al. 1992) and enhances adherence and uptake by intestinal epithelial cells derived from the colon and duodenum (Sartingen et al. 2000). In a catheter-induced rabbit endocarditis model, rabbits infected with a strain expressing aggregation substance displayed increased heart valve vegetation weight (Chow et al. 1993). However, in an *E. faecalis* endophthalmitis infection model, aggregation substance did not affect the ability of enterococci to attach to membranous structures within the vitreous (Jett et al. 1998), highlighting the importance of other adhesins in this infection.

Pheromone-responsive plasmids also encode virulence factors extrinsic to the transfer machinery. The enterococcal cytolysin is a toxin that exhibits both hemolytic and bactericidal activities, and is frequently encoded by pheromone-responsive plasmids, the prototype being pAD1 (Clewell 1993). The *E. faecalis* cytolysin represents the archetype of a novel class of bacterial toxins related to streptolysin S and to lantibiotic-type bacteriocins. The cytolysin is heterodimeric, consisting of a large and small subunit, both of which are required for hemolytic and bactericidal activity (Gilmore et al. 1994). Both subunits have been shown to possess lanthionine residues, the hallmark of lantibiotic bacteriocins (Booth et al. 1996). These posttranslational modifications require the involvement of a modification gene contained within the cytolysin operon (Gilmore et al. 1994). Both cytolysin subunits are secreted through a dedicated ATP-binding cassette transporter (Gilmore et al. 1990). Secretion of each subunit is accompanied by a proteolytic processing event (Booth et al. 1996). Once extracellular, both subunits require an additional proteolytic removal of six residues from the amino terminus for activity (Booth et al. 1996). The final activating cleavage is accomplished by a subtilisin-class serine protease also encoded by the cytolysin operon (Segarra et al. 1991). A recently identified gene, *cylI*, located at the extreme 3′ end of the operon, encodes a factor that confers immunity to the bacteriocin effects of the cytolysin to cytolysin-producing bacterial cells (Coburn et al. 1999). Recent data suggests that two open reading frames, 5′ to the cytolysin structural genes, and divergently transcribed, are involved in a quorum-sensing mode of autoregulation and have been termed *cylR1* and *cylR2* (W. Haas, personal communication). The small cytolysin subunit, $CylL_S$, appears to autoinduce expression of the cytolysin operon (W. Haas, personal communication).

Cytolysin expression is common among clinical isolates of *E. faecalis* (Huycke and Gilmore 1995; Ike et al. 1987) and has been associated with acutely terminal outcome (Huycke et al. 1991). A variety of animal studies utilizing isogenic mutants of the cytolysin have provided direct proof of the role of this virulence factor as a key determinant of disease severity (Chow et al. 1993; Ike et al. 1984; Jett et al. 1992).

Cytolysin and aggregation substance act synergistically in contributing to the virulence of *E. faecalis*. Chow et al. (1993) examined strains of *E. faecalis* defective in expression of aggregation substance and/or cytolysin in a catheter-induced rabbit endocarditis model, and found that infections with strains expressing either factor singly were not significantly lethal. In contrast, 55% of animals infected with an isogenic strain expressing both factors died. The basis for synergy probably relates to the role of aggregation substance in positioning the bacterium on the surface of a target cell and/or in causing bacterial aggregation promoting quorum-sensing dependent expression of the broad-spectrum cytolysin.

Recent studies have also found the cytolysin operon to be associated with a putative surface adhesin, termed Esp (N. Shankar, personal communication). Clinical isolates of *E. faecalis* have been identified that possess the cytolysin adjacent to Esp in an element that possesses both IS elements, putative transposases, and other functions that may be associated with niche control. The strain of *E. faecalis* for which the genome sequence is being determined appears to have undergone a spontaneous deletion of a partially defective form of this element; a second otherwise identical isolate from the same patient (Sahm et al. 1989) possesses the 17-kb element. These observations illustrate the ability of functions with synergistic (or for Esp, putatively synergistic) activities to associate on the genome of *E. faecalis* and highlight the mobility of these elements. Whether the Esp/cytolysin complex represents an evolving transposon, or a bona fide pathogenicity island remains to be determined.

6 Conjugative Transposons

Conjugative transposons are promiscuous mobile genetic elements that frequently harbor antibiotic resistance determinants. These elements are capable of transposition from one DNA molecule to another within the same cell or of transferring to a DNA molecule within another cell, potentially a cell of a different species. Conjugative transposons share several features, namely the ability to excise from a donor DNA molecule, the ability to integrate into a recipient molecule, and the production of a circular intermediate in the process (Bedzyk et al. 1992; Salyers et al. 1995; Scott 1992; Scott and Churchward 1995; Scott et al. 1988). Conjugative transposons typically display little target site specificity, other than for AT-rich regions (Scott et al. 1994; Trieu-Cuot et al. 1993).

The process of conjugative transposon excision and integration follows discrete steps (Caparon and Scott 1989; Salyers et al. 1995; Scott and Churchward 1995). The initial event involves endonucleolytic cleavage of the ends of the transposon. Cleavage of one strand occurs six bases from the end of the transposon and immediately adjacent to the transposon on the opposite strand. Identical cleavage events occur at the opposite end of the transposon. This event generates six base pair overhangs at the transposon termini that are referred to as coupling sequences. Both the donor and excised transposon are then covalently closed. However, since the six base pair coupling sequences are noncomplementary, the joint in both the donor molecule and the transposon are mismatched. This mismatch is apparently resolved by replication in the donor molecule but remains unresolved in the transposon due to lack of replication. Staggered endonucleolytic cleavage of both the circular, covalently closed intermediate and a new target occurs, followed by ligation of the transposon to the target molecule. A six base pair sequence of noncomplementarity results at the junctions of the transposon and target that is resolved by replication of the recipient molecule (CAPARON and SCOTT 1989; SALYERS et al. 1995; SCOTT and CHURCHWARD 1995). These processes are mediated by the products of the *int* and *xis* genes that are also encoded within the transposon (FLANNAGAN et al. 1994; POYART-SALMERON et al. 1989; POYART-SALMERON et al. 1990; STORRS et al. 1991).

The relevance of conjugative transposons to the current review is their similarity to temperate bacteriophages (indeed, they may be remnants of phage genomes that have lost the genes encoding structural and coat proteins) and that they encode resistance determinants that have significantly impacted the ability of gram-positive bacteria (particularly *E. faecium*) to colonize and infect. The excision and integration events are similar in both conjugative transposons and phages, and integrases of conjugative transposons are related to phage integrases (POYART-SALMERON et al. 1989; POYART-SALMERON et al. 1990). Like converting phages, transposon insertion may also modulate the expression of infection-relevant genes. Insertion into a member of an operon may result in polar effects on genes 3' to the insertion site, as was shown for the expression of the cytolysin immunity gene due to insertion of Tn917 into the immediately 5' gene for the cytolysin activator protease (COBURN et al. 1999), and has been observed for inactivation of the cytolysin transporter in the V583 sibling strain, V586 (SAHM et al. 1989). Transposon insertion may also result in the upregulation of genes located adjacent to the site of insertion, as was shown for Tn916. It has been demonstrated by Northern blot analysis that outward reading transcripts, initiated from promoters located near the end of Tn916 containing the *tet* M gene, the *xis* and *int* genes, can extend into the host chromosome (CELLI and TRIEU-CUOT 1998), potentially conferring resistance and upregulating expression of virulence-relevant traits.

The prototype conjugative transposon, Tn916, was discovered in *E. faecalis* strain DS16. This 18.5-kb transposon possesses the *tetM* gene (FRANKE and CLEWELL 1981; GAWRON-BURKE and CLEWELL 1982). A related element, designated Tn5253, has been identified in *S. pneumoniae* and represents a composite possessing the Tn916-like element Tn5251 inserted within another element, Tn5252 (AYOUBI et al. 1991; SHOEMAKER et al. 1980). COURVALIN and CARLIER (1986) characterized a conjugative transposon, designated Tn1545, capable of conjugation and chromosomal integration into a variety of streptococcal species, *S. aureus*, and *L. monocytogenes*. This element encoded resistances to kanamycin and related aminoglycosides, members of the macrolide-lincosamide-streptogramin B class of antibiotics, and tetracycline (COURVALIN and CARLIER 1986).

Of considerable clinical concern are conjugal transposons carrying glycopeptide resistance determinants that potentially could be transferred from enterococci to *S. aureus*. The elements Tn*1547* (QUINTILIANI and COURVALIN 1996) and Tn*5382* (CARIAS et al. 1998) have been demonstrated to specify the *vanB* resistance determinant, and more recently, another conjugative transposon, Tn*1549*, was shown to carry the *vanB2* operon and to be organized in a similar fashion to Tn*916* (GARNIER et al. 2000).

Other complex conjugative transposons mediating antibiotic resistance have also been described. Tn*5385*, a 65-kb element found in the clinical *E. faecalis* strains CH19 and CH116, appears to be a conglomeration of a number of elements, including the conjugative transposon Tn*5381*, the composite transposon Tn*5384*, staphylococcal elements Tn*4001* and Tn*552*, as well as staphylococcal and enterococcal insertion sequence (IS) elements IS*256*, IS*257*, and IS*1216*. This 65-kb composite transposon specifies a large number of resistances, including erythromycin, gentamicin, mercuric chloride, streptomycin, tetracycline-minocycline, and penicillin. As a result, this conjugative element is capable of converting highly adapted GI tract commensal enterococci into multiple antibiotic resistant strains in a single event (BONAFEDE et al. 1997; RICE and CARIAS 1998).

7 Conclusion

Mobile elements, including bacteriophages, conjugative plasmids, and conjugative transposons are capable of influencing the evolution of gram-positive pathogens by the dissemination of potentially beneficial traits in a more rapid time course than mutation alone. The occurrence of genes, such as toxins, on phages or other mobile or variable elements clearly shows that natural selection has favored variation, itself, among a population; otherwise, strains with these toxins firmly integrated into the chromosome would have outpopulated those lacking such traits. Horizontal transfer of virulence and antibiotic resistance traits via conjugation and transduction provides a mechanism for the rapid dissemination of such elements to the broader population in environments where such traits confer a selective advantage. This transfer appears to account for much of the explosive increase in the occurrence of antibiotic-refractory gram-positive infections, and genera, such as enterococci, appear to serve as reservoirs for such elements.

References

Ayoubi P, Kilic AO, Vijayakumar MN (1991) Tn*5253*, the pneumococcal omega (cat tet) BM6001 element, is a composite structure of two conjugative transposons, Tn*5251* and Tn*5252*. J Bacteriol 173:1617–1622

Barksdale L, Arden SB (1974) Persisting bacteriophage infections, lysogeny, and phage conversions. Annu Rev Microbiol 28:265–299

Barksdale W, Pappenheimer A (1954) Phage-host relationships in nontoxigenic and toxigenic diphtheria bacilli. J Bacteriol 56:220–232

Bedzyk LA, Shoemaker NB, Young KE, Salyers AA (1992) Insertion and excision of Bacteroides conjugative chromosomal elements. J Bacteriol 174:166–172

Bensing BA, Dunny GM (1993) Cloning and molecular analysis of genes affecting expression of binding substance, the recipient-encoded receptor(s) mediating mating aggregate formation in *Enterococcus faecalis*. J Bacteriol 175:7421–7429

Bernheimer HP, Tiraby JG (1976) Inhibition of phage infection by pneumococcus capsule. Virology 73:308–309

Betley MJ, Mekalanos JJ (1985) Staphylococcal enterotoxin A is encoded by phage. Science 229:185–187

Bonafede ME, Carias LL, Rice LB (1997) Enterococcal transposon Tn*5384*: evolution of a composite transposon through cointegration of enterococcal and staphylococcal plasmids. Antimicrob Agents Chemother 41:1854–1858

Booth MC, Bogie CP, Sahl H-G, Siezen RJ, Hatter KL, Gilmore MS (1996) Structural analysis and proteolytic activation of *Enterococcus faecalis* cytolysin, a novel lantibiotic. Mol Microbiol 21:1175–1184

Cantacuzene J, Boncieu O (1926) Modifications subies par des streptococques d'origine non-scarlatineuse qu contact des produits scarlatineux filtres. CR Acad Sci 182:1185

Caparon MG, Scott JR (1989) Excision and insertion of the conjugative transposon Tn*916* involves a novel recombination mechanism. Cell 59:1027–1034

Carias LL, Rudin SD, Donskey CJ, Rice LB (1998) Genetic linkage and co-transfer of a novel, vanB-containing transposon (Tn*5382*) and a low-affinity penicillin-binding protein 5 gene in a clinical vancomycin-resistant *Enterococcus faecium* isolate. J Bacteriol 180:4426–4434

Celli J, Trieu-Cuot P (1998) Circularization of Tn*916* is required for expression of the transposon-encoded transfer functions: characterization of long tetracycline-inducible transcripts reading through the attachment site. Mol Microbiol 28:103–117

Chow JW, Thal LA, Perri MB, Vazquez JA, Donabedian SM, Clewell DB, Zervos MJ (1993) Plasmid-associated hemolysin and aggregation substance production contribute to virulence in experimental enterococcal endocarditis. Antimicrob Agents Chemother 37:2474–2477

Clewell DB (1993) Bacterial sex pheromone-induced plasmid transfer. Cell 73:9–12

Coburn PS, Hancock LE, Booth MC, Gilmore MS (1999) A novel means of self-protection, unrelated to toxin activation, confers immunity to the bactericidal effects of the *Enterococcus faecalis* cytolysin. Infect Immun 67:3339–3347

Cohen S, Sweeney HM (1970) Transduction of methicillin resistance in *Staphylococcus aureus* dependent on an unusual specificity of the recipient strain. J Bacteriol 104:1158–1167

Coleman DC, Arbuthnott JP, Pomeroy HM, Birkbeck TH (1986) Cloning and expression in *Escherichia coli* and *Staphylococcus aureus* of the beta-lysin determinant from *Staphylococcus aureus*: evidence that bacteriophage conversion of beta-lysin activity is caused by insertional inactivation of the beta-lysin determinant. Microb Pathog 1:549–564

Coleman D, Knights J, Russell R, Shanley D, Birkbeck TH, Dougan G, Charles I (1991) Insertional inactivation of the *Staphylococcus aureus* beta-toxin by bacteriophage phi 13 occurs by site- and orientation-specific integration of the phi 13 genome. Mol Microbiol 5:933–939

Coleman DC, Sullivan DJ, Russell RJ, Arbuthnott JP, Carey BF, Pomeroy HM (1989) *Staphylococcus aureus* bacteriophages mediating the simultaneous lysogenic conversion of beta-lysin, staphylokinase and enterotoxin A: molecular mechanism of triple conversion. J Gen Microbiol 135:1679–1697

Couch JL, Soltis MT, Betley MJ (1988) Cloning and nucleotide sequence of the type E staphylococcal enterotoxin gene. J Bacteriol 170:2954–2960

Courvalin P, Carlier C (1986) Transposable multiple antibiotic resistance in *Streptococcus pneumoniae*. Mol Gen Genet 205:291–297

Dunny GM, Craig RA, Carron RL, Clewell DB (1979) Plasmid transfer in *Streptococcus faecalis*: production of multiple sex pheromones by recipients. Plasmid 2:454–465

Ehrenfeld EE, Kessler RE, Clewell DB (1986) Identification of pheromone-induced surface proteins in *Streptococcus faecalis* and evidence of a role for lipoteichoic acid in formation of mating aggregates. J Bacteriol 168:6–12

Eklund MW, Poysky FT (1969) Growth and toxin production of *Clostridium botulinum* types E, nonproteolytic B, and F in nonirradiated and irradiated fisheries products in the temperature range of 38 degrees to 50 degrees F. TID-25231. TID Rep 1–33

Eklund MW, Poysky FT, Boatman ES (1969) Bacteriophages of *Clostridium botulinum* types A, B, E, and F and nontoxigenic strains resembling type E. J Virol 3:270–274

Eklund MW, Poysky FT, Reed SM, Smith CA (1971) Bacteriophage and the toxigenicity of *Clostridium botulinum* type C. Science 172:480–482

Flannagan SE, Zitzow LA, Su YA, Clewell DB (1994) Nucleotide sequence of the 18-kb conjugative transposon Tn*916* from *Enterococcus faecalis*. Plasmid 32:350–354

Fourel G, Phalipon A, Kaczorek M (1989) Evidence for direct regulation of diphtheria toxin gene transcription by an Fe^{2+}-dependent DNA-binding repressor, DtoxR, in *Corynebacterium diphtheriae*. Infect Immun 57:3221–3225

Franke AE, Clewell DB (1981) Evidence for a chromosome-borne resistance transposon (Tn916) in *Streptococcus faecalis* that is capable of "conjugal" transfer in the absence of a conjugative plasmid. J Bacteriol 145:494–502

Freeman V (1951) Studies on the virulence of bacteriophage-infected strains of *Corynebacterium diphtheriae*. J Bacteriol 61:675–688

Galli D, Wirth R, Wanner G (1989) Identification of aggregation substances of *Enterococcus faecalis* cells after induction by sex pheromones. An immunological and ultrastructural investigation. Arch Microbiol 151:486–490

Garnier F, Taourit S, Glaser P, Courvalin P, Galimand M (2000) Characterization of transposon Tn*1549*, conferring VanB-type resistance in *Enterococcus* spp. Microbiology 146:1481–1489

Gawron-Burke C, Clewell DB (1982) A transposon in *Streptococcus faecalis* with fertility properties. Nature 300:281–284

Gill DM, Uchida T, Singer RA (1972) Expression of diphtheria toxin genes carried by integrated and nonintegrated phage beta. Virology 50:664–668

Gilmore MS, Segarra RA, Booth MC (1990) An HlyB-type function is required for expression of the *Enterococcus faecalis* hemolysin/bacteriocin. Infect Immun 58:3914–3923

Gilmore MS, Segarra RA, Booth MC, Bogie CP, Hall LR, Clewell DB (1994) Genetic structure of the *Enterococcus faecalis* plasmid pAD1-encoded cytolytic toxin system and its relationship to lantibiotic determinants. J Bacteriol 176:7335–7344

Gindreau E, Lopez R, Garcia P (2000) MM1, a temperate bacteriophage of the type 23F Spanish/USA multi-resistant epidemic clone of *Streptococcus pneumoniae*: structural analysis of the site-specific integration system. J Virol 74:7803–7813

Goshorn SC, Schlievert PM (1989) Bacteriophage association of streptococcal pyrogenic exotoxin type C. J Bacteriol 171:3068–3073.

Greenfield L, Bjorn MJ, Horn G, Fong D, Buck GA, Collier RJ, Kaplan DA (1983) Nucleotide sequence of the structural gene for diphtheria toxin carried by corynebacteriophage beta. Proc Natl Acad Sci USA 80:6853–6857

Groman N (1953) The relation of bacteriophage to the change of *Corynebacterium diphtheriae* from avirulence to virulence. Science 117:297–299

Groman NB (1984) Conversion by corynephages and its role in the natural history of diphtheria. J Hyg (Lond) 93:405–417

Hacker J, Blum-Oehler G, Muhldorfer I, Tschape H (1997) Pathogenicity islands of virulent bacteria: structure, function and impact on microbial evolution. Mol Microbiol 23:1089–1097

Hirt H, Wirth R, Muscholl A (1996) Comparative analysis of 18 sex pheromone plasmids from *Enterococcus faecalis*: detection of a new insertion element on pPD1 and implications for the evolution of this plasmid family. Mol Gen Genet 252:640–647

Holmes RK (1976) Characterization and genetic mapping of nontoxinogenic (*tox*) mutants of coryne-bacteriophage beta. J Virol 19:195–207

Holmes RK (2000) Biology and molecular epidemiology of diphtheria toxin and the *tox* gene. J Infect Dis 181 Suppl 1:S156–167

Huycke MM, Gilmore MS (1995) Frequency of aggregation substance and cytolysin genes among enterococcal endocarditis isolates. Plasmid 34:152–156

Huycke MM, Spiegel CA, Gilmore MS (1991) Bacteremia caused by hemolytic, high-level gentamicin-resistant *Enterococcus faecalis*. Antimicrob Agents Chemother 35:1626–1634

Hynes WL, Hancock L, Ferretti JJ (1995) Analysis of a second bacteriophage hyaluronidase gene from *Streptococcus pyogenes*: evidence for a third hyaluronidase involved in extracellular enzymatic activity. Infect Immun 63:3015–3020

Ike Y, Hashimoto H, Clewell DB (1984) Hemolysin of *Streptococcus faecalis* subspecies *zymogenes* contributes to virulence in mice. Infect Immun 45:528–530

Ike Y, Hashimoto H, Clewell DB (1987) High incidence of hemolysin production by *Enterococcus* (*Streptococcus*) *faecalis* strains associated with human parenteral infections. J Clin Microbiol 25:1524–1528

Inoue K, Iida H (1971) Phage-conversion of toxigenicity in *Clostridium botulinum* types C and D. Jpn J Med Sci Biol 24:53–56

Ivanovics G, Gaal V, Pragai B (1974) Lysogenic conversion to phospholipase A production in *Bacillus cereus*. J Gen Virol 24:349–358

Jett BD, Jensen HG, Nordquist RE, Gilmore MS (1992) Contribution of the pAD1-encoded cytolysin to the severity of experimental *Enterococcus faecalis* endophthalmitis. Infect Immun 60:2445–2452

Jett BD, Atkuri RV, Gilmore MS (1998) *Enterococcus faecalis* localization in experimental endophthalmitis: role of plasmid-encoded aggregation substance. Infect Immun 66:843–848

Johnson LP, Schlievert PM (1984) Group A streptococcal phage T12 carries the structural gene for pyrogenic exotoxin type A. Mol Gen Genet 194:52–56

Johnson LP, Tomai MA, Schlievert PM (1986) Bacteriophage involvement in group A streptococcal pyrogenic exotoxin A production. J Bacteriol 166:623–627

Kaneko J, Kimura T, Kawakami Y, Tomita T, Kamio Y (1997) Panton-Valentine leukocidin genes in phage-like particle isolated from mitomycin C-treated *Staphylococcus aureus* V8 (ATCC 49775). Biosci Biotechnol Biochem 61:1960–1962

Kapur V, Nelson K, Schlievert PM, Selander RK, Musser JM (1992) Molecular population genetic evidence of horizontal spread of two alleles of the pyrogenic exotoxin C gene (*speC*) among pathogenic clones of *Streptococcus pyogenes*. Infect Immun 60:3513–3517

Katayama Y, Ito T, Hiramatsu K (2000) A new class of genetic element, Staphylococcus cassette chromosome *mec*, encodes methicillin resistance in *Staphylococcus aureus*. Antimicrob Agents Chemother 44:1549–1555

Kondo I, Fujise K (1977) Serotype B staphylococcal bacteriophage singly converting staphylokinase. Infect Immun 18:266–272

Kreft B, Marre R, Schramm U, Wirth R (1992) Aggregation substance of *Enterococcus faecalis* mediates adhesion to cultured renal tubular cells. Infect Immun 60:25–30

Kreiswirth BN, Projan SJ, Schlievert PM, Novick RP (1989) Toxic shock syndrome toxin-1 is encoded by a variable genetic element. Rev Infect Dis 11:S75–S82

Laird W, Groman N (1976a) Prophage map of converting corynebacteriophage beta. J Virol 19:208–219

Laird W, Groman N (1976b) Orientation of the *tox* gene in the prophage of corynebacteriophage beta. J Virol 19:228–231

Lee CY, Iandolo JJ (1986) Lysogenic conversion of staphylococcal lipase is caused by insertion of the bacteriophage L54a genome into the lipase structural gene. J Bacteriol 166:385–391

Lindsay JA, Ruzin A, Ross HF, Kurepina N, Novick RP (1998) The gene for toxic shock toxin is carried by a family of mobile pathogenicity islands in *Staphylococcus aureus*. Mol Microbiol 29:527–543

Marciel AM, Kapur V, Musser JM (1997) Molecular population genetic analysis of a *Streptococcus pyogenes* bacteriophage-encoded hyaluronidase gene: recombination contributes to allelic variation. Microb Pathog 22:209–217

Matsuda M, Barksdale L (1966) Phage-directed synthesis of diphtherial toxin in non-toxinogenic *Corynebacterium diphtheriae*. Nature 210:911–913

Matsuda M, Barksdale L (1967) System for the investigation of the bacteriophage-directed synthesis of diphtherial toxin. J Bacteriol 93:722–730

McShan WM, Ferretti JJ (1997) Genetic diversity in temperate bacteriophages of *Streptococcus pyogenes*: Identification of a second attachment site for phages carrying the erythrogenic toxin A gene. J Bacteriol 179:6509–6511

McShan WM, Tang YF, Ferretti JJ (1997) Bacteriophage T12 of *Streptococcus pyogenes* integrates into the gene encoding a serine tRNA. Mol Microbiol 23:719–728

Miao EA, Miller SI (1999) Bacteriophages in the evolution of pathogen-host interactions. Proc Natl Acad Sci USA 96:9452–9454

Musser JM, Hauser AR, Kim MH, Schlievert PM, Nelson K, Selander RK (1991) *Streptococcus pyogenes* causing toxic-shock-like syndrome and other invasive diseases: Clonal diversity and pyrogenic exotoxin expression. Proc Natl Acad Sci USA 88:2668–2672

Nelson K, Schlievert PM, Selander RK, Musser JM (1991) Characterization and clonal distribution of four alleles of the speA gene encoding pyrogenic exotoxin A (scarlet fever toxin) in *Streptococcus pyogenes*. J Exp Med 174:1271–1274

Nida SK, Ferretti JJ (1982) Phage influence on the synthesis of extracellular toxins in group A streptococci. Infect Immun 36:745–750

Nordmann P, Keller M, Espinasse F, Ronco E (1994) Correlation between antibiotic resistance, phage-like particle presence, and virulence in *Rhodococcus equi* human isolates. J Clin Microbiol 32:377–383

Podbielski A, Woischnik M, Pohl B, Schmidt KH (1996) What is the size of the group A streptococcal *vir* regulon? The Mga regulator affects expression of secreted and surface virulence factors. Med Microbiol Immunol (Berl) 185:171–181

Popovic T, Mazurova IK, Efstratiou A, Vuopio-Varkila J, Reeves MW, De Zoysa A, Glushkevich T, Grimont P (2000) Molecular epidemiology of diphtheria. J Infect Dis 181 Suppl 1:S168–177

Poyart-Salmeron C, Trieu-Cuot P, Carlier C, Courvalin P (1989) Molecular characterization of two proteins involved in the excision of the conjugative transposon Tn*1545*: homologies with other site-specific recombinases. EMBO J 8:2425–2433

Poyart-Salmeron C, Trieu-Cuot P, Carlier C, Courvalin P (1990) The integration-excision system of the conjugative transposon Tn*1545* is structurally and functionally related to those of lambdoid phages. Mol Microbiol 4:1513–1521

Quintiliani R Jr., Courvalin P (1996) Characterization of Tn*1547*, a composite transposon flanked by the IS*16* and IS*256*-like elements, that confers vancomycin resistance in *Enterococcus faecalis* BM4281. Gene 172:1–8

Ramirez M, Severina E, Tomasz A (1999) A high incidence of prophage carriage among natural isolates of *Streptococcus pneumoniae*. J Bacteriol 181:3618–3625

Rappuoli R, Ratti G (1984) Physical map of the chromosomal region of *Corynebacterium diphtheriae* containing corynephage attachment sites *attB1* and *attB2*. J Bacteriol 158:325–330

Ratti G, Covacci A, Rappuoli R (1997) A tRNA (2Arg) gene of *Corynebacterium diphtheriae* is the chromosomal integration site for toxinogenic bacteriophages [letter]. Mol Microbiol 25:1179–1181

Rice LB, Carias LL (1998) Transfer of Tn*5385*, a composite, multi-resistance chromosomal element from *Enterococcus faecalis*. J Bacteriol 180:714–721

Sahm DF, Kissinger J, Gilmore MS, Murray PR, Mulder R, Solliday J, Clarke B (1989) In vitro susceptibility studies of vancomycin-resistant *Enterococcus faecalis*. Antimicrob Agents Chemother 33:1588–1591

Sako T, Sawaki S, Sakarui T, Ito S, Yoshizawa Y, Kondo I (1983) Cloning and expression of the staphylokinase gene of *Staphylococcus aureus* in *Escherichia coli*. Mol Gen Genet 190:271–277

Salyers AA, Shoemaker NB, Stevens AM, Li LY (1995) Conjugative transposons: an unusual and diverse set of integrated gene transfer elements. Microbiol Rev 59:579–590

Sartingen S, Rozdzinski E, Muscholl-Silberhorn A, Marre R (2000) Aggregation substance increases adherence and internalization but not translocation, of *Enterococcus faecalis* through different intestinal epithelial cells in vitro. Infect Immun 68:6044–6047

Schmitt MP, Holmes RK (1993) Analysis of diphtheria toxin repressor-operator interactions and characterization of a mutant repressor with decreased binding activity for divalent metals. Mol Microbiol 9:173–181

Scott JR (1992) Sex and the single circle: conjugative transposition. J Bacteriol 174:6005–6010

Scott JR, Churchward GG (1995) Conjugative transposition. Annu Rev Microbiol 49:367–397

Scott JR, Kirchman PA, Caparon MG (1988) An intermediate in transposition of the conjugative transposon Tn*916*. Proc Natl Acad Sci USA 85:4809–4813

Scott JR, Bringel F, Marra D, Van Alstine G, Rudy CK (1994) Conjugative transposition of Tn*916*: preferred targets and evidence for conjugative transfer of a single strand and for a double-stranded circular intermediate. Mol Microbiol 11:1099–1108

Segarra RA, Booth MC, Morales DA, Huycke MM, Gilmore MS (1991) Molecular characterization of the *Enterococcus faecalis* cytolysin activator. Infect Immun 59:1239–1246

Shoemaker NB, Smith MD, Guild WR (1980) DNase-resistant transfer of chromosomal cat and tet insertions by filter mating in *Pneumococcus*. Plasmid 3:80–87

Soltis MT, Mekalanos JJ, Betley MJ (1990) Identification of a bacteriophage containing a silent staphylococcal variant enterotoxin gene (*sezA*$^+$). Infect Immun 58:1614–1619

Stevens DL, Tanner MH, Winship J, Swarts R, Ries KM, Schlievert PM, Kaplan E (1989) Severe group A streptococcal infections associated with a toxic shock-like syndrome and scarlet fever toxin A. N Engl J Med 321:1–7

Storrs MJ, Poyart-Salmeron C, Trieu-Cuot P, Courvalin P (1991) Conjugative transposition of Tn*916* requires the excisive and integrative activities of the transposon-encoded integrase. J Bacteriol 173:4347–4352

Tao X, Murphy JR (1992) Binding of the metalloregulatory protein DtxR to the diphtheria *tox* operator requires a divalent heavy metal ion and protects the palindromic sequence from DNAse I digestion. J Biol Chem 267:21761–21764

Tao X, Boyd J, Murphy JR (1992) Specific binding of the diphtheria *tox* regulatory element DtxR to the *tox* operator requires divalent heavy metal ions and a 9-base-pair interrupted palindromic sequence. Proc Natl Acad Sci USA 89:5897–5901

Trieu-Cuot P, Poyart-Salmeron C, Carlier C, Courvalin P (1993) Sequence requirements for target activity in site-specific recombination mediated by the Int protein of transposon Tn*1545*. Mol Microbiol 8:179–185

Uchida T, Gill DM, Pappenheimer AM Jr. (1971) Mutation in the structural gene for diphtheria toxin carried by temperate phage. Nat New Biol 233:8–11

van der Vijver JC, van Es-Boon M, Michel MF (1972) Lysogenic conversion in *Staphylococcus aureus* to leucocidin production. J Virol 10:318–319

Weeks CR, Ferretti JJ (1984) The gene for type A streptococcal exotoxin (erythrogenic toxin) is located in bacteriophage T12. Infect Immun 46:531–536

Weeks CR, Ferretti JJ (1986) Nucleotide sequence of the type A streptococcal exotoxin (erythrogenic toxin) gene from *Streptococcus pyogenes* bacteriophage T12. Infect Immun 52:144–150

Winkler KC, de Waart J, Grootsen C (1965) Lysogenic conversion of staphylococci to loss of beta-toxin. J Gen Microbiol 39:321–333

Wirth R (1994) The sex pheromone system of *Enterococcus faecalis*. More than just a plasmid-collection mechanism? Eur J Biochem 222:235–246

Wirth R, Marcinek H (1995) In vivo gene transfer by *Enterococcus faecalis*. Dev Biol Stand 85:51–54

Yoshizawa Y, Sakurada J, Sakurai S, Machida K, Kondo I, Masuda S (2000) An exfoliative toxin A-converting phage isolated from *Staphylococcus aureus* strain ZM. Microbiol Immunol 44:189–191

Zabriskie J (1964) The role of temperate bacteriophage in the production of erythrogenic toxin by group A streptococci. J Exp Med 119:761–779

Genome Structure and Evolution
of the *Bacillus cereus* Group

A.-B. Kolstø[1], D. Lereclus[2], and M. Mock[3]

1 Introduction

Bacillus species are among the best characterized and genetically amenable Gram-positive bacteria and are widely used in the biotechnological, pharmaceutical, and food industries. First described by Ferdinand Cohn in 1872, the genus *Bacillus* is the largest of the family *Bacillaceae*, including more than 65 described species. *Bacillus subtilis* is registered as the type species, and members of the genus *Bacillus* are aerobic or facultative anaerobic, usually motile, endospore-forming rods that are ubiquitous in the environment, commonly found in soil, air, dust and water. The members exhibit both a remarkable metabolic diversity and an ability to secrete very efficiently large amounts of metabolites to the growth medium, making the bacteria commercially useful for the production of enzymes, antibiotics, insecticides, and fine biochemicals, such as flavour enhancers and food supple-

[1] Biotechnology Centre of Oslo and Institute of Pharmacy, University of Oslo, PB 1125, 0316 Oslo, Norway
[2] Department des Biotechnologies, Unite de Biochimie Microbienne, 25, rue du Dr Roux, 75724 Paris cedex 15, France
[3] Toxines et Pathogenie Bacteriennes, Institut Pasteur, 28, rue du Dr Roux, 75724 Paris cedex 15, France

ments. *Bacillus subtilis* 168 was the first genome of a Gram-positive bacterium to be completely sequenced, involving a consortium of 151 scientists from Europe and Japan (KUNST et al. 1997). The *B. subtilis* genome is of fundamental importance to science and industry.

The *Bacillus cereus* group is a subdivision of the *Bacillus* genus and includes the closely related species *B. anthracis*, *B. cereus*, and *B. thuringiensis*. Although other species, like *B. mycoides*, are also closely related, this species is less studied and is not included in the present review.

The characteristic feature of *B. thuringiensis* is its ability to produce insecticidal crystal toxins (δ-endotoxins) of different specificity (*Lepidoptera*, *Coleoptera*, Diptera) inside the cell during sporulation or stationary phase (SCHNEPF et al. 1998). For this reason *B. thuringiensis* has, for a number of years, been the most widely used biopesticide, being used commercially to combat insects that damage to crops or that are vectors for diseases, such as malaria or yellow fever. It is, therefore, of high economic importance for the agricultural industry, with more than 200 products registered in the United States by 1998 (for complete reviews on these subjects see CHARLES et al. 2000). The genes encoding entomopathogenic proteins in *B. thuringiensis* are most frequently located extrachromosomally on conjugative plasmids (GONZALES et al. 1982; GONZALEZ et al. 1981). The pheno-typical traits employed for the identification of *B. thuringiensis* may thus be lost, making the strains indistinguishable from strains of *B. cereus*.

B. anthracis has been identified as a non-haemolytic, non-motile, penicillin-sensitive, encapsulated bacterium causing the potentially lethal disease anthrax. It is endemic or hyper-endemic in Africa, Asia, and South-America. Anthrax-like infections have been described in ancient literature dating back more than 2,000 years and have been claimed to be responsible for enormous domestic livestock losses in Europe from the seventeenth throughout the nineteenth century. The bacterium is also considered a potential weapon in biological warfare (reviewed by INGLESBY et al. 1999). The genes causing the lethal effect of anthrax are located on two large virulence plasmids, pXO1 encoding the three anthrax toxin subunits and their regulatory elements (UCHIDA et al. 1993) and pXO2 encoding the poly-D-glutamate capsule (LEPPLA 1991).

Bacillus cereus is a major cause of food-borne infections due to its production of an emetic toxin and one or more enterotoxins. It is an opportunistic pathogen causing several types of infections in man (DROBNIEWSKI 1993), including serious eye infections that may result in blindness (HEMADY et al. 1990). When *B. cereus* strains receive plasmids encoding crystal toxin or capsule formation, they are transformed into Cry+ or Cap+ variants that would be identified as *B. thuringiensis* and *B. anthracis*, respectively.

The bacterium is frequently isolated as a contaminant in foods, including milk products, rice, meat, eggs, potatoes, vegetables, and fruit. The symptoms of *B. cereus* food poisoning include abdominal pain, vomiting and/or diarrhoea within 1–12h after intake. Cases of death in hospitalized individuals caused by food-related *B. cereus* infection have been reported (LUND et al. 2000). It is thus an important determinant of food-borne diseases, mainly caused by three properties:

its ability to form extremely heat- and chemical-resistant spores that can survive pasteurization and the psychrophilic (cold-tolerant) properties of many strains, especially those isolated from dairy products.

2 Virulence Factors

The three species may produce virulence factors that are unique or common to at least two of the species.

2.1 Species-Specific Virulence Factors

Virulence factors that are specific for one species include the *B. anthracis* toxins and the insecticidal toxins from *B. thuringiensis* (Table 1).

The insecticidal properties of *B. thuringiensis* are due to the production of various larvicidal toxins: the Cry, Cyt and Vip proteins (SCHNEPF et al. 1998). The Cry and Cyt toxins are synthesized during the sporulation (or the stationary phase) and accumulate in the mother cell to form the crystal inclusion, which is the major distinctive trait of *B. thuringiensis*. The Cry toxins constitute a large family of proteins comprising about 200 different members distributed in 32 classes sharing less than 45% sequence identity (for review see CRICKMORE et al. 1998 and see also http://www.biols.susx.ac.uk/Home/Neil_Crickmore/Bt/toxins.html for the most recent update of the *cry* gene nomenclature). The Cry toxins bind to specific receptors located in the insect midgut. The insertion of the toxins into the apical membrane of the epithelial cells results in the formation of pores causing cell lysis. The Cyt proteins have cytolytic properties, which may synergize the activity of the Cry proteins. The Vip toxins (for vegetative insecticidal proteins) are produced during the vegetative phase of growth and during early stages of stationary phase

Table 1. Species-specific virulence factors

Virulence factor	Bacterial species			
	B. anthracis	*B. thuringiensis*	*B. cereus*	
Capsule	+	–	–	Genes on pXO2 (UCHIDA et al. 1993)
Lethal toxin	+	–	–	Genes on pXO1 (LEPPLA 1991)
Oedema toxin	+	–	–	Genes on pXO1 (LEPPLA 1991)
Cry proteins	–	+	–[a]	Genes on plasmids (LERECLUS et al. 1993)
Cyt proteins	–	+	–	Genes on plasmids (LERECLUS et al. 1993)
Vip proteins	–	+	+	Localization not determined (ESTRUCH et al. 1996)

[a] By definition a *B. cereus* strain is acrystalliferous. Indeed, a *B. cereus* strain carrying a functional *cry* gene is considered as a *B. thuringiensis* strain.

(ESTRUCH et al. 1996). They do not accumulate in the cell, but are secreted into the culture medium. The ingestion of Vip proteins by susceptible insects results in gut paralysis, disruption of the gut epithelium and death (YU et al. 1997).

No virulence factor specific for *B. cereus* has yet been identified. Proteins that previously were associated with *B. cereus*, have more recently been found also in certain *B. thuringiensis* strains (for review, see SCHNEPF et al. 1998). These include phospholipases, hemolysins, collagenases and enterotoxins (see below).

Several *B. thuringiensis* strains produce a heat stable component, the β-exotoxin, which is an ATP analogue acting as an inhibitor of RNA polymerase. Due to its mode of action, this component has a broad activity spectrum against insects. A correlation between β-exotoxin production and the presence of a large plasmid was established (LEVINSON et al. 1990). However, the genes involved in β-exotoxin production are not determined, and their distribution within the strains of the *B. cereus* group is not known.

The capsule, polymer of γ-D-glutamic acid (ZWARTOUW and SMITH 1956), is currently considered to be one of two major virulence factors of *B. anthracis* (THORNE 1993 and references herein). The capsule contributes to pathogenicity by enabling the bacteria to evade the host immune defenses and provoke septicaemia. Indeed, the *B. anthracis* capsule inhibits phagocytosis (MAKINO et al. 1989; PREISZ 1909; ZWARTOUW and SMITH 1956) and is a monotonous linear polymer only very weakly immunogenic (GOODMAN and NITECKI 1967). The genes necessary for capsule synthesis *cap*B, *cap*C and *cap*A, are encoded by the plasmid pXO2 (GREEN et al. 1985).

Toxins that play a key role in the pathogenesis of anthrax are composed of three proteins, acting in binary combinations (STANLEY and SMITH 1961), which are now termed: protective antigen (PA) for its ability to elicit a protective immune response against anthrax (GLADSTONE 1946); lethal factor (LF); and oedema factor (EF). Intravenous injection of PA + LF (LeTx, lethal toxin) provokes death of the animal (BEALL et al. 1962), whereas intradermal injection of PA + EF (EdTx, edema toxin) produces edema in the skin (STANLEY and SMITH 1961). Separately, none of these proteins is toxic. They represent a unique variation of the A-B toxins (LEPPLA 1995). PA is the common cell-binding domain (B) able to interact with two different enzyme domains (A), EF and LF, that elicit cell damage.

In the past decade, an enormous amount of work has addressed the structural and functional analysis of these three secreted protein toxins and focused on the role of EdTx and LeTx in pathogenesis. The structural genes *pagA*, *lef*, *cya*, encoding PA, LF, and EF, respectively, are all located on pXO1. The three genes have been cloned (MOCK et al. 1988; ROBERTSON and LEPPLA 1986; VODKIN and LEPPLA 1983) and sequenced (BRAGG and ROBERTSON 1989; ESCUYER et al. 1988; WELKOS et al. 1988).

2.2 Other Virulence Factors

Several putative virulence factors have been described and appear to be common both in *B. cereus* and *B. thuringiensis*. These factors are, for the most part, probably not present, or at least not active even if the gene is present, in *B. anthracis*.

However, these questions will only be answered when the complete sequence of *B. anthracis* and closely related strains are fully sequenced.

2.2.1 *B. cereus* and *B. thuringiensis*

Both species may produce at least two diarrhoeogenic enterotoxins of protein nature, the necrotizing, enterotoxic haemolysin BL (HBL) (BEECHER and MAC-MILLAN 1991; HEINRICHS et al. 1993; RYAN et al. 1997) and a non-hemolytic enterotoxin (NHE) (GRANUM et al. 1999; LUND and GRANUM 1997). The two species also produce a range of other proteins that may be important pathogenic determinants in non-gastrointestinal and infections, including membrane-active and tissue-degrading enzymes such as phospholipases, proteases, collagenases and haemolysins (DROBNIEWSKI 1993). The production of the toxins and accessory proteins possibly promoting tissue invasion may, along with bacterial multiplication, contribute to the range of diseases observed. Recently, a cytotoxin (CytK) has been isolated from a *B. cereus* strain that caused severe food poisoning (LUND et al. 2000).

Several of the putative virulence factors are regulated by PlcR, a transcriptional regulator first shown to be active as a regulator of PI-PLC in *B. thuringiensis* (LERECLUS et al. 1996) and later shown to be present and active both in *B. cereus* and *B. thuringiensis* (AGAISSE et al. 1999), stimulating transcription of several putative exported virulence factors. The disruption of the *plcR* gene in *B. thuringiensis* or *B. cereus* greatly reduces the haemolytic activity of the strains, and results in a loss of pathogenicity, both against insect larvae and mice (SALAMITOU et al. 2000). This suggests that the opportunistic pathogenicity of *B. cereus* and *B. thuringiensis* is due, at least in part, to the *plcR* regulon. The loss of the haemolytic properties might result from the non-expression of two PlcR-regulated genes: *hblC* and *plcB*, encoding components of the HBL enterotoxin and of the cereolysin AB, respectively (AGAISSE et al. 1999; ØKSTAD et al. 1999). The products of these two genes have haemolytic properties (GILMORE et al. 1989; LINDBÄCK et al. 1999) and are involved in the virulence of *B. cereus* endophthalmitis (BEECHER et al. 2000). Interestingly, plcR is not present in *B. subtilis* or any other *Bacillus* species. PlcR recognizes a 17-bp sequence, located a varying distance upstream of the transcription start sites in the target genes. The PlcR-regulated genes are frequently grouped in pairs and transcribed divergently from a unique PlcR box (AGAISSE et al. 1999; ØKSTAD et al. 1999). However, analysis of their distribution indicates that they are not clustered in a pathogenicity island but scattered throughout the chromosome (AGAISSE et al. 1999).

2.2.2 *B. anthracis*

Although the *plc*R gene is present in *B. anthracis*, the gene is mutated, making *B. anthracis* unable to form a functional protein (AGAISSE et al. 1999). This is probably the reason *B. anthracis* strains do not produce any phospholipase C and haemolytic activity, even though the corresponding genes are present. The virulence genes controlled by the *plc*R regulon are not expressed in *B. anthracis* strains. *B. anthracis* contains genes for NHE (the non-haemolytic enterotoxin), but not for the HBL (the haemolytic enterotoxin), similar results have been reported in *B. cereus* strains closely related to *B. anthracis* (HELGASON et al. 2000).

3 Genome Structure

Complex genome structures are not uncommon in bacteria (KOLSTØ 1999). They may contain two circular chromosomes, or one linear and one circular. In addition, bacteria may harbour several plasmids of variable sizes, and these plasmids may be circular, linear, or both. The plasmids may contain housekeeping genes and, therefore, be impossible to cure, and such plasmids that carry housekeeping genes may thus be called "secondary chromosomes" (KOLSTØ 1997).

The degree of genome structure conservation appears to vary broadly in bacteria. Gene order may be highly conserved or highly rearranged in strains apparently of the same species (FONSTEIN and HASELKORN 1995).

3.1 *B. cereus* and *B. thuringiensis*

Comparison of physical maps of chromosomes of *B. cereus* and *B. thuringiensis* strains indicates that these bacteria have variable chromosomes, where gene order appears to be conserved in one part of the chromosome and variable in another part of the chromosome (CARLSON et al. 1994, 1996; CARLSON and KOLSTØ 1994; ØKSTAD et al. 1999). Sequences in the variable part of the chromosome may, in other strains, be part of large plasmids or a "secondary chromosome".

The sequencing projects of bacterial genomes have confirmed that, in general, genome organization in closely related species may be very conserved, like in *Mycoplasma genitalium* and *Mycoplasma pneumonia* (HIMMELREICH et al. 1997). The genomes of two strains of *Helicobacter pylori* were highly similar in their gene organization, yet they contained a hypervariable plasticity zone, which would influence apparent genomic and allelic diversity (ALM et al. 1999). *B. thuringiensis* and *B. cereus* strains usually have one or more plasmids, and their sizes may vary from a few kb to several hundred kb (CARLSON et al. 1994). Several strains contain linear plasmids as well, and phages are common within this group of bacteria. Plasmids may be transferred between strains, and transfer mechanisms have been studied, although the detailed mechanisms may not be completely understood (WILCKS et al. 1999). Plasmids may not only carry determinants of phenotypes used for species definition within the group (crystal toxin, capsule formation etc.), but may also specify additional elements important to virulence. A *B. cereus* strain is being sequenced by Complete Genomics, USA.

3.2 *B. anthracis*

The chromosome of the *B. anthracis* Ames strain is being sequenced by TIGR, while the two large plasmids pXO1 and pXO2 are fully sequenced (OKINAKA et al. 1999) (AF188935, Okinaka, personal communication). Probably within the next year comparative information about the genomes of several members of the *B. cereus* group will become available.

4 Pathogenicity Islands in the *B. cereus* Group

Pathogenicity islands (PAIs) are clusters of genes coding for proteins associated with pathogenicity, and such clusters may integrate at various sites within a genome (for review see HACKER and KAPER 2000). Commonly used integration sites are tRNA genes.

To our knowledge, there is no information yet about pathogenicity islands in *B. cereus* strains. There is a region flanking the *hbl* operon that appears to be conserved in several other *B. cereus* and *B. thuringiensis* strains containing the *hbl* locus, but lacking in *B. cereus* strains (and *B. anthracis*) that do not contain the *hbl* operon. More sequence is obviously needed to determine whether *hbl* or any of the other enterotoxin gene loci are part of pathogenicity islands. Such analysis is under way in the laboratory of one of the authors.

4.1 *B. thuringiensis*

The *cry* genes are often flanked by transposable elements, including insertion sequences (IS) and class II transposons (Tn). The first studies on the genetic environment of the lepidopteran-active *cry1 A* genes revealed that these toxin genes were flanked by two sets of inverted repeated sequences (Fig. 1) (KRONSTAD and WHITELEY 1984; LERECLUS et al. 1984). These DNA sequences were subsequently identified as IS, and designated IS*231* and IS*232* (MAHILLON et al. 1985; MENOU et al. 1990). They belong to the IS*4* and to the IS*21* families of insertion sequences, respectively (MAHILLON and CHANDLER 1998). A large number of IS*231* variants were found in various *B. thuringiensis* strains, as well as in *B. cereus*, *B. anthracis* and *B. mycoides* (HENDERSON et al. 1995; LEONARD et al. 1997). The IS*232* element is less prevalent than IS*231* in these bacterial species.

Analysis of the genetic environment of the *cry4* genes in *B. thuringiensis* *israelensis* showed that these genes were also flanked by inverted repeated sequences, which were subsequently characterized and designated IS*240* (Fig. 1) (BOURGOUIN et al. 1988; DELÉCLUSE et al. 1989). The IS *240* elements belong to the widely spread IS*6* family (MAHILLON and CHANDLER 1998). An exhaustive mapping of the IS elements harboured by the 137-kb plasmid of the *israelensis* strain has been published (ROSSO et al. 2000).

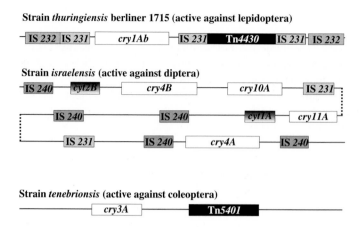

Fig. 1. Examples of genetic organization of *cry* genes in *B. thuringiensis* strains

Several other IS were found in *B. thuringiensis*; an element belonging to the IS*3* family was found between the *cry1C* and *cry1D* genes in *aizawai* strains (SMITH et al. 1994); a DNA sequence, presenting similarity with the transposase of IS*605*, is located downstream from the *vip3A* gene (accession number L48811). However, this sequence appears truncated in comparison to the transposase gene of the IS*605* element.

The first transposable element identified in *B. thuringiensis* was isolated in vivo during the course of a conjugation experiment (LERECLUS et al. 1983). This element fulfilled the characteristics of a transposon belonging to the Tn*3* family and was designated Tn*4430* (LERECLUS et al. 1986; MAHILLON and LERECLUS 1988). Tn*4430* tranposes by a replicative mechanism involving the formation of a cointegrate between the donor and the recipient molecules. This transposable element is frequently found in the vicinity of *cry1A* genes (Fig. 1) and is also found in *B. cereus* strains (CARLSON et al. 1994). A transposable element related to Tn*4430* was isolated from a coleopteran-active *B. thuringiensis tenebrionis* strain (BAUM 1994). This transposon (Tn*5401*) is located downstream from the *cry3A* toxin gene (Fig. 1).

The close association between the insecticidal toxin genes of *B. thuringiensis* and transposable elements suggests that most of the *cry* genes constitute complex genetic structures similar to composed transposons. The function of these transposable elements is not clearly demonstrated. However, it is reasonable to hypothesize that they are involved in the vertical and horizontal dissemination of the toxin genes within a given strain and within the *B. thuringiensis–B. cereus* species. Conjugation experiments between various bacteria belonging to the *B. cereus* group showed that Tn*4430* is able to mediate the transfer of non-conjugative plasmids by a conduction process (GREEN et al. 1989). Similar phenomena might also be mediated by the IS*240* elements. Indeed, it was shown that the members of the IS*6* family transpose via a replicative mechanism leading to the formation of cointegrates (MAHILLON and CHANDLER 1998).

4.2 *B. anthracis*

pXO1 carries the structural toxin genes, *pagA*, *lef*, and *cya*, regulatory elements, a resolvase, and a transposase, and *gerX*, a three-gene germination operon (GUIDI-RONTANI et al. 1999). All these genes map within a 44.8-kbp region flanked by inverted IS*1627* elements; this region has been termed a "pathogenicity island" (Fig. 2). It appears to be able to transpose, since its inversion has been reported once in a laboratory strain (THORNE 1993). The plasmid also carries DNA topo-isomerase (FOUET et al. 1994) and 15 ORFs, possibly involved in horizontal transfer. Long before the discovery of plasmids, attempts to attenuate the virulence of anthrax strains for vaccine purposes led to plasmid curing. The various atten-uated strains obtained by Louis Pasteur had lost either one or both plasmids. Strains can be cured of plasmids by various laboratory conditions, such as growth at 43°C or in the presence of antibiotics. Curing of pXO1 is rare, and its sponta-neous loss in environmental samples has not been reported. Various phenotypes, in addition to toxin production (MIKESELL et al. 1983), have been linked to the presence of pXO1 (THORNE 1993). Cured cells sporulate earlier and at higher fre-quencies; they grow more poorly on certain minimal media and are more sensitive to some bacteriophages. pXO1$^-$ strains are also less capsulated. Unlike pXO1, pXO2 is easily and spontaneously lost. pXO1$^+$, pXO2$^-$ strains have been found in environmental samples and among virulent strains (TURNBULL et al. 1992). The only phenotype thus far associated with pXO2 is capsulation, which is easy to detect by observing colony morphology. However, among pXO2$^+$ strains uncap-sulated mutants can be found at rather high frequency (GREEN et al. 1985). Thus, pXO2 may be more susceptible to rearrangements than pXO1. Interestingly, pXO2 can be associated with the differences in virulence between wild-type strains (WELKOS 1991; WELKOS et al. 1993).

5 The Evolution of the *B. cereus* Group

The species status of the members of the *B. cereus* group is questionable. It has been suggested that the members of the group should be considered as belonging to the same species, *B. anthracis* and *B. thuringiensis* being classified as variants of *B. cereus* (GORDON et al. 1973). Determination of mol% (G+C) and DNA reas-sociation experiments are consistent with this conclusion (PRIEST 1981), and rRNA sequences of strains of the four variants are clearly within the range of variation

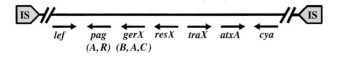

Fig. 2. Genetic organization of the 45-kb pathogenicity island in *B. anthracis* plasmid pXO1

seen in single species (ASH et al. 1991). Neither multi-locus enzyme electrophoresis nor comparison of physical maps could distinguish between the two species (CARLSON et al. 1994), and 75% of examined *B. thuringiensis* strains have been found positive for *B. cereus* enterotoxin. From the comparisons of physical chromosome maps, *B. cereus* and *B. thuringiensis* strains apparently exhibit a high genome flexibility (CARLSON et al. 1996). A 142-bp repeated element, *bcr1*, has been identified in multiple copies in the *B. cereus*, *B. anthracis* and *B. thuringiensis* genomes (ØKSTAD et al. 1999). *bcr1* is, however, not present in *B. subtilis* and may be specific to the *B. cereus* group. Most, perhaps all, of the strains from the *B. cereus* group contain one large chromosome and a collection of extrachromosomal elements. None of the larger plasmids has been completely sequenced yet. Analysis of the replication region of a large conjugative plasmid of *B. thuringiensis* subsp. *kurstaki* HD73 shows that the plasmid belongs to the pAMbeta1 family of theta-replicating plasmids (WILCKS et al. 1999), with the pXO2 from *B. anthracis* as the closest relative, when the ParA plasmid genes were compared (GERDES et al. 2000).

Analysis of the genetic relationship using multi-locus enzyme electrophoresis (MEE) shows great variation between strains isolated from soil samples from various parts of Norway (HELGASON et al. 1998). Similar results were obtained when amplified fragment length polymorphism (AFLP) was used (Jackson et al. submitted). Analysis of *B. cereus*, *B. thuringiensis* and *B. anthracis* by multi-locus enzyme electrophoresis or by sequencing fragments of housekeeping genes clearly showed that some strains of *B. cereus*, as well as strains of *B. thuringiensis*, were more closely related to *B. anthracis* than they were to strains within their own species (HELGASON et al. 2000). Sequencing of both the 16S rRNA gene and the spacer region between 16S rRNA and 23S rRNA genes show a similar relationship.

Although there is no information yet about the development of the members of the *B. cereus* group members, it seems likely from the lack of variation within the *B. anthracis* species that this species has evolved rather recently. Perhaps when we

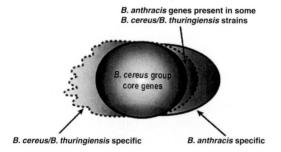

B. anthracis genes present in some
B. cereus/B. thuringiensis strains

B. cereus group
core genes

B. cereus/B. thuringiensis specific   **B. anthracis specific**

Fig. 3. *B. cereus* core genes are present in all *B. cereus*, *B. thuringiensis* and *B. anthracis* strains. *B. cereus/ B. thuringiensis* strains may have additional genes on their chromosomes as well as on the large plasmids, which will contribute to the variability within these species. Such *B. cereus/B. thuringiensis* specific genes are not present in all strains. *B. anthracis* specific genes are present on the plasmids pXO1 and pXO2, and perhaps also on the chromosome, although chromosomally located unique *B. anthracis* genes have not yet been identified. *B. anthracis* genes present in some strains of *B. cereus/B. thuringiensis* are most likely present within the chromosomes of strains that are most closely related to *B. anthracis*

have more sequence information of several chromosomes and large number of plasmids, we may understand some of the underlying mechanisms for the evolution of the group. Much work is needed before we can increase our knowledge beyond what is illustrated in Fig. 3: There is a set of genes common to all members of the *B. cereus* strains. Then there are genes that are strictly specific to *B. anthracis*; also there are genes that are shared by some strains of *B. cereus*, *B. thuringiensis* and *B. anthracis*, and finally there are genes that are present in a varying number of *B. cereus* and *B. thuringiensis* strains, with an unknown number of these genes present on extrachromosomal elements.

References

Agaisse H, Gominet M, Okstad OA, Kolsto AB, Lereclus D (1999) PlcR is a pleiotropic regulator of extracellular virulence factor gene expression in *Bacillus thuringiensis*. Mol Microbiol 32:1043–1053

Alm RA, Ling LS, Moir DT, King BL, Brown ED, Doig PC, Smith DR, Noonan B, Guild BC, deJonge BL, Carmel G, Tummino PJ, Caruso A, Uria-Nickelsen M, Mills DM, Ives C, Gibson R, Merberg D, Mills SD, Jiang Q, Taylor DE, Vovis GF, Trust TJ (1999) Genomic-sequence comparison of two unrelated isolates of the human gastric pathogen *Helicobacter pylori*. Nature 397:176–180

Ash C, Farrow JA, Dorsch M, Stackebrandt E, Collins MD (1991) Comparative analysis of *Bacillus anthracis*, *Bacillus cereus*, and related species on the basis of reverse transcriptase sequencing of 16S rRNA. Int J Syst Bacteriol 41:343–346

Baum JA (1994) Tn5401, a new class II transposable element from *Bacillus thuringiensis*. J Bacteriol 176:2835–2845

Beall FA, Taylor MJ, Thorne CB (1962) Rapid lethal effects in rats of a third component found upon fractionating the toxin of *Bacillus anthracis*. J Bacteriol 83:1274–1280

Beecher DJ, Macmillan JD (1991) Characterization of the components of hemolysin BL from *Bacillus cereus*. Infect Immun 59:1778–1784

Beecher DJ, Olsen TW, Somers EB, Wong AC (2000) Evidence for contribution of tripartite hemolysin BL, phosphatidylcholine-preferring phospholipase C, and collagenase to virulence of *Bacillus cereus* endophthalmitis. Infect Immun 68:5269–5276

Bourgouin C, Delecluse A, Ribier J, Klier A, Rapoport G (1988) A *Bacillus thuringiensis* subsp. *israelensis* gene encoding a 125-kilodalton larvicidal polypeptide is associated with inverted repeat sequences. J Bacteriol 170:3575–3583

Bragg TS, Robertson DL (1989) Nucleotide sequence and analysis of the lethal factor gene (*lef*) from *Bacillus anthracis*. Gene 81:45–54

Carlson CR, Kolstø AB (1994) A small (2.4 Mb) *Bacillus cereus* chromosome corresponds to a conserved region of a larger (5.3 Mb) *Bacillus cereus* chromosome. Mol Microbiol 13:161–169

Carlson CR, Caugant D, Kolstø A-B (1994) Genotypic diversity among *Bacillus cereus* and *Bacillus thuringiensis* strains. Appl Eviron Microbiol 60:1719–1725

Carlson CR, Johansen T, Kolstø AB (1996) The chromosome map of *Bacillus thuringiensis* subsp. *canadensis* HD224 is highly similar to that of the *Bacillus cereus* type strain ATCC 14579. FEMS Microbiol Lett 141:163–167

Charles J-F, Delécluse A, Nielsen-LeRoux C (2000) Entomopathogenic Bacteria: from Laboratory to Field Application. Kluwer Academic Publishers, Dordrecht, The Netherlands.

Crickmore N, Zeigler DR, Feitelson J, Schnepf E, Van Rie J, Lereclus D, Baum J, Dean DH (1998) Revision of the nomenclature for the *Bacillus thuringiensis* pesticidal crystal proteins. Microbiol Mol Biol Rev 62:807–813

Delécluse A, Bourgouin C, Klier A, Rapoport G (1989) Nucleotide sequence and characterization of a new insertion element, IS240, from *Bacillus thuringiensis israelensis*. Plasmid 21:71–78

Drobniewski FA (1993) *Bacillus cereus* and related species. Clin Microbiol Rev 6:324–338

Escuyer V, Duflot E, Sezer O, Danchin A, Mock M (1988) Structural homology between virulence-associated bacterial adenylate cyclases. Gene 71:293–298

Estruch JJ, Warren GW, Mullins MA, Nye GJ, Craig JA, Koziel MG (1996) Vip3 A, a novel *Bacillus thuringiensis* vegetative insecticidal protein with a wide spectrum of activities against lepidopteran insects. Proc Natl Acad Sci USA 93:5389–5394

Fonstein M, Haselkorn R (1995) Physical mapping of bacterial genomes. J Bacteriol 177:3361–3369

Fouet A, Sirard JC, Mock M (1994) *Bacillus anthracis* pXO1 virulence plasmid encodes a type 1 DNA topoisomerase. Mol Microbiol 11:471–479

Gerdes K, Moller-Jensen J, Bugge Jensen R (2000) Plasmid and chromosome partitioning: surprises from phylogeny. Mol Microbiol 37:455–466

Gilmore MS, Cruz-Rodz AL, Leimeister-Wachter M, Kreft J, Goebel W (1989) A *Bacillus cereus* cytolytic determinant, cereolysin AB, which comprises the phospholipase C and sphingomyelinase genes: nucleotide sequence and genetic linkage. J Bacteriol 171:744–753

Gladstone GP (1946) Immunity of anthrax: protective antigen present in cell-free culture filtrates. Br J Exp Pathol 27:393–410

Gonzalez JM, Dulmage HT, Carlton BC (1981) Correlation between specific plasmids and δ-endotoxin production in *Bacillus thuringiensis*. Plasmid 5:352–365

Gonzales JMJ, Brown BS, Carlton BC (1982) Transfer of *Bacillus thuringiensis* plasmids coding for δ-endotoxin among strains of *Bacillus thuringiensis* and *Bacillus cereus*. Proc Natl Acad Sci USA 79:6951–6955

Goodman JW, Nitecki DE (1967) Studies on the relation of a prior immune response to immunogenicity. Immunology 13:577–583

Gordon RE, Haynes WC, Pang CH-N. (1973) The genus *Bacillus*. United States Department of Agriculture, Washington DC

Granum PE, O'Sullivan K, Lund T (1999) The sequence of the non-haemolytic enterotoxin operon from *Bacillus cereus*. FEMS Microbiol Lett 177:225–229

Green BD, Battisti L, Koehler TM, Thorne CB, Ivins BE (1985) Demonstration of a capsule plasmid in *Bacillus anthracis*. Infect Immun 49:291–297

Green BD, Battisti L, Thorne CB (1989) Involvement of Tn*4430* in transfer of *Bacillus anthracis* plasmids mediated by *Bacillus thuringiensis* plasmid pXO12. J Bacteriol 171:104–113

Guidi-Rontani C, Pereira Y, Ruffie S, Sirard JC, Weber-Levy M, Mock M (1999) Identification and characterization of a germination operon on the virulence plasmid pXO1 of *Bacillus anthracis*. Mol Microbiol 33:407–414

Hacker J, Kaper JB (2000) Pathogenicity islands and the evolution of microbes. Annu Rev Microbiol 54:641–679

Heinrichs JH, Beecher DJ, MacMillan JD, Zilinskas BA (1993) Molecular cloning and characterization of the *hblA* gene encoding the B component of hemolysin BL from *Bacillus cereus*. J Bacteriol 175:6760–6766

Helgason E, Caugant DA, Lecadet MM, Chen Y, Mahillon J, Lövgren A, Hegna I, Kvaløy K, Kolstø AB (1998) Genetic diversity of *Bacillus cereus/B. thuringiensis* isolates from natural sources. Curr Microbiol 37:80–87

Helgason E, Okstad OA, Caugant DA, Johansen HA, Fouet A, Mock M, Hegna I, Kolsto (2000) *Bacillus anthracis*, *Bacillus cereus*, and *Bacillus thuringiensis* – one species on the basis of genetic evidence. Appl Environ Microbiol 66:2627–2630

Hemady R, Zaltas M, Paton B, Foster CS, Baker AS (1990) *Bacillus*-induced endophthalmitis: new series of 10 cases and review of the literature. Br J Ophthalmol 74:26–29

Henderson I, Yu D, Turnbull PC (1995) Differentiation of *Bacillus anthracis* and other '*Bacillus cereus* group' bacteria using IS*231*-derived sequences. FEMS Microbiol Lett 128:113–118

Himmelreich R, Plagens H, Hilbert H, Reiner B, Herrmann R (1997) Comparative analysis of the genomes of the bacteria *Mycoplasma pneumoniae* and *Mycoplasma genitalium*. Nucleic Acids Res 25:701–712

Inglesby TV, Henderson DA, Bartlett JG, Ascher MS, Eitzen E, Friedlander AM, Hauer J, McDade J, Osterholm MT, O'Toole T, Parker G, Perl TM, Russell PK, Tonat K (1999) Anthrax as a biological weapon: medical and public health management. Working Group on Civilian Biodefense. JAMA 281:1735–1745

Kolstø AB (1997) Dynamic bacterial genome organization. Mol Microbiol 24:241–248

Kolstø AB (1999) Time for a fresh look at the bacterial chromosome. Trends Microbiol 7:223–226

Kronstad JW, Whiteley HR (1984) Inverted repeat sequences flank a *Bacillus thuringiensis* crystal protein gene. J Bacteriol 160:95–102

Kunst F, Ogasawara N, Moszer I, Albertini AM, Alloni G, Azevedo V, Bertero MG, Bessieres P, Bolotin A, Borchert S, Borriss R, Boursier L, Brans A, Braun M, Brignell SC, Bron S, Brouillet S, Bruschi

CV, Caldwell B, Capuano V, Carter NM, Choi SK, Codani JJ, Connerton IF, Danchin A, et al. (1997) The complete genome sequence of the gram-positive bacterium *Bacillus subtilis*. Nature 390:249–256

Leonard C, Chen Y, Mahillon J (1997) Diversity and differential distribution of IS*231*, IS*232* and IS*240* among *Bacillus cereus*, *Bacillus thuringiensis* and *Bacillus mycoides*. Microbiology 143:2537–2547

Leppla SH (1991) Purification and characterization of adenylyl cyclase from *Bacillus anthracis*. Methods Enzymol 195:153–168

Leppla S (1995) Anthrax toxins. In: Moss J, Iglewski B, Vaughan M, Tu AT (eds) Bacterial Toxins and Virulence Factors in Disease. Handbook of Natural Toxins. New York, Basel, Hong Kong, pp 543–572

Lereclus D, Menou G, Lecadet MM (1983) Isolation of a DNA sequence related to several plasmids from *Bacillus thuringiensis* after a mating involving the *Streptococcus faecalis* plasmid pAMβ1. Mol Gen Genet 191:307–313

Lereclus D, Ribier J, Klier A, Menou G, Lecadet MM (1984) A transposon-like structure related to the δ-endotoxin gene of *Bacillus thuringiensis*. EMBO J 3:2561–2567

Lereclus D, Mahillon J, Menou G, Lecadet MM (1986) Identification of Tn*4430*, a transposon of *Bacillus thuringiensis* functional in *Escherichia coli*. Mol Gen Genet 204:52–57

Lereclus D, Delécluse A, Lecadet M-M (1993) Diversity of *Bacillus thuringiensis* toxins and genes. In: Entwistle P, Cory JS, Bailey MJ, Higgs S (eds) *Bacillus thuringiensis* an Environmental Biopesticide: Theory and Practice. John Wiley & Sons, Ltd, Chichester, UK, pp 37–69

Lereclus D, Agaisse H, Gominet M, Salamitou S, Sanchis V (1996) Identification of a *Bacillus thuringiensis* gene that positively regulates transcription of the phosphatidylinositol-specific phospholipase C gene at the onset of the stationary phase. J Bacteriol 178:2749–2756

Levinson BL, Kasyan KJ, Chiu SS, Currier TC, Gonzalez JM (1990) Identification of beta-exotoxin production, plasmids encoding beta-exotoxin, and a new exotoxin in *Bacillus thuringiensis* by using high-performance liquid chromatography. J Bacteriol 172:3172–3179

Lindbäck T, Økstad OA, Rishovd AL, Kolstø AB (1999) Insertional inactivation of *hblC* encoding the L2 component of Bacillus cereus ATCC 14579 haemolysin BL strongly reduces enterotoxigenic activity, but not the haemolytic activity against human erythrocytes. Microbiology 145:3139–3146

Lund T, Granum PE (1997) Comparison of biological effect of the two different enterotoxin complexes isolated from three different strains of *Bacillus cereus*. Microbiology 143:3329–3336

Lund T, De Buyser ML, Granum PE (2000) A new cytotoxin from *Bacillus cereus* that may cause necrotic enteritis. Mol Microbiol 38:254–261

Mahillon J, Chandler M (1998) Insertion sequences. Microbiol Mol Biol Rev 62:725–774

Mahillon J, Lereclus D (1988) Structural and functional analysis of Tn*4430*: identification of an integrase-like protein involved in the co-integrate-resolution process. EMBO J 7:1515–1526

Mahillon J, Seurinck J, van Rompuy L, Delcour J, Zabeau M (1985) Nucleotide sequence and structural organization of an insertion sequence element (IS*231*) from *Bacillus thuringiensis* strain berliner 1715. EMBO J 4:3895–3899

Makino S, Uchida I, Terakado N, Sasakawa C, Yoshikawa M (1989) Molecular characterization and protein analysis of the *cap* region, which is essential for encapsulation in *Bacillus anthracis*. J Bacteriol 171:722–730

Menou G, Mahillon J, Lecadet MM, Lereclus D (1990) Structural and genetic organization of IS*232*, a new insertion sequence of *Bacillus thuringiensis*. J Bacteriol 172:6689–6696

Mikesell P, Ivins BE, Ristroph JD, Dreier TM (1983) Evidence for plasmid-mediated toxin production in *Bacillus anthracis*. Infect Immun 39:371–376

Mock M, Labruyere E, Glaser P, Danchin A, Ullmann A (1988) Cloning and expression of the calmodulin-sensitive *Bacillus anthracis* adenylate cyclase in *Escherichia coli*. Gene 64:277–284

Okinaka RT, Cloud K, Hampton O, Hoffmaster AR, Hill KK, Keim P, Koehler TM, Lamke G, Kumano S, Mahillon J, Manter D, Martinez Y, Ricke D, Svensson R, Jackson PJ (1999) Sequence and organization of pXO1, the large *Bacillus anthracis* plasmid harboring the anthrax toxin genes. J Bacteriol 181:6509–6515

Økstad OA, Gominet M, Purnelle B, Rose M, Lereclus D, Kolstø AB (1999) Sequence analysis of three *Bacillus cereus* loci carrying PIcR-regulated genes encoding degradative enzymes and enterotoxin. Microbiology 145:3129–3138

Preisz H (1909) Experimentelle Studien über Virulenz, Empfänglichkeit und Immunität beim Milzbrand. Zeitschr. Immunität.-Forsch 5:341–452

Priest FG (1981) DNA homology in the genus Bacillus. In: Berkeley RCW, Goodfellow M (eds) The Aerobic Endospore-forming Bacteria: Classification and Identification. Academic Press, New York, pp 33–57

Robertson DL, Leppla SH (1986) Molecular cloning and expression in *Escherichia coli* of the lethal factor gene of *Bacillus anthracis*. Gene 44:71–78

Rosso M-L, Mahillon J, Deléclus A (2000) Genetic and genomic context of toxin genes. In: Charles J-F, Delécluse A, Nielsen-LeRoux C (eds) Entomopathogenic Bacteria: from Laboratory to Field Application. Kluwer Academic Publishers, Dordrecht, The Netherlands

Ryan PA, Macmillan JD, Zilinskas BA (1997) Molecular cloning and characterization of the genes encoding the L1 and L2 components of hemolysin BL from *Bacillus cereus*. J Bacteriol 179:2551–2556

Salamitou S, Ramisse F, Brehelin M, Bourguet D, Gilois N, Gominet M, Hernandez E, Lereclus D (2000) The *plcR* regulon is involved in the opportunistic properties of *Bacillus thuringiensis* and *Bacillus cereus* in mice and insects. Microbiology 146:2825–2832

Schnepf E, Crickmore N, Van Rie J, Lereclus D, Baum J, Feitelson J, Zeigler DR, Dean DH (1998) *Bacillus thuringiensis* and its pesticidal crystal proteins. Microbiol Mol Biol Rev 62:775–806

Smith GP, Ellar DJ, Keeler SJ, Seip CE (1994) Nucleotide sequence and analysis of an insertion sequence from *Bacillus thuringiensis* related to IS*150*. Plasmid 32:10–18

Stanley JL, Smith H (1961) Purification of factor I and recognition of a third factor of the anthrax toxin. J Gen Microbiol 26:49–66

Thorne CB (1993) *Bacillus anthracis*. In: Sonenshein AL, Hoch JA, Losick R (eds) *Bacillus subtilis* and Other Gram-positive Bacteria. American Society of Microbiologists, Washington, DC, pp 113–124

Turnbull PC, Hutson RA, Ward MJ, Jones MN, Quinn CP, Finnie NJ, Duggleby CJ, Kramer JM, Melling J (1992) *Bacillus anthracis* but not always anthrax. J Appl Bacteriol 72:21–28

Uchida I, Hornung JM, Thorne CB, Klimpel KR, Leppla SH (1993) Cloning and characterization of a gene whose product is a trans-activator of anthrax toxin synthesis. J Bacteriol 175:5329–5338

Vodkin MH, Leppla SH (1983) Cloning of the protective antigen gene of *Bacillus anthracis*. Cell 34:693–697

Welkos SL (1991) Plasmid-associated virulence factors of non-toxigenic (pX01-) *Bacillus anthracis*. Microb Pathog 10:183–198

Welkos SL, Lowe JR, Eden-McCutchan F, Vodkin M, Leppla SH, Schmidt JJ (1988) Sequence and analysis of the DNA encoding protective antigen of *Bacillus anthracis*. Gene 69:287–300

Welkos SL, Vietri NJ, Gibbs PH (1993) Non-toxigenic derivatives of the Ames strain of *Bacillus anthracis* are fully virulent for mice: role of plasmid pX02 and chromosome in strain-dependent virulence. Microb Pathog 14:381–388

Wilcks A, Smidt L, Økstad OA, Kolstø A-B, Mahillon J, Andrup L (1999) Replication mechanism and sequence analysis of the replicon of pAW63, a conjugative plasmid from *Bacillus thuringiensis*. J Bacteriol 181:3193–3200

Yu CG, Mullins MA, Warren GW, Koziel MG, Estruch JJ (1997) The *Bacillus thuringiensis* vegetative insecticidal protein Vip3 A lyses midgut epithelium cells of susceptible insects. Appl Environ Microbiol 63:532–536

Zwartouw HT, Smith H (1956) Polyglutamic acid from *Bacillus anthracis* grown in vivo: structure and aggressin activity. Biochem J 63:437–454

Pathogenicity Islands and Other Virulence Elements in *Listeria*

J. Kreft[1], J.-A. Vázquez-Boland[2], S. Altrock[1], G. Dominguez-Bernal[2], and W. Goebel[1]

1 Introduction

Listeria spp. are short, gram-positive rods, asporogenic, aerobic and facultatively anaerobic. They multiply between pH 6 and pH 9 and over a remarkably broad temperature range (1–45°C). Their cryotolerance is related to their ability to grow at high osmolarities. The genus comprises six species (Rocourt 1999); the hemolytic *L. monocytogenes* and *L. ivanovii* are pathogenic for humans and/or animals, a third hemolytic species, *L. seeligeri*, normally is nonvirulent, the three nonhemolytic species *L. innocua*, *L. welshimeri* and *L. grayi* are harmless saprophytes. Their natural habitat is decaying plant material in soil, where they are ubiquitous, although normally in low numbers. The plant material is the source of contamination of animal feed and human food. Consequently, *Listeriae* are also found in the intestine of asymptomatic animals and humans. From soil and faeces they gain access to sewage and water, where they survive for extended periods of time but may also contaminate improperly sanitized processing facilities for milk and meat

[1] Theodor-Boveri-Institut (Biozentrum) der Universität Würzburg, Lehrstuhl für Mikrobiologie, Am Hubland, 97074 Würzburg, Germany
[2] Universidad Complutense, Facultad de Veterinaria, Grupo de Patogénesis Molecular Bacteriana, Avda. Puerto de Hierro s/n, 28040 Madrid, Spain

products. Due to their cryotolerance, *Listeriae* are able to multiply even in refrigerated food (for reviews on these aspects see SEELIGER 1961; JONES 1990; SCHUCHAT et al. 1991; FARBER and PETERKIN 1991; FENLON 1999). The disease caused by the pathogenic species, listeriosis, is rare (in humans 1/100,000 per year, significantly higher in immunocompromised individuals) but with a high mortality rate. Its clinical manifestations range from cutaneous lesions, influenza-like illness, febrile gastroenteritis, septicaemia, abortion, abscesses to a severe syndrome of newborns (granulomatosis infantiseptica) and meningoencephalitis (SEELIGER 1961; JONES 1990; LORBER 1997). Except for the cutaneous and transplacentally transmitted forms, the route of infection is via uptake of contaminated food (FARBER and PETERKIN 1991). To reach deeper organs, *Listeria* has to breach the intestinal barrier and eventually the blood–brain or placental barrier, respectively. Clearance of and resistance to listeriosis is predominantly, but not exclusively, cell mediated (MACKANESS 1962; EDELSON and UNANUE 2000). These traits are directly related to the fact that pathogenic *Listeriae*, similar to *Shigella*, *Salmonella*, *Legionella*, etc., are facultative intracellular bacteria, i.e. they can invade eukaryotic host cells and multiply therein. Because of this, they also exploit normal functions and mechanisms of these cells (COSSART et al. 1996; FINLAY and COSSART 1997; MITCHELL 2000). In the case of pathogenic *Listeriae*, the intracellular life cycle involves the following steps:

1. Adherence to the target cell
2. Uptake of the bacterium, either by normal phagocytosis (if the host cell is phagocytic) or by bacterium-triggered phagocytosis, in case the target cell is not a professional phagocyte, e.g. a hepatocyte, an epithelial or endothelial cell
3. Escape from the primary phagosome
4. Cytosolic replication
5. Recruitment of host cell actin to the bacterial surface, formation of an actin tail at one bacterial pole and intracellular bacterial movement
6. Formation of bacteria-containing pseudopods of the host cell
7. Phagocytosis of these protrusions by neighbouring cells
8. Escape from the double-membrane phagosome, followed by another round of cytosolic multiplication and cell-to-cell spread (reviewed in TILNEY and PORTNOY 1989; COSSART and LECUIT 1998; COSSART and PORTNOY 2000)

Depending on the nature of the host cell and on the particular *Listeria* strain or species, the infected host cell may survive for extended periods of time or become necrotic or apoptotic, respectively, thus releasing the bacteria. The clinical and molecular biological aspects of *Listeria* virulence are extensively outlined in a recent review (VAZQUEZ-BOLAND et al. 2001a); therefore, they will be only briefly described and referenced in the paragraphs below. Most of the listerial genes identified up to now as being involved in the infectious cycle are clustered on the bacterial chromosome, either in large, multi-component units or in groups of two to four genes. The first one of these characterized was the PrfA-dependent virulence gene cluster (PORTNOY et al. 1992; SHEEHAN et al. 1994), now referred to as LIPI-1 (VAZQUEZ-BOLAND et al. 2001b). Later on, more such clustered determinants were found in *Listeriae*; they all fulfil at least one essential criterium of so-called "pathogenicity islands (PAIs)", namely their presence in pathogenic species only, whereas close, but avirulent, relatives are devoid of them. The concept of PAIs, originally developed for *Escherichia coli* and then extended to other bacteria, by Hacker and colleagues (e.g. BLUM et al. 1994; HACKER et al. 1997; MCDANIEL and KAPER 1997; HACKER and KAPER 2000), also applies to *Listeria* (KREFT et al. 1999) and has given momentum to investigations into the evolution of virulence in this bacterial genus (CHAKRABORTY et al. 2000; VAZQUEZ-BOLAND et al. 2001b; NG et al. 2001).

2 LIPI-1 (PrfA-Dependent Virulence Gene Cluster)

This gene cluster is present with an identical structure in the two pathogenic *Listeria* species, *L. monocytogenes* and *L. ivanovii* (PORTNOY et al. 1992; HAAS et al. 1992; GOUIN et al. 1994; LAMPIDIS et al. 1994; SHEEHAN et al. 1994; NG et al. 2001). It comprises six genes (Fig. 1), the products of which are required for crucial steps in the intracellular life cycle of these bacteria. Located between the housekeeping genes *prs* (for phosphoribosyl synthetase) and *ldh* (for lactate dehydrogenase) and in the central part of the cluster is the gene for a cholesterol-binding, pore-forming cytolysin (ALOUF 1999), *hly* (gene product listeriolysin O [LLO]) in *L. monocytogenes*. This cytolysin is essential for the rapid escape of the bacteria (within

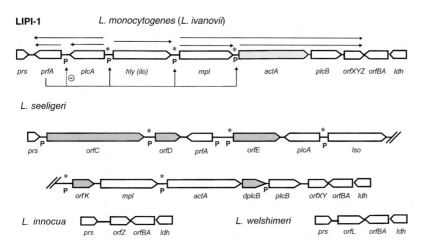

Fig. 1. Structure of LIPI-1 and the corresponding genomic regions of *L. innocua* and *L. welshimeri*. For gene names, functions of the gene products and regulation, see text. An *asterisk* denotes a "PrfA-box"; *P*: promoter. *Arrows* above the gene boxes indicate the different transcripts. Additional orfs present in *L. seeligeri* are *shaded*. Combined and modified from PORTNOY et al. (1992), BREHM et al. (1996), KREFT et al. (1999) and unpublished results from the authors laboratories; the structures for *L. innocua/ L. welshimeri* are according to CHAKRABORTY et al. (2000)

> 30min) from the primary phagosome after uptake into the target cell. Mutants defective in this gene are avirulent and are rapidly destroyed in phagocytes. The products of the *plc*A and *plc*B genes, a phosphatidylinositol-specific phospholipase C (PI-PLC) and a broad-range phospholipase C (lecithinase), respectively, have accessory roles in this process. PlcB is essential for the release of the bacteria from the double-membrane phagosome formed after pseudopode ingestion by neighbouring cells. The two phospholipases have partially redundant functions in the bacterial escape from the primary phagosome, but it has been shown that PlcA (and LLO) has an additional function in modulating the host cell response to infection (GOLDFINE et al. 2000). The product of the *mpl* gene is a metalloprotease, which in vitro is required for the maturation of the prepro-form of PlcB. Its in vivo role is unclear. The product of the *act*A gene induces the recruitment of host cell actin and the formation of the propulsive actin tail; it is necessary for intracellular motility and cell-to-cell spread and, hence, for virulence. Interestingly, the ActA proteins of *L. monocytogenes* and *L. ivanovii*, although functionally equivalent, exhibit only a limited similarity in their amino acid sequence (KREFT et al. 1995). Furthermore, a considerable variability of Acta within the species *L. monocytogenes* has been demonstrated (e.g. SOKOLOVIC et al. 1996).

Like PlcA and LLO, ActA is a multifunctional protein, also involved in invasion and host cell response. The product of the *prf*A (positive regulatory factor A) gene is a transcriptional activator of all the genes in LIPI-1. Its synthesis and activity is influenced by a number of environmental parameters (e.g. temperature) and is upregulated after uptake of *Listeria* into mammalian host cells. The target sequence of PrfA is a 14-bp palindrome (PrfA-box) in the promoter region of the transcription units of the cluster. The transcription of *prf*A itself is subject to a complex regulatory circuit. On the one hand, PrfA enhances the synthesis of the bicistronic *plc*A/*prf*A mRNA. On the other hand, it represses the synthesis of its own monocistronic mRNA (Fig. 1), thus creating an autoregulatory loop. In addition, the activity of PrfA is modulated by a not yet precisely characterised listerial factor (BÖCKMANN et al. 2000) and possibly also by components of the host cell (RENZONI et al. 1999). It has to be noted that there are additional genes dispersed on the chromosome that are also positively or negatively regulated by PrfA (see Sect. 4). Taken together, the complex and not yet completely understood PrfA system seems to ensure a temporally and spatially regulated expression of genes involved in the intracellular life of *Listeria* (for reviews on this issue, see BREHM et al. 1996; GOEBEL et al., 2000; VAZQUEZ-BOLAND et al. 2001a). Downstream of *plc*B, several open reading frames of unknown function (orfs XYZ and BA) are present. In *L. seeligeri*, which is non-virulent at least for man and mammals, a considerably modified cluster is found (KREFT et al. 1999; NG et al. 2001; R. Lampidis et al., in preparation). As shown in Fig. 1, there are not only two additional open reading frames between *prs* and *prf*A but, most importantly, there is one open reading frame inserted, and with a divergent transcriptional direction, between *plc*A and *prf*A, thus interrupting the autoregulatory loop required for full transcriptional activation of *prf*A. This results in a very low [in the case of the *hly* gene product of *L. seeligeri*, seeligerolysin (LSO)] to undetectable expression of the genes of the virulence cluster. Complementation experiments have shown that this is the cause for the incapability of *L. seeligeri* to escape from the phagosome of mammalian cells. The apparent inability of the *L. seeligeri* ActA to induce actin polymerisation in such cells is another reason for the observed avirulence of this listerial species for man and mammals (KARUNASAGAR et al. 1997). In the apathogenic species *L. innocua* and *L. welshimeri*, none of the above mentioned virulence genes are found between *prs* and *ldh* (Fig. 1); rather, there are only the orfsBA, which obviously are an integral part of the *Listeria* genome, plus orfZ (modified) or an orfL, respectively (CHAKRABORTY et al. 2000; NG et al. 2001).

3 Internalin Islets and Islands

As mentioned in the introduction, pathogenic *Listeriae* are able to efficiently invade normally non-phagocytic cells by triggering an induced phagocytosis. This capability is a prerequisite for breaching epithelial, endothelial and placental barriers, respectively, and, hence, for establishing sytemic infections. ActA and the bifunctional protein p60 (*iap* gene product) are involved in the invasion of some cell types (reviewed in KUHN and GOEBEL 2000; VAZQUEZ-BOLAND et al. 2001a), but clearly the most important listerial factors involved in uptake by host cells are the internalin proteins. These proteins are encoded on a multi-gene family, the first two have been detected in the *inl*AB operon. The additional *inl*C2DE and *inl*F loci were described subsequently (DRAMSI et al. 1997), as well as a modified form of *inl*C2DE, the *inl*GHE determinant (RAFFELSBAUER et al. 1998) (Fig. 2A). The *inl*C2DE cluster has been described for a particular isolate of *L. monocytogenes* EGD, *inl*GHE have been found in another EGD isolate and several other strains. Sequence analyses revealed that *inl*H obviously arose by recombination between the ancestral *inl*C2 and *inl*D genes; presumably the *inl*C2DE cluster is also preceeded by *inl*G (RAFFELSBAUER et al. 1998). Although the *inl*AB operon is partially regulated by PrfA, it is mainly expressed outside of host cells, *inl*C2DE/GHE and *inl*F are PrfA-independent. The products of all these genes are rather large proteins with a characteristic structure: At their N-terminus, a canonical export-mediating sequence, the signal peptide, is found, followed by a stretch of 6–16 leucine-rich repeats (LRRs) (depending on the respective protein and also on the definition of the LRR; see MARINO et al. 2000). These are blocks of, in the case of *Listeria*, 22 amino acids with a characteristic signature of leucines; the repeat units together forming a right-handed parallel beta-helix. This structure presumably is involved in protein-protein interactions and was first described for eukaryotes, including plants. So far they have only rarely been found in prokaryotes (reviewed in KAJAVA 1998). The LRR-domain is separated by an interrepeat region of variable length from another repeat region (2–3 B-repeats) in the C-terminal half of the protein. Close to the C-terminus, all these internalins, except InlB, contain an LPXTG motif (or LPXAG in some of them, see Fig. 2A) preceding a stretch of about 20

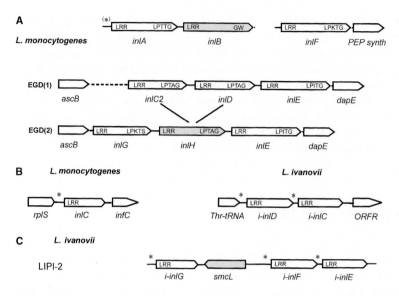

Fig. 2A–C. Structure of internalin islets and islands. **A** Large internalins of *L. monocytogenes*; **B** small, secreted internalins; **C** LIPI-2. An *asterisk* indicates a "PrfA-box"; LRR a leucine-rich repeat domain; the pentapeptide of the different cell wall anchor motifs is given in one letter code. For internalin names and functions see text. *PEP synth*, phosphoenolpyruvate synthase; *asc*B, 6-phospho-beta-glucosidase; *dap*E, succinyl-diaminopimelate desuccinylase; *rpl*S, ribosomal protein L19; *inf*C, initiation factor IF3; *smc*L, sphingomyelinase. Combined and modified from DRAMSI et al. (1997), ENGELBRECHT et al. (1998a), KUHN and GOEBEL (2000), KREFT et al. (1999)

hydrophobic amino acids, followed by a short tail of positively charged residues. This structure serves to anchor the internalins to the cell wall (DHAR et al. 2000). In internalin B, this particular C-terminal structure is missing; rather, there are tandem repeats starting with glycine-tryptophan, and evidence has been presented that these GW-repeats associate with lipoteichoic acid in the cell wall (see COSSART and LECUIT 1998). The functions of the surface-exposed proteins InlA and InlB have been well characterized, InlA being required for uptake by cells with human-type E-cadherin on their surface, e.g. enterocytes. InlB is essential for invasion of other cells, e.g. brain microvascular endothelial cells (reviewed in COSSART and LECUIT 1998; KUHN and GOEBEL 2000). Recently, the InlB receptor has been identified as the Met receptor tyrosine kinase (SHEN et al. 2000). Binding of InlA or InlB to their target cell receptors triggers signal transduction events in the host cell, which ultimately lead to cytoskeleton rearrangements, invagination of the host cell membrane and zipper-type phagocytosis of the bacterium. The function of the additional internalins C2-H has not yet clearly been elucidated.

In addition to these large, cell wall-associated internalins (l-Inls), a number of considerably smaller proteins also containing LRRs have been found. These proteins lack the C-terminal cell wall anchor and are secreted by the bacteria, at least some of them predominantly inside the host cell and have, therefore, been termed s-Inls. In *L. monocytogenes*, only inlC has been found so far (ENGELBRECHT et al.

1996). In *L. ivanovii* a large number of highly similar genes is present, among them i-inlDC (ENGELBRECHT et al. 1998a) (Fig. 2B). A mutant defective in *inl*C was severely impaired in its in vivo virulence when tested in mice; however, the function of InlC or i-InlDC is unknown to date. There is no evidence so far that any of them has a role in internalization of the bacteria into eukaryotic host cells. The designation "small internalins" has been retained due to the striking similarity of their LLR region to that of the large internalins. In contrast to the l-Inls the expression of all s-Inls is strictly PrfA-dependent, which corresponds well to their preferential expression in the host cell (see Sect. 1).

Recently, it has been found that the previously described *i-inl*FE genes, encoding two typical s-Inls (ENGELBRECHT et al. 1998b), are part of a large (about 22kb) virulence gene cluster of *L. ivanovii*. Such a cluster is not found in other *Listeria* species; it shows several characteristics of a PAI and has, therefore, been termed LIPI-2 (Fig. 2C). In addition to *i-inl*FE, it comprises the gene *smc*L, encoding a sphingomyelinase C (GONZALEZ-ZORN et al. 1999) plus a number of genes for new sInls, e.g. *i-inl*G. The *smc*L gene is located in between the region ending with *i-inl*G and the *i-inl*FE locus, with respect to the *i-inl*s, it is transcribed in the opposite direction, and in contrast to the *i-inl* genes, its expression is not controlled by PrfA (Fig. 2C). Non-polar mutants, in which either *i-inl*F, *i-inl*E or both have been deleted, were drastically reduced in their virulence in vivo (ENGELBRECHT et al. 1998b); deletion of *smc*L attenuated the virulence for mice and impaired the intracellular replication of *L. ivanovii* in a bovine cell line (GONZALEZ-ZORN et al. 1999). As decribed above, at least one *s-inl* gene is also present in *L. monocytogenes*. A sphingomyelinase gene, however, is not found there or in other *Listeria* species. Interestingly, this region can be deleted spontaneously from the chromosome, albeit at a low frequency. Together with some genomic islands of *S. aureus* (LINDSAY et al. 1998; FITZGERALD et al. 2001), LIPI-2 is one of the few examples of an unstable virulence gene cluster in gram-positive bacteria. A detailed analysis of the structure and function of LIPI-2 is in progress in the authors' laboratories.

4 Evolution of Virulence in *Listeria*

It is generally accepted that evolution of prokaryotes is driven, to a large extent, by "horizontal" or "lateral" gene transfer between different species or even genera (for recent reviews, see DOOLITTLE 1999; DE LA CRUZ and DAVIES 2000; OCHMAN et al. 2000). This applies, in particular, to the evolution of bacterial pathogenicity and virulence. The original concept of PAIs stated that typically these entities are "foreign" to the ancestral chromosome where they are found now. This notion is supported by the fact that often these regions differ in molecular terms (e.g. G + C content, codon usage) from the rest of the chromosome and that they often contain genes or structures implicated in mobility of DNA elements (transposases, integrases, phage-like genes, repeat structures). Furthermore, mobile elements such as conjugative transposons (SALYERS et al. 1995) or bacteriophages (CHEETHAM and KATZ 1995), to mention only some, have roles in the evolution and transfer of virulence traits. In the following text, the virulence gene clusters of *Listeria* will be analysed with respect to the criteria and phenomena just mentioned. In this context, it must be kept in mind that, on the one hand, it has been shown that *L. monocytogenes* is clonally rather stable (e.g. RASMUSSEN et al. 1995; WIEDMANN et al. 1997), but that a considerable intraspecies diversity is seen as well. Furthermore, mobile genetic elements such as lysogenic and transducing bacteriophages are quite common in *Listeria* (LOESSNER et al. 2000; HODGSON 2000), and parts of conjugative transposons have also been found here (RICE 1998). Together this indicates that in *Listeria*, too, horizontal gene transfer is taking place.

4.1 Evolution of LIPI-1

Based on rRNA analyses, the genus *Listeria* can be divided into three (phylo-) genetic groups, one comprising *L. monocytogenes* and the completely avirulent *L. innocua*, a second one including the animal pathogen *L. ivanovii*, the normally avirulent species *L. seeligeri* and the apathogenic *L. welshimeri*, the harmless *L. grayi* forming the third branch (COLLINS et al. 1991; SALLEN et al. 1996; NG et al. 2001). Interestingly LIPI-1 is found in two of these genetic groups, in the *L. monocytogenes* lineage as well in the *L. ivanovii/L. seeligeri* one and is always found at exactly the same chromosomal location (see Section 2). Both of these groups, however, have members (*L. innocua* and *L. welshimeri*, respectively) that do not contain this cluster of virulence genes; rather, the orfs BA plus either a derivative of orfZ or the unrelated orfL (Fig. 1) is found between *prs* and *ldh* (CHAKRABORTY et al. 2000; VAZQUEZ-BOLAND et al. 2001b; NG et al. 2001). The orfsBA, therefore, have to be considered an integral part of the genus' chromosome. The fact that LIPI-1 is found at the same location within members of two distinct phylogenetic groups of *Listeria* and is missing in other members of the same groups clearly indicates that LIPI-1 has been acquired by or evolved in a common ancestor of the present *Listeria* species and has been deleted from the chromosome of *L. innocua* and *L. welshimeri*, respectively (NG et al. 2001). The finding that *L. seeligeri*, which has to be regarded as avirulent for mammals, contains all the genes of the "canonical" LIPI-1 structurally intact is intriguing. If these genes were of no use at all for *L. seeligeri*, they certainly would have suffered from mutations and deletions during evolution. In this context, the finding that not only *L. monocytogenes* but also *L. seeligeri* survives quite well in bacteriovorous protozoa, like *Tetrahymena* (LY and MÜLLER 1990), is of particular interest. It is tempting to speculate that the modified LIPI-1 of *L. seeligeri* is at least sufficiently expressed there for survival in these organisms, yet to date there are no experimental data available to support this assumption. However, the observations made for *L. monocytogenes* and *L. seeligeri* lends support to the hypothesis that either the common ancestor of today's *Listeriae* (with the possible exception of *L. grayi*) was primarily adapted for a life in protozoa, a capability that was then lost again by some members of the genus or that those *Listeria* that are pathogenic for warm-blooded animals can also exist as commensals in water-living unicellular organisms (BARKER and BROWN 1994). In any case, the modified LIPI-1 of *L. seeligeri* can be regarded as an ancestral form, which became optimised, in the sense of "patho-adaptive mutations" (SOKURENKO et al. 1999) for the infection of and the survival in warm-blooded animals during the evolution of *L. monocytogenes* and *L. ivanovii*. If LIPI-1 had originally been acquired by horizontal gene transfer (see Sect. 4.1), the loss of the additional orfs present in *L. seeligeri* and interrupting transcriptional units being contiguous in *L. monocytogenes* and *L. ivanovii*, can be regarded as steps in operon evolution (LAWRENCE 1999).

4.2 Evolution of the Internalin Islets and Islands

As described above, the large cell wall-associated internalins of *L. monocytogenes* are mostly encoded by clusters of two to four closely related genes. It is evident that such highly homologous sequences have a tendency to recombine. In fact, the *inl*H gene of one EGD strain (and a number of other strains) evolved by recombination of the *inl*C2/*inl*D genes (Fig. 2A) (RAFFELSBAUER et al. 1998). In addition to the large internalin genes, *L. monocytogenes* contains the gene for InlC, which differs from the large internalins by the absence of the C-terminal B-repeats and the cell wall anchor motif. In *L. ivanovii*, the closely related *i-inl*C is found, preceded by *i-inl*D (Fig. 2B). In addition, *L. ivanovii* contains a large number of other more or less similar genes for s-Inls in LIPI-2 (see Sect. 4.2). It is not clear if the i-*inl*DC locus (note that it is located next to a tRNA gene, something that is regarded as typical for PAIs) has been mobilized into *L. monocytogenes*, where i-*inl*D was then deleted. Alternatively *inl*C originated in *L. monocytogenes*, then became integrated into *L. ivanovii*, where it underwent duplication (yielding *i-inl*DC), transposition and further amplification (LIPI-2). An analysis of the respective gene loci, where in *L. monocytogenes* or *L. ivanovii* either l-Inl or s-Inl genes are found, in other *Listeria* species revealed that these loci are devoid of any internalin genes (NG et al. 2001). Although the idea that similar genes are present at other locations in those species cannot be excluded, these findings make it rather unlikely that such genes, in particular those encoding l-Inls, were already present in this form in a common ancestor. As mentioned, in addition to *i-inl*DC, *L. ivanovii* contains LIPI-2, a large cluster of s-Inl genes; furthermore, this cluster carries the *smc*L gene (sphingomy-elinase), which is not found in other *Listeria* species. This gene cluster has not yet completely been characterised, but it is clearly involved in *L. ivanovii* pathogenicity. In *L. ivanovii*, it is flanked on one side by housekeeping genes; the corresponding region of the *L. monocytogenes* chromosome lacks such a cluster. Several inde-pendent isolates of *L. ivanovii* all contain LIPI-2 at the same location and with a basically identical structure. The s-Inl genes in LIPI-2 are highly similar to *i-inl*DC, but the evolutionary relationship between these two loci is not yet clear. The *smc*L gene obviously is a later acquisition, since it is the only gene in LIPI-2 that is not under PrfA control and is transcribed in the opposite direction with respect to the s-Inls (GONZALEZ-ZORN et al. 1999). The chromosomal region containing LIPI-2 is structurally unstable. As spontaneous deletion occurs there with low frequency, the mechanism underlying the deletion event is unknown.

Leucine-rich repeat proteins of the s-Inl type have been found in a wide variety of different organisms, including bacteria (KAJAVA 1998). Also cell wall-anchored proteins with an LPXTG motif are present in several other gram-positive bacteria (NAVARRE and SCHNEEWIND 1999). However, the particular combination of these two domains in one protein, so far, has only been described for *L. monocytogenes*. This makes it plausible to assume that l-Inls evolved by recombination (plus duplication) between originally unlinked and functionally unrelated genes of an ancestral *Listeria* species to adapt to the special requirements of a later facultative intracellular parasite, which needs to trigger its own uptake by non-phagocytic cells.

4.3 Evolution of the PrfA Regulon

The question of how the PrfA regulon of *L. monocytogenes*, *L. ivanovii*, and *L. seeligeri* may have evolved deserves some special attention. This regulon comprises not only LIPI-1, where the *prf*A gene itself is located, but a number of other genes. This was first noticed by the analysis of surface-associated proteins of *L. monocytogenes* (SOKOLOVIC et al. 1993) and of *L. ivanovii* (LAMPIDIS et al. 1994). All the s-Inl genes are under strict PrfA control. The *inl*AB operon is partially PrfA-dependent, and several more of the PrfA-regulated genes have been identified, too (RIPIO et al. 1997, 1998; MICHEL et al. 1998). If one assumes that LIPI-1 had been acquired by horizontal gene transfer from other organisms (see Sect. 4.1), the fact that the genes comprising today's PrfA regulon are found dispersed over the chromosome may be explained in two different ways. One possibility is that *prf*A itself and most of the PrfA-regulated genes, except the virulence factor genes (*hly*, *plc*A/B, etc.) now found on LIPI-1, were already part of the ancestral genome and that this primordial PrfA regulon co-opted a horizontally transferred virulence gene cluster. A similar phenomenon has been described for the PhoPQ regulon of *Salmonella* and the ToxRS regulon of *V. cholerae* (COTTER and DIRITA 2000). Alternatively, *prf*A may already have been an integral part of a horizontally transmitted virulence gene cluster, and a number of genes on the ancestral chromosome slowly and independently evolved binding sites for PrfA, their expression thus becoming optimised for a facultative intracellular lifestyle and for virulence. A third alternative is that the entire PrfA regulon evolved directly in *Listeria*, including rearrangements, duplications and also, presumably, exchange of individual components with other bacteria.

4.4 Possible Origin of Virulence Genes

As discussed above, the large family of internalins presumably evolved within *Listeria*. This does not exclude a horizontal acquisition of individual components

(LRR and/or LPXTG protein genes) at the beginning. As also mentioned, the *smc*L gene in LIPI-2 shows signs of a rather late addition from outside; this view is supported by the high similarity of its gene product to sphingomyelinases from other bacteria (Table 2). A detailed analysis of LIPI-1, with respect to traces of a horizontal transfer, gave the following results. The G + C content of this cluster is 36% in *L. monocytogenes*, 37% and 34.5%, respectively, in *L. ivanovii* and *L. seeligeri*. This is very similar to the G + C content of the respective chromosomes (38%, 37% and 32%) but does not exclude acquisition from organisms with similar nucleotide composition. The dinucleotide relative abundance of a genome or of larger sections of it is regarded as a more reliable parameter than the mere G + C content to detect a possible foreign origin of particular chromosomal regions (KARLIN and BURGE 1995). As shown in Table 1, the dinucleotide relative abundance of LIPI-1 from *L. monocytogenes* shows the same characteristic pattern as 38kb of DNA sequences outside of the cluster, which have been compiled from the public database. The deviations seen for *act*A and the internalins are explained by the biased amino acid composition of their gene products (repeat proteins), in

Table 1. Characteristic dinucleotide relative abundance in the *Listeria* genome (based on 38kb of sequences in the EMBL database) compared to virulence-associated genes

Gene	GpG	ApG	TpG	CpG	ApA	TpA	ApT	TpT	CpT	GpC	ApC	TpC	CpC
Genome	0.94	0.84	1.17	1.10	1.17	0.75	0.93	1.24	0.98	1.29	0.94	0.92	0.87
Vir-clu	1.08	0.86	1.13	1.02	1.14	0.78	0.97	1.22	0.97	1.38	0.86	0.98	0.98
lmact A	0.82	1.06	1.05	0.98	1.12	0.75	0.85	1.51	1.03	1.23	0.81	0.95	1.26
*inl*AB	1.22	0.88	1.03	0.90	1.11	0.94	0.88	1.24	1.04	1.21	1.09	0.74	1.02
*inl*C2DE	1.22	0.91	1.16	0.87	1.12	0.93	0.93	1.24	1.01	1.23	1.06	0.77	1.05
inl C	0.96	1.03	1.12	0.56	1.17	0.88	0.90	1.09	1.16	1.28	0.93	0.90	1.07

Calculated according to KARLIN and BURGE 1995. Relative abundance values with high (> 1.23) or low (< 0.79) compositional extremes are significant.

Table 2. Similarity of virulence-associated *Listeria* proteins to proteins of same or related function/structure in other gram-positive bacteria (first value: percent identity; second value: percent similarity)

Species	PrfA[a]	PlcA	LLO	Mpl	PlcB	SmcL	InlA[b] (LRR-region)	InlC[b]
B. subtilis	22/45	n.p.	n.p.	42/57	n.p.	n.p.	n.p.	n.p.
B. cereus[c]	n.e.	28/42	40/62	32/45	38/58	54/66	n.e.	n.e.
B. anthracis[d]	25/46	29/44	41/64[e]	31/47	39/59	55/67	30/49	28/46
S. aureus	25/44	27/48	n.p.	41/58	20/44	55/70	23/40	n.p.
S. pyogenes	27/52	n.p.	41/65	n.p.	n.p.	n.p.	27/50	25/49
E. faecalis	25/47	n.p.	n.p.	29/49	n.p.	n.p.	32/49	24/37

[a] Similarity to Crp/Fnr family proteins; [b] similarity to leucine-rich repeat proteins; [c] no genome sequence available; [d] unfinished genome sequence; [e] note that *B. anthracis* is described as non-hemolytic; n.p.: not present; n.e.: no entry in database. The unfinished genome sequence of *B. anthracis* and the complete sequences of *S. aureus*, *S. pyogenes* and *E. faecalis* were searched at www.tigr.org, the complete genome sequence of *B. subtilis* at mips.gsf.de; additional searches have been done at wit.integratedgenomics.com/IGwit. PrfA: Positive regulator A; PlcA: Phosphatidylinositol-specific phospholipase C; LLO: Listeriolysin O; Mpl: Metalloprotease; PlcB: Lecithinase; SmcL: Sphingomyelinase; InlA: Internalin A; InlC: Internalin C.

conjuction with the codon preference for the amino acids overrepresented in these proteins. No significant difference in codon usage could be detected between LIPI-1 and 38kb of sequences outside (data not shown). Furthermore, no extended inverted or direct repeat structures were detectable at the ends of LIPI-1 (NG et al. 2001). Thus, LIPI-1 in its present form perfectly matches the molecular features of the rest of the chromosome. If it has originally been acquired by horizontal gene transfer, no clear traces of such an event are left. Possible mechanisms of horizontal gene transfer are conjugative transposition, phage transduction or uptake of DNA via transformation. So far, no competence state could be demonstrated for *Listeria*; however, homologues of *mec*A and *com*K, involved in competence of *B. subtilis*, have been found in *L. monocytogenes* (BOREZEE et al. 2000; LOESSNER et al. 2000). So the lack of transformability may only reflect that the appropriate conditions have not yet been found. A similar problem existed for *Bacillus cereus* until a special protocol was developed (SABELNIKOV and ULYASHOVA 1990). Regardless of whether the virulence genes found in LIPI-1 have been acquired as a larger unit or individually from other organisms or if they spread from *Listeria* to other bacteria, it seems worthwhile to have a closer look at similar genes, respectively, gene products of related mainly pathogenic gram-positives.

Table 2 shows the major results of an extensive database search. In addition to the species listed in the table, the available genome sequences of about ten other bacteria have been searched without yielding significant homologies. In accordance with previous reports, no proteins with significant similarity to the entire ActA have been found. It has been reported that two domains of ActA show similarity to the eukaryotic proteins zyxin and vinculin, and it has been speculated that the respective coding sequences have been acquired from host cells (reviewed in COSSART and LECUIT 1998). With respect to the additional orfs present in LIPI-1 of *L. seeligeri*, the orfC product is rather similar to the C protein alpha-antigen of *Streptococcus agalactiae*. OrfD clearly is a L-ribulose-5-ph-4-epimerase, for OrfE no hit was found in the entire database. Not surprisingly, regulators of the Crp/Fnr family have been found in most cases; none of them had the particular features of PrfA (i.e. a C-terminal leucine zipper and a putative second helix-turn-helix motif at the N-terminus). Likewise, a number of leucine-rich repeat proteins is present in other gram-positives (the largest number was found in *Clostridium acetobutylicum*, results of a database search, not shown), but the characteristics of the large internalins from *Listeria*, i.e. the fusion of LRRs with a cell wall anchor structure, could not be detected. Concerning cholesterol-binding cytolysins of the LLO type and phospholipases (PlcA and PlcB) as well as an Mpl-like metalloprotease, a striking similarity was found between *Listeria* and *Bacillus anthracis*. As far as could be deduced from the unfinished genome sequence of *B. anthracis*, these genes are not contiguous there. No genome sequence for *B. cereus* is available to date; therefore, the comparison had to remain incomplete. Other possible sources (or recipients) of virulence genes include streptococci and enterococci. Up to now, the only finished and completely annotated genome sequence of a related, low G + C gram-positive bacterium is that of *Bacillus subtilis*. This has been considered a good reason to use this organism often as a reference. However, the current phylogeny of

Listeria and relatives (Fig. 3) shows that *Listeriae* are more closely related to the *B. cereus/B. anthracis* and *B. thuringiensis* branch than to *B. subtilis*. It has been shown that the former ones may even belong to a single species (HELGASON et al. 2000) and that the genome organization is not conserved between *B. subtilis* and *B. cereus* (OKSTAD et al. 1999). Future comparisons of the complete genomes of *Listeria* species to those of *B. anthracis/B. cereus* might reveal a much closer relationship than anticipated. In this context, it is interesting to note that *B. anthracis/B. cereus* share the soil habitat with *Listeria*. Furthermore, *B. cereus* is often found as a food contaminant, similar to *Listeria* (and enterococci), and may cause a number of extra-intestinal infections (reviewed in DROBNIEWSKI 1993).

5 Perspectives

The ongoing genome sequencing projects will replace the fragmentary information available to date. This will shed new light on the phylogenetic relationship between the pathogens discussed above, as well as on their evolution, in particular with respect to virulence and the role of horizontal gene transfer therein. Furthermore, this development will make it possible to address more precisely new questions, like the role of specific metabolic adaptations of facultative intracellular parasites to replicate in the cytoplasm of eukaryotic host cells (GOEBEL and KUHN 2000). This also includes the role of "housekeeping genes" in the context of the interaction between a pathogen and its host. In the long range, comparative and functional genomics, bioinformatics, and mathematical modelling should even make it possible to evaluate the contribution to pathogens' virulence potential of factors that are, at first glance, not so obviously involved in pathogenicity like toxins, etc., but have a high impact on evolutionary plasticity. Such factors as efficacy of lateral gene transfer systems and also, for example, the fitness to survive in multiple, sometimes harsh, environments, can, in this way, be considered complementary or "meta-virulence factors".

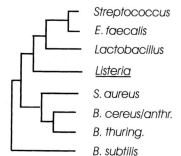

Fig. 3. Phylogeny of *Listeria* and related gram-positive bacteria. Modified from RÖSSLER et al. (1991) and ZINDER (1998)

References

Alouf JE (1999) Introduction to the family of the structurally related cholesterol-binding cytolysins ("sulfhydryl-activated" toxins). In: Alouf JE, Freer JH (eds) The Comprehensive Sourcebook of Bacterial Protein Toxins, 2nd edn. Academic Press, London

Barker J, Brown MRW (1994) Trojan horses of the microbial world: protozoa and the survival of bacterial pathogens in the environment. Microbiology 140:1253–1259

Blum G, Ott M, Lischewski A, Ritter A, Imrich H, Tschäpe H, Hacker J (1994) Excision of large DNA-regions termed pathogenicity islands from tRNA-specific loci in the chromosome of an *Escherichia coli* wild-type pathogen. Infect Immun 62:606–614

Böckmann R, Dickneite C, Goebel W, Sokolovic Z (2000) PrfA mediates specific binding of RNA polymerase to PrfA-dependent virulence gene promoters resulting in a transcriptionally active complex. Mol Microbiol 36:487–497

Borezee E, Msadek T, Durant L, Berche P (2000) Identification in *Listeria monocytogenes* of MecA, a homologue of the *Bacillus subtilis* competence regulatory protein. J Bacteriol 182:5931–5934

Brehm K, Kreft J, Ripio MT, Vazquez-Boland JA (1996) Regulation of virulence gene expression in pathogenic *Listeria*. Microbiologia 12:219–236

Chakraborty T, Hain T, Domann E (2000) Genome organization and the evolution of the virulence gene locus in *Listeria* species. Int J Med Microbiol 290:167–174

Cheetham BF, Katz ME (1995) A role for bacteriophages in the evolution and transfer of bacterial virulence determinants. Mol Microbiol 18:201–208

Collins MD, Wallbanks S, Lane DJ, Shah J, Nietupski R, Smida J, Dorsch M, Stackebrandt E (1991) Phylogenetic analysis of the genus *Listeria* based on reverse transcriptase sequencing of 16 S rRNA. Int J Syst Bacteriol 41:240–246

Cossart P, Lecuit M (1998) Interaction of *Listeria monocytogenes* with mammalian cells during entry and actin-based movement: bacterial factors, cellular ligands and signaling. EMBO J 17:3797–3806

Cossart P, Portnoy D (2000) The cell biology of invasion and intracellular growth by *Listeria monocytogenes*. In: Fischetti VA, Novick RP, Ferretti JJ, Portnoy DA, Rood JI (eds) Gram-positive Pathogens. American Society for Microbiology, Washington DC, pp 507–515

Cossart P, Boquet P, Normark S, Rappuoli R (1996) Cellular microbiology emerging. Science 271: 315–316

Cotter PA, DiRita VJ (2000) Bacterial virulence gene regulation: an evolutionary perspective. Annu Rev Microbiol 54:519–565

De la Cruz F, Davies J (2000) Horizontal gene transfer and the origin of species: lessons from bacteria. Trends Microbiol 8:128–133

Dhar G, Faull KF, Schneewind O (2000) Anchor structure of cell wall surface proteins in *Listeria monocytogenes*. Biochemistry 39:3725–3733

Doolittle WF (1999) Lateral genomics. Trends Genet 15:M5–M8

Dramsi S, Dehoux P, Lebrun M, Goossens PL, Cossart P (1997) Identification of four new members of the internalin multigene family of *Listeria monocytogenes* EGD. Infect Immun 65:1615–1625

Drobniewski FA (1993) *Bacillus cereus* and related species. Clin Microbiol Rev 6:324–338

Edelson BT, Unanue ER (2000) Immunity to *Listeria* infection. Curr Opin Immunol 12:425–431

Engelbrecht F, Chun SK, Ochs C, Hess J, Lottspeich F, Goebel W, Sokolovic Z (1996) A new PrfA-regulated gene of *Listeria monocytogenes* encoding a small, secreted protein, which belongs to the family of internalins. Mol Microbiol 21:823–837

Engelbrecht F, Dickneite C, Lampidis R, Götz M, DasGupta U, Goebel W (1998a) Sequence comparison of the chromosomal regions encompassing the internalin C genes (*inlC*) of *Listeria monocytogenes* and *Listeria ivanovii*. Mol Gen Genet 257:186–197

Engelbrecht F, Dominguez-Bernal G, Dickneite C, Hess J, Greiffenberg L, Lampidis R, Raffelsbauer D, Kaufmann SHE, Kreft J, Vazquez-Boland JA, Goebel W (1998b) A novel PrfA-regulated chromosomal locus of *Listeria ivanovii* encoding two small, secreted internalins is essential for virulence in mice. Mol Microbiol 30:405–417

Farber JM, Peterkin PI (1991) *Listeria monocytogenes*, a food-borne pathogen. Microbiol Rev 55: 476–511

Fenlon DR (1999) *Listeria monocytogenes* in the natural environment. In: Ryser ET, Marth EH (eds) *Listeria*, Listeriosis, and Food Safety, 2nd edn. Marcel Dekker Inc., New York

Finlay BB, Cossart P (1997) Exploitation of mammalian host cell functions by bacterial pathogens. Science 276:718–725

Fitzgerald JR, Monday SR, Foster TJ, Bohach GA, Hartigan PJ, Meaney WJ, Smyth CJ (2001) Characterization of a putative pathogenicity island from bovine *Staphylococcus aureus* encoding multiple superantigens. J Bacteriol 183:63–70

Goebel W, Kuhn M (2000) Bacterial replication in the host cell cytosol. Curr Opin Microbiol 3:49–53

Goebel W, Kreft J, Böckmann R (2000) Regulation of virulence genes in pathogenic *Listeria*. In: Fischetti VA, Novick RP, Ferretti JJ, Portnoy DA, Rood JI (eds) Gram-positive Pathogens. American Society for Microbiology, Washington DC, pp 499–506

Goldfine H, Wadsworth SJ, Johnston NC (2000) Activation of host phospholipases C and D in macrophages after infection with *listeria monocytogenes*. Infect Immun 68:5735–5741

González-Zorn B, Dominguez-Bernal G, Suarez M, Ripio MT, Vega Y, Novella S, Vázquez-Boland JA (1999) The *smc*L gene of *Listeria ivanovii* encodes a sphingomyelinase C that mediates bacterial escape from the phagocytic vacuole. Mol Microbiol 33:510–523

Gouin E, Mengaud J, Cossart P (1994) The virulence gene cluster of *Listeria monocytogenes* is also present in *Listeria ivanovii*, an animal pathogen, and *Listeria seeligeri*, a nonpathogenic species. Infect Immun 62:3550–3553

Haas A, Dumbsky M, Kreft J (1992) Listeriolysin genes: complete sequence of *ilo* from *Listeria ivanovii* and of *lso* from *Listeria seeligeri*. Biochim Biophys Acta 1130:81–84

Hacker J, Kaper JB (2000) Pathogenicity islands and the evolution of microbes. Annu Rev Microbiol 54:641–679

Hacker J, Blum-Oehler G, Mühldorfer I, Tschäpe H (1997) Pathogenicity islands of virulent bacteria: structure, function and impact on microbial evolution. Mol Microbiol 23:1089–1097

Helgason E, Okstad OA, Caugant DA, Johansen HA, Fouet A, Mock M, Hegna I, Kolsto AB (2000) *Bacillus anthracis*, *Bacillus cereus*, and *Bacillus thuringiensis* – one species on the basis of genetic evidence. Appl Environ Microbiol 66:2627–2630

Hodgson DA (2000) Generalized transduction of serotype 1/2 and serotype 4b strains of *Listeria monocytogenes*. Mol Microbiol 35:312–323

Jones D (1990) Foodborne listeriosis. Lancet 336:1171–1174

Kajava AV (1998) Structural diversity of leucine-rich repeat proteins. J Mol Biol 277:519–527

Karlin S, Burge C (1995) Dinucleotide relative abundance extremes: a genomic signature. Trends Genet 11:283–290

Karunasagar I, Lampidis R, Goebel W, Kreft J (1997) Complementation of *Listeria seeligeri* with the *plc*A-*prf*A genes from *L. monocytogenes* activates transcription of seeligerolysin and leads to bacterial escape from the phagosome of infected mammalian cells. FEMS Microbiol Lett 146:303–310

Kreft J, Dumbsky M, Theiss S (1995) The actin-polymerization protein from *Listeria ivanovii* is a large repeat protein, which shows only limited amino acid sequence homology to ActA from *Listeria monocytogenes*. FEMS Microbiol Lett 126:113–122

Kreft J, Vazquez-Boland JA, Ng E, Goebel W (1999) Virulence gene clusters and putative pathogenicity islands in *Listeria*. In: Kaper J, Hacker J (eds) Pathogenicity Islands and Other Mobile Virulence Elements. American Society for Microbiology, Washington, DC

Kuhn M, Goebel W (2000) Internalization of *Listeria monocytogenes* by nonprofessional and professional phagocytes. Subcell Biochem 33:411–436

Lampidis R, Gross R, Sokolovic Z, Goebel W, Kreft J (1994) The virulence regulator protein of *Listeria ivanovii* is highly homologous to PrfA from *Listeria monocytogenes* and both belong to the Crp-Fnr family of transcription regulators. Mol Microbiol 13:141–151

Lawrence J (1999) Selfish operons: the evolutionary impact of gene clustering in prokaryotes and eukaryotes. Curr Opin Genet Dev 9:642–648

Lindsay JA, Ruzin A, Ross HF, Kurepina N, Novick RP (1998) The gene for toxic shock toxin is carried by a family of mobile pathogenicity islands in *Staphylococcus aureus*. Mol Microbiol 29:527–543

Loessner MJ, Inman RB, Lauer P, Calendar R (2000) Complete nucleotide sequence, molecular analysis and genome structure of bacteriophage A118 of *Listeria monocytogenes*: implications for phage evolution. Mol Microbiol 35:324–340

Lorber B (1997) Listeriosis. Clin Infect Dis 24:1–11

Ly TMC, Müller HE (1990) Interactions of *Listeria monocytogenes*, *Listeria seeligeri*, and *Listeria innocua* with protozoans. J Gen Appl Microbiol 36:143–150

Mackaness GB (1962) Cellular resistance to infection. J Exp Med 116:381–406

Marino M, Braun L, Cossart P, Ghosh P (2000) A framework for interpreting the leucine-rich repeats of *Listeria* internalins. Proc Natl Acad Sci USA 97:9784–8788

McDaniel TK, Kaper JB (1997) A cloned pathogenicity island from enteropathogenic *Escherichia coli* confers the attaching and effacing phenotype on *E. coli* K-12. Mol Microbiol 23:399–407

Michel E, Mengaud J, Galsworthy S, Cossart P (1998) Characterization of a large motility gene cluster containing the *cheR*, *motAB* genes of *Listeria monocytogenes* and evidence that PrfA downregulates motility genes. FEMS Microbiol Lett 169:341–347

Mitchell TJ (2000) Cellular microbiology: an integrated approach to understanding pathogenesis of infection. J Cell Sci 113:3355–3356

Navarre WW, Schneewind O (1999) Surface proteins of gram-positive bacteria and mechanisms of their targeting to the cell wall envelope. Microbiol Mol Biol Rev 63:174–229

Ng E, Schmid M, Wagner M, Goebel W (2001) Pathogenic capability has been lost at least twice within the genus *Listeria*. Inf Genet Evol (submitted)

Ochman H, Lawrence JG, Groisman EA (2000) Lateral gene transfer and the nature of bacterial innovation. Nature 405:299–304

Okstad OA, Hegna I, Lindbäck T, Rishovd AL, Kolsto AB (1999) Genome organization is not conserved between *Bacillus cereus* and *Bacillus subtilis*. Microbiology 145:621–631

Portnoy DA, Chakraborty T, Goebel W, Cossart P (1992) Molecular determinants of *Listeria monocytogenes* pathogenesis. Infect Immun 60:1263–1267

Raffelsbauer D, Bubert A, Engelbrecht F, Scheinpflug J, Simm A, Hess J, Kaufmann SHE, Goebel W (1998) The gene cluster *inl*C2DE of *Listeria monocytogenes* contains additional new internalin genes and is important for virulence in mice. Mol Gen Genet 260:144–158

Rasmussen OF, Skouboe P, Dons L, Rossen L, Olsen JE (1995) *Listeria monocytogenes* exists in at least three evolutionary lines: evidence from flagellin, invasive associated protein and listeriolysin O genes. Microbiology 141:2053–2061

Renzoni A, Cossart P, Dramsi S (1999) PrfA, the transcriptional activator of virulence genes, is upregulated during interaction of *Listeria monocytogenes* with mammalian cells and in eukaryotic cell extracts. Mol Microbiol 34:552–561

Rice LB (1998) Tn916 family conjugative transposons and dissemination of antimicrobial resistance determinants. Antimicrob Agents Chemother 42:1871–1877

Ripio MT, Brehm K, Lara M, Suárez M, Vázquez-Boland JA (1997) Glucose-1-phosphate utilization by *Listeria monocytogenes* is PrfA dependent and coordinately expressed with virulence factors. J Bacteriol 197:7174–7180

Ripio MT, Vazquez-Boland JA, Vega Y, Nair S, Berche P (1998) Evidence for expressional crosstalk between the central virulence regulator PrfA and the stress response mediator ClpC in *Listeria monocytogenes*. FEMS Microbiol Lett 158:45–50

Rocourt J (1999) The genus *Listeria* and *Listeria monocytogenes*: phylogenetic position, taxonomy, and identification. In: Ryser ET, Marth EH (eds) *Listeria*, Listeriosis, and Food Safety, 2nd edn. Marcel Dekker Inc., New York

Rössler D, Ludwig N, Schleifer KH, Lin C, McGill TJ, Wisotzkey JD, Jurtshuk P Jr, Fox GE (1991) Phylogenetic diversity in the genus *Bacillus* as seen by 16 S rRNA sequencing studies. Syst Appl Microbiol 14:266–269

Sabelnikov AG, Ulyashova LV (1990) Plasmid transformation of *Bacillus cereus* on cellophane membranes. FEMS Microbiol Lett 60:123–126

Sallen BA, Rajoharison S, Desverenne S, Quinn F, Mabilat C (1996) Comparative analysis of 16 S and 23 S rRNA sequences of *Listeria* species. Int J Syst Bacteriol 46:669–674

Salyers AA, Shoemaker NB, Stevens AM, Li LY (1995) Conjugative transposons: an unusual and diverse set of integrated gene transfer elements. Microbiol Rev 59:579–590

Schuchat A, Swaminathan B, Broome CV (1991) Epidemiology of human listeriosis. Clin Microbiol Rev 4:169–183

Seeliger HPR (1961) Listeriosis. Karger, Basel, New York

Sheehan B, Kocks C, Dramsi S, Gouin E, Klarsfeld AD, Mengaud J, Cossart P (1994) Molecular and genetic determinants of the *Listeria monocytogenes* infectious process. Curr Top Microbiol Immunol 192:187–216

Shen Y, Naujokas M, Park M, Ireton K (2000) InlB-dependent internalization of Listeria is mediated by the Met receptor tyrosine kinase. Cell 103:501–510

Sokolovic Z, Riedel J, Wuenscher M, Goebel W (1993) Surface-associated, PrfA-regulated proteins of *Listeria monocytogenes* synthesized under stress conditions. Mol Microbiol 8:219–227

Sokolovic Z, Schuller S, Bohne J, Baur A, Rdest U, Dickneite C, Nichterlein T, Goebel W (1996) Differences in virulence and in expression of PrfA and PrfA-regulated virulence genes of *Listeria monocytogenes* strains belonging to serogroup 4. Infect Immun 64:4008–4019

Sokurenko EV, Hasty DL, Dykhuizen DE (1999) Pathoadaptive mutations: gene loss and variation in bacterial pathogens. Trends Microbiol 7:191–195

Tilney LG, Portnoy DA (1989) Actin filaments and the growth, movement, and spread of the intracellular bacterial parasite, *Listeria monocytogenes*. J Cell Biol 109:1597–1608

Vázquez-Boland JA, Kuhn M, Berche P, Chakraborty T, Domínguez-Bernal G, Goebel W, Gonzalez-Zorn B, Wehland J, Kreft J (2001a) *Listeria* pathogenesis and molecular virulence determinants. Clin Microbiol Rev 14:584–640

Vázquez-Boland JA, Dominguez-Bernal G, Gonzalez-Zorn B, Kreft J, Goebel W (2001b) Pathogenicity islands and virulence evolution in *Listeria*. Microbes Infect 3:1–14

Wiedmann M, Bruce JL, Keating C, Johnson AE, McDonough PL, Batt CA (1997) Ribotypes and virulence gene polymorphism suggest three distinct Listeria monocytogenes lineages with differences in pathogenic potential. Infect Immun 65:2707–2716

Zinder SH (1998) Bacterial diversity. In: Collier L, Balows A, Sussman M (eds) Microbiology and Microbial Infections, Vol 2. Arnold-Oxford University Press, London, New York, pp 125–147

Pathogenicity Islands and Virulence Plasmids of Bacterial Plant Pathogens

J.F. Kim[1] and J.R. Alfano[2]

1 Introduction

Numerous microorganisms inhabit plants. Diverse endophytic bacteria grow in the vascular system and within the intercellular spaces of plant cells. Bacteria live on plant surfaces or in the soil adjacent to plant roots. Although most of these plant-

[1] Microbial Genomics Laboratory, Genome Research Center, Korea Research Institute of Bioscience and Biotechnology, P.O. Box 115, Yusong, Taejon 305-600, Republic of Korea
[2] Plant Science Initiative and the Department of Plant Pathology, University of Nebraska – Lincoln, N315 Beadle Center for Genetic Research, 1901 Vine Street, Lincoln, NE 68588-0665, USA

associated bacteria are either symbiotic or commensal with plants, a handful have
evolved the ability to exploit the plants to gain nutrients and in the process cause
diseases (AGRIOS 1997). These select bacteria include proteobacterial genera of
Agrobacterium, *Brenneria*, *Erwinia*, *Pantoea*, *Pectobacterium*, *Pseudomonas*,
Burkholderia, *Ralstonia*, *Xanthomonas*, and *Xylella*, and Gram-positive genera of
Clavibacter, *Rhodococcus*, *Streptomyces*, *Spiroplasma*, and '*Candidatus* Phytoplasma'. They cause a wide variety of diseases with a bewildering array of symptoms
(Table 1). Some of these symptoms are localized necrotic lesions associated with the
spot, speck, canker, blast, and blight diseases occurring on stems, leaves, or fruits.
Other symptoms of bacterial plant pathogens result in the blockage of the vascular
system of plants, resulting in "wilt" diseases or the complete loss of tissue integrity,
the so-called "soft rots". Pathogens in the genus *Agrobacterium* deliver genetic

Table 1. Virulence systems of major plant pathogenic bacteria

Bacterial species	Plant host	Disease or symptom	Major virulence systems
α-Proteobacteria			
Agrobacterium tumefaciens	Dicots	Crown gall	Type IV secretion; hormone
β-Proteobacteria			
Burkholderia cepacia	Onion	Sour skin	Not known
Ralstonia solanacearum	Solanaceous plants	Southern bacterial wilt	Type III secretion; EPS[a]
Enterobacteriaceae			
Erwinia amylovora	Rosaceous trees and shrubs (apple, pear)	Fire blight	Type III secretion; Dsp; EPS
Erwinia stewartii (*Pantoea stewartii*)	Corn	Stewart's wilt	Type III secretion; Dsp; EPS
Erwinia herbicola pathovars (*Pantoea agglomerans*)	Gypsophila (baby's breath), beet	Gall formation	Type III secretion; hormone
Soft-rot erwinias (*Pectobacterium* species)	Dicots	Soft rot	Type I, II & III secretion; enzymes
Pseudomonads			
Pseudomonas aeruginosa	*Arabidopsis thaliana*	Soft rot	Exotoxin, phospholipase
Pseudomonas syringae pathovars	Monocots and dicots	Spot, speck, blight, canker, gall	Type III secretion; Avr; toxin; hormone
Xanthomonads			
Xanthomonas species pathovars	Monocots and dicots	Spot, blight, and rot	Type II & III secretion; Avr; EPS
Xylella fastidiosa	Monocots and dicots	Pierce's disease, chlorosis, leaf scorch	Not known
Gram-positive bacteria			
Clavibacter michiganensis	Solanaceous plants	Rot, canker, wilt	Not known
Rhodococcus fascians	Monocots and dicots	Leafy gall	Hormone
Streptomyces scabies	Potato	Scab	Toxin
Spiroplasma citri	Monocots and dicots	Stubborn, stunt	Not known
'*Candidatus* Phytoplasma'	Monocots and dicots	Yellows, witches' broom	Not known

[a] Exoploysaccharides.

material into plant cells and transform them resulting in the formation of tumors or galls.

These varied disease syndromes result from different sets of pathogenicity or virulence systems that each plant pathogenic species possess. Proteins and protein-secretion systems play a key role in the ability of a pathogen to infect plants. These include proteases secreted by a type I protein-secretion system, a variety of plant cell wall-degrading pectic enzymes secreted by a type II secretion system, effector proteins secreted via type III secretion systems, or the T-DNA-protein complex that is delivered into plant cells via a type IV secretion system. Nonproteinaceous factors are also important in the bacterial pathogenesis of plants. These include exopolyssacharides, phytotoxins, plant hormones and iron-scavenging systems (Table 1; ALFANO and COLLMER 1996). Because bacterial plant pathogens share the ability of acquiring horizontally transferred foreign DNA with animal pathogens, perhaps it is not surprising that plant pathogenic bacteria also carry many virulence genes within pathogenicity islands (PAIs) and on virulence plasmids. While the presence of virulence factors on plasmids of plant pathogens is well established, the existence of virulence determinants in PAIs is a relatively recent development. The purpose of this review is to highlight several examples of PAIs and virulence plasmids in bacterial plant pathogens along with a brief summary of what proteins these genes encode to favor pathogenesis. Because of the importance of type III protein secretion systems in bacterial-plant interactions, these are covered in more detail than other PAIs, virulence plasmids, or pathogenicity determinants, and we refer the reader to other reviews on topics in bacterial plant pathogenicity (ALFANO and COLLMER 1996; EXPERT et al. 1996; HUGOUVIEUX-COTTE-PATTAT et al. 1996; LORIA et al. 1997; BENDER et al. 1999; DOW and DANIELS 2000; HIRANO and UPPER 2000; KEEN et al. 2000; LEE et al. 2000; VANNESTE 2000; ZHU et al. 2000a).

2 Hrp Pathogenicity Islands

2.1 The Hrp Type III Protein Delivery System Is Commonly Used to Interact with Plant Hosts

Several gram-negative plant pathogens use type III protein secretion systems to deliver bacterial proteins inside plant cells (for reviews, see ALFANO and COLLMER 1997; MUDGETT and STASKAWICZ 1998; GALÁN and COLLMER 1999; CORNELIS and VAN GIJSEGEM 2000; KJEMTRUP et al. 2000). The genes encoding type III secretion systems were originally isolated from several bacterial plant pathogens when transposon mutagenesis screens isolated a mutant class in several different species of plant pathogens that were defective in the ability to elicit a hypersensitive response (HR) in resistant plants and cause disease in susceptible plants (for recent reviews, see ALFANO and COLLMER 1997; LINDGREN 1997). These genes were named *hrp* genes for *HR* and *p*athogenicity. The HR is a programmed cell death of plant tissue associated with defense. Because the HR phenotype is much easier to score than pathogenesis phenotypes, the HR was useful in the discovery of *hrp* genes. Often the eliciting of plant defenses in resistant plants is due to the presence of resistance (*R*) genes that make products that can recognize specific avirulence (*avr*) gene products from a pathogen. These so-called gene-for-gene interactions between an *R* gene and an *avr* gene are well described in plant pathology (KEEN 1990; BAKER et al. 1997; BONAS and VAN DEN ACKERVEKEN 1999). Currently, most Avr proteins in gram-negative bacterial plant pathogens appear to be type III-secreted proteins that are translocated into plant cells, where the recognition event occurs in plants that are resistant (MUDGETT and STASKAWICZ 1999; ROSSIER et al. 1999; VAN DIJK et al. 1999). In susceptible plants that cannot recognize these Avr proteins, it seems all but certain that these proteins contribute to parasitism (BOGDANOVE et al. 1998; JACKSON et al. 1999; EZRA et al. 2000; SHAN et al. 2000; TSIAMIS et al. 2000; YANG et al. 2000). However, specific roles of type III-secreted proteins in bacterial-plant interactions remain unclear (WHITE et al. 2000).

hrp genes are clustered and are usually contained in the chromosome of the pathogen. The *hrp* genes encoding proteins that are widely distributed in the type III systems of animal pathogens were renamed *hrc* for *HR* and conserved and given the last-letter designation of their orthologs in the prototypical type III systems present in *Yersinia* species (with the exception of *hrcV*) (BOGDANOVE et al. 1996; HUECK 1998; CORNELIS and VAN GIJSEGEM 2000). *hrp/hrc* clusters of plant pathogens fall into two distinct groups based on their similarities. Group I *hrp/hrc* clusters, such as those present in *Pseudomonas syringae* pathovars and in *Erwinia* species share a similar operon structure and are regulated with the help of a sigma factor, HrpL, which belongs to the ECF (extracytoplasmic function) subfamily (XIAO et al. 1994; WEI and BEER 1995). *Ralstonia solanacearum* (*Pseudomonas solanacearum*) and *Xanthomonas* species are well-characterized representatives of pathogens having Group II *hrp/hrc* clusters. Members of this group share similar operon structure and are regulated, at least in part, by a positive regulatory protein homologous to the AraC family of regulatory proteins (GENIN et al. 1992; WENGELNIK and BONAS 1996). The two groups of *hrp/hrc* clusters share the nine *hrc* genes between each group and at least two other genes that also share similarity with the *ysc* genes of the *Yersinia* spp. type III system. In addition, each group shares genes in common, which are not present in members of the other group (ALFANO and COLLMER 1997). Among the plant-associated non-pathogens that have been recognized to have a type III system, *Pseudomonas fluorescens* has a group I *hrp/hrc* cluster (RAINEY 1999), and *Sinorhizobium fredii*, *Rhizobium* sp. NGR234 and *Bradyrhizobium japonicum* have type III gene clusters distantly related to group II *hrp/hrc* clusters (MEINHARDT et al. 1993; FREIBERG et al. 1997; GOTTFERT et al. 2001). Interestingly, a type III system closely related to the group II *hrp/hrc* system is present in the opportunistic human pathogen *Burkholderia pseudomallei* (WINSTANLEY et al. 1999).

The large majority of the proteins encoded by the *hrp/hrc* cluster of plant pathogens make-up the Hrp type III apparatus itself or are secreted proteins that help in the delivery of other secreted proteins across the plant cell wall and plasma membrane. Other proteins that are secreted by the type III pathway are the actual effector proteins that are delivered into plant cells, where they are predicted to modify the plant cell to favor pathogenesis. A subset of these proteins is the Avr proteins that were identified because they were recognized by resistant plants' anti-parasite surveillance system. Proteins belonging to this class that do not have Avr characteristics are being cataloged and are being referred to as Hop proteins for *H*rp-dependent *o*uter *p*rotein (VAN DIJK et al. 1999). Recent sequence analysis of the regions flanking the *hrp/hrc* clusters of *E. amylovora* and *P. syringae* revealed that these clusters are parts of PAIs, which have been termed Hrp PAIs (ALFANO et al. 2000; J.F. Kim and S.V. Beer, submitted).

2.2 Hrp PAIs in the Plant Pathogenic Enterobacteria

Plant pathogenic bacteria in the family *Enterobacteriaceae* contain closely related *hrp/hrc* gene clusters and the overall gene organization is almost identical, except for a few intergenic insertions that appear unrelated to type III secretion (Fig. 1). However, the flanking regions are quite dissimilar and contain genes predicted to encode proteins with diverse functions. The *hrp/hrc* clusters of *E. amylovora* and *Erwinia* (*Pectobacterium*) *chrysanthemi* are present in the chromosome, whereas the *hrp/hrc* cluster is contained on a 150-kb plasmid called pPATH in plant pathogenic

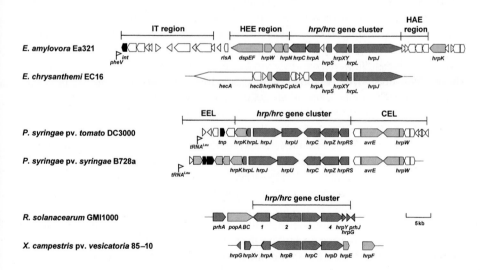

Fig. 1. Hrp PAIs of plant pathogenic bacteria. Genes or operons names (in the case of the *hrp/hrc* gene clusters) are indicated underneath *arrow boxes*, which depict predicted direction of transcription. Arrow boxes associated with the Hrp function are *shaded*. Integrase/transposase genes or ORFs similar to those found in other mobile elements are depicted as *black arrow boxes*. The *open flags* represent tRNA genes, which have been implicated in the establishment of many PAIs. *IT*, island transfer; *HEE*, Hrp effectors and elicitors; *HAE*, Hrp-associated enzymes; *EEL*, exchangeable effector locus; *CEL*, conserved effector locus

strains of *Erwinia herbicola* (*Pantoea agglomerans*) (NIZAN et al. 1997). The Hrp
PAI of the fire-blight pathogen *E. amylovora* Ea321 is approximately 60kb and is
adjacent to a tRNA gene, *pheV* (Fig. 1; J.F. Kim and S.V. Beer, submitted). It
consists of the main *hrp/hrc* gene cluster (KIM and BEER 2000), a region (HEE, Hrp
effectors and elicitors) containing two harpin genes (*hrpN* and *hrpW*; WEI et al.
1992; KIM and BEER 1998), an *avrRxv/yopJ* homolog and the *dspEF* locus (DspE is
an Hrp-secreted pathogenicity/avirulence protein; BOGDANOVE et al. 1998), and a
region (HAE, Hrp-associated enzymes) containing genes that contain HrpL-dependent promoter motifs and encode enzymes possibly involved in phytotoxin
biosynthesis. In addition, in the left flank of the Hrp PAI of *E. amylovora*, there is a
region (IT, island transfer) of varied G + C content that contains homologs of
phage-related genes, and an integrase gene at the *pheV*-proximal end (Fig. 1). These
homologs of mobile DNA elements provide a possible mechanism for introduction
of the Hrp PAI into the *E. amylovora* genome.

   hrp/hrc gene clusters almost identical to that of *E. amylovora* have been partially characterized from *Erwinia stewartii* (*Pantoea stewartii*) (COPLIN et al. 1992),
pathovars of *E. herbicola* (NIZAN et al. 1997; MOR et al. 2001), and *E. chrysanthemi*
(Fig. 1; HAM et al. 1998). Thus, they are likely to be contained in PAIs. While the
genes encoding the type III apparatus appear to be conserved throughout the plant
pathogenic enterobacteria, there are some differences in terms of conservation of
genes that encode type III-secreted products. For example, both *E. stewartii* and
E. herbicola are missing the *hrpW* gene and the *avrRxv/yopJ* homolog (MOR et al.
2001; D.L. Coplin et al. unpublished), both of which encode secreted products and
are carried in the *E. amylovora* Hrp PAI in between *hrpN* and *dspEF*. Instead, in
E. stewartii a homolog of *P. syringae* pv. *pisi avrPpiB*, a plasmid protein gene *repA*,
and transposase genes are located next to *wtsF* (*dspF*) (D.L. Coplin et al.,
unpublished). In *E. herbicola,* two virulence determinants *hsvG* and *pthG*, which
have HrpL-dependent promoter motifs, are found in this location on pPATH
(VALINSKY et al. 1998; EZRA et al. 2000). Other differences between the suite of
proteins that travel these closely related Hrp pathways will become apparent as the
Hrp PAIs are fully characterized in these other species.

   One emerging theme with the Hrp PAIs of the plant pathogenic enterobacteria is
that in the regions flanking the *hrp/hrc* clusters, there are virulence-associated genes
that are seemingly unrelated to the Hrp system. For example, *rlsA* encoding a regulator
of levan production is located next to *dspF* of *E. amylovora* (ZHANG and GEIDER 1999).
In *E. stewartii*, flanking the *hrp/hrc* cluster there is an open reading frame (ORF)
encoding a methyl-accepting chemotaxis protein (D.L. Coplin et al. unpublished).
Most strikingly, a DNA region flanking the *hrp/hrc* cluster in *E. chrysanthemi* contains
a phospholipase gene and homologs of hemolysin/adhesin genes and associated ac-
tivator/transporter genes (Fig. 1; KIM et al. 1998b; A. Collmer et al., unpublished).
Whether these examples are anomalies or mark an early trend is an open question.
Nevertheless, a stretch of DNA containing multiple mobile DNA elements and a
mosaic of recombination events as Hrp PAIs often possess would probably be capable
of receiving horizontally transferred DNA unassociated with type III systems. Currently, a genome sequencing project is in progress for *E. chrysanthemi* 3937 by

University of Wisconsin-Madison, The Institute for Genomic Research and University of California-Riverside. Completion of this project would provide valuable information and allow for the identification of all genes involved in the Hrp pathogenicity and the full tally of PAIs in the genome.

2.3 Hrp PAIs of *P. syringae* Pathovars Have a Tripartite Mosaic Structure

The Hrp PAI of *P. syringae* is located in the chromosome and has a tripartite mosaic structure (Fig. 1; COLLMER et al. 2000). Near its center are the conserved *hrp/hrc* genes. These genes have been sequenced in at least three different *P. syringae* strains (*P. s. tomato* DC3000 and *P. s. syringae* strains B728a and 61) where they are conserved and arranged with similar operon structure. To the right of the *hrp/hrc* cluster is another region that is conserved in *P. syringae* pathovars and has been known for years to contain the well-characterized *avr* gene *avrE* and the *hrpW* gene (LORANG and KEEN 1995; CHARKOWSKI et al. 1998). HrpW and a homolog of AvrE, DspE, from *E. amylovora* have been shown to be type III secreted proteins. Several other operons in this region have *hrp/avr* boxes in their promoter regions indicating that they are positively regulated by the sigma factor HrpL and are likely to encode effectors. Because this region appears to encode predominately type III-secreted proteins, it was named the conserved effector locus (CEL) of the *P. syringae* Hrp PAI (Fig. 1). A *P. s. tomato* DC3000 mutant with a large deletion in the CEL maintained its ability to elicit an HR and secrete AvrPto via the type III system but was unable to produce disease symptoms in the tomato, and bacterial multiplication *in planta* was strongly reduced (ALFANO et al. 2000). This suggests that the one or more of the genes that were deleted in the mutant encode effector proteins required for pathogenesis in the tomato.

To the left of the *hrp/hrc* cluster in *P. syringae* is a region that is completely dissimilar between different *P. syringae* pathovars. The DNA sequence similarities stops immediately after the *hrpK* gene on the edge of the *hrp/hrc* cluster. Based on the nucleotide sequence in three different strains of *P. syringae*, the region is rich in effector genes and appears particularly adept at genetic exchange due to the presence of several remnants of mobile DNA. Because of this, the region was named the exchangeable effector locus (EEL) of the *P. syringae* Hrp PAI. In the EEL of *P. s. syringae* 61 is the gene *hopPsyA*, which was shown to act as an *avr* gene on tobacco and encode a protein secreted by the *P. syringae* Hrp system (ALFANO et al. 1997; VAN DIJK et al. 1999). The EEL of *P. s. syringae* B728a contains ORFs with predicted products that share similarity to known Avr proteins from other plant pathogens (Fig. 1). The *P. s. tomato* DC3000 EEL contains several ORFs that have *hrp/avr* boxes and one ORF that has been shown to encode a protein that is secreted via the type III pathway (J.R. Alfano et al. unpublished data) (Fig. 1). A *P. s. tomato* DC3000 EEL deletion mutant was only slightly affected in its ability to grow in tomato plants (ALFANO et al. 2000). Thus, the *P. syringae* Hrp PAI consists of a conserved set of *hrp/hrc* genes that encode the type III apparatus, a conserved

CEL rich in effector genes, and a variable EEL, also rich in effector genes, which may represent a fluid region of the Hrp PAI seemingly poised for genetic recombination. To a certain extent the G + C content supports this because the EEL has a significantly lower G + C content than the rest of the Hrp PAI, suggesting that it was acquired sometime after the acquisition of the *hrp/hrc* cluster and the CEL. The complete genome sequence of *P. s. tomato* DC3000 is near completion as part of a U.S.-funded project to study the functional genomics of the *P. s. tomato* DC3000-tomato pathosystem. This will greatly facilitate the isolation of all genes related to the Hrp system and will allow a better understanding *P. syringae* pathogenesis.

2.4 *hrp/hrc* Gene Clusters of *R. solanacearum* and *Xanthomonas* Species

R. solanacearum and *Xanthomonas* species possess *hrp/hrc* gene clusters almost identical to each other. The *hrp/hrc* cluster of *X. campestris* pv. *vesicatoria* 85-10 is located in the main chromosome and that of *R. solanacearum* GMI1000 on a megaplasmid (BONAS 1994; BOUCHER et al. 1992). *R. solanacearum* belongs to the β-subdivision of proteobacteria, while the genus *Xanthomonas* belongs to the γ-subdivision. This observation suggests that at least one of these *hrp/hrc* clusters might have been horizontally transferred. The *hrp/hrc* gene cluster of *R. solanacearum* has been extensively characterized (Fig. 1; for recent papers, see ALDON et al. 2000; GUENERON et al. 2000; VAN GIJSEGEM et al. 2000). Unlike the other plant pathogens that have a type III system, *R. solanacearum* is not known to contain any genes with homology to *avr* genes although it does have *popA,* which encodes a type III-secreted protein (ARLAT et al. 1994). Because the indirect evidence for translocation of Hop/Avr proteins into plant cells is based on the induction of an *avr/R* gene-dependent HR, it is unclear which *R. solanacearum* proteins are delivered into plant cells. Nonetheless, two proteins secreted in culture via the *R. solanacearum* type III system are good candidates to act inside plant cells: PopB contains functional nuclear localization signals and PopC contains leucine-rich repeats (LRR) that match the consensus LRRs found in plant resistance proteins (GUENERON et al. 2000). An area that researchers studying the *R. solanacearum* type III system have made significant progress on is the contact-dependent nature of transcription of *hrp/hrc* genes. The transcription of several *hrp/hrc* genes is induced when the bacteria are co-cultured with plant suspension cells, and this induction is dependent on the putative sensor protein PrhA (MARENDA et al. 1998; ALDON et al. 2000). The genes encoding PrhA, PopB, and PopC are located flanking the *hrp/hrc* cluster and other type III-associated genes will probably be discovered in these flanking regions. Even though the region associated with the type III cluster in *R. solanacearum* has not been completely characterized, it is likely that this region represents a bona fide PAI. The complete genome sequence of *R. solanacearum* GMI1000 has been determined (C. Boucher et al. unpublished; home page: http://sequence.toulouse.inra.fr/R.solanacearum). Undoubtedly, the number of PAIs present in the genome of *R. solanacearum* will be revealed when the nucleotide sequence of the genome is reported.

In *X. campestris* pv. *vesicatoria*, *hrp/hrc* genes are clustered in a ca. 23-kb region of the chromosome (Fig. 1; BONAS 1994). The flanking regions of the *hrp/hrc* cluster in *X. c. vesicatoria* have not been completely characterized. A recent report indicated that there is at least one gene flanking the *hrp/hrc* cluster that encodes a type III-secreted protein. *hrpF* is located to the right of the *hrp/hrc* cluster in *X. c. vesicatoria* 85-10 and encodes a protein that is secreted in culture and required for translocation of another type III-secreted protein, AvrBs3, into plant cells (ROSSIER et al. 2000). In addition, one gene unique to group II *hrp/hrc* clusters, HrpB2, is secreted via the type III pathway, and its secretion is required for the type III secretion in culture of other proteins (ROSSIER et al. 2000). Other proteins secreted via the type III system of *X. c. vesicatoria* are the Avr proteins AvrBs2 and AvrRxv (MUDGETT et al. 2000; ROSSIER et al. 1999).

Analysis of DNA adjacent to the *hrp/hrc* cluster in the rice pathogen *X. oryzae* pv. *oryzae* identified several genes likely to encode type III-secreted proteins (ZHU et al. 2000b). *hpa1* and *hpa2* (for *hrp*-associated) are located to the left of the *hrp/hrc* cluster's *hrpA* in *X. o. oryzae*. *hpa1* shares characteristics with PopA and other harpins from several plant pathogens, which appear to act as extracellular helper proteins. *hpa2* encodes a lysozyme-like protein found in type III secretion systems, including that of *P. syringae* and *E. chrysanthemi* (ALFANO et al. 2000; A. Collmer et al., unpublished), as well as other secretion systems in gram-negative bacteria and is predicted to act in the periplasm (MUSHEGIAN et al. 1996; ZHU et al. 2000b). Also associated with this region is an IS element, although it may not be responsible for integration of *hpa2* or the *hrp/hrc* cluster (ZHU et al. 2000b). On the other side of the *hrp/hrc* cluster in *X. o. oryzae* between *hpaB* and *hrpF* lie IS elements and transposase genes (S. Heu et al., unpublished; Genbank accession no. AB045312). Next to *hrpF* is an ORF similar to *popC* of *R. solanacearum* and other genes containing LRRs reminiscent of plant disease-resistance proteins (S. Heu et al., unpublished). The fact that multiple LRR-containing proteins are now known to be associated with group II Hrp systems suggests that *Xanthomonas* spp. and *R. solanacearum* use proteins to directly interact with R proteins inside plant cells to confound the plant-defense response. Nucleotide sequences of the corresponding regions in *X. c.* pv. *glycines* identified ORFs similar to *Brucella suis vir* genes, *Xanthomonas* avirulence genes of the *avrBs3* family, and transposase genes, as well as orthologs of *hpa2* and *popC* (S. Heu et al., unpublished; B.K. Park and I. Hwang, unpublished). Further characterization of these regions flanking the *hrp/hrc* cluster will likely reveal genes that encode other type III-secreted products and continue to compile the evidence suggesting that this represents a PAI. Presently, there are several genome projects on xanthomonads. The genomes of *X. axonopodis* pv. *citri*, a pathogen of citrus trees, and two more *Xanthomonas* strains are being sequenced by the Organization for Nucleotide Sequencing and Analysis (ONSA) (homepage: http://genoma4.iq.usp.br/xanthomonas/) in São Paulo, Brazil, and a genome project is under way on *X. c. campestris* by the Chinese Academy of the Sciences. Also in Korea and in Japan, genome-sequencing efforts are in progress for strains of *X. o. oryzae*. Comparative genomics on multiple xanthomonads will greatly enhance the understanding of its pathogenesis and help identify PAIs and other virulence associated loci.

3 Avirulence Gene Pathogenicity Islets

3.1 *avr* Genes Are Often Associated with Mobile Elements

Over 40 *avr* genes have been isolated from different bacterial plant pathogens, especially *P. syringae* pathovars and *Xanthomonas* species (DANGL 1994; LEACH and WHITE 1996; VIVIAN and GIBBON 1997). Although expression of many *avr* genes is induced by *hrp* regulatory genes, and several Avr proteins are secreted via the type III protein secretion machine, only a few *avr* or *avr*-like genes are physi-

Table 2. Association of virulence/avirulence effector genes with sequences of mobile elements

Name	Source organism	Mobile sequence element	Reference[b]
avrA	*P. syringae* pv. *glycinea*	Transposable element	KIM et al. 1998
avrB	*P. syringae* pv. *glycinea*	Transposable element	KIM et al. 1998
avrC	*P. syringae* pv. *glycinea*	Plasmid, transposable element	KIM et al. 1998
avrD	*P. syringae* pv. *glycinea*, pv. *lachrymans*, pv. *phaseolicola*, pv. *tomato*	Plasmid	KOBAYASHI et al. 1989; YUCEL et al. 1994a
avrE	*P. syringae* pv. *tomato*	Hrp PAI	ALFANO et al. 2000
avrPphB	*P. syringae* pv. *phaseolicola*	PAI	JACKSON et al. 2000
avrPphC	*P. syringae* pv. *phaseolicola*	Plasmid, transposable element	YUCEL et al. 1994b; KIM et al. 1998
avrPphE	*P. syringae* pv. *phaseolicola*	Hrp PAI	GenBank accession no. U16817
avrPphF	*P. syringae* pv. *phaseolicola*	Plasmid, PAI	TSIAMIS et al. 2000
avrPpiA	*P. syringae* pv. *pisi*	Plasmid, transposable element, bacteriophage	GIBBON et al. 1997; KIM et al. 1998; ARNOLD et al. 2000
avrPpiB	*P. syringae* pv. *pisi*	Plasmid	COURNOYER et al. 1995
avrPto	*P. syringae* pv. *tomato*	Bacteriophage	KIM et al. 1998
avrRps4	*P. syringae* pv. *pisi*	Plasmid	HINSCH and STASKAWICZ 1996
avrRpm1	*P. syringae* pv. *maculicola*	Plasmid, transposable element	KIM et al. 1998
dspE	*E. amylovora*	Hrp PAI	Kim and Beer submitted
hopPsyA (*hrmA*)	*P. syringae* pv. *syringae*	Hrp PAI	ALFANO et al. 2000
hsvG	*E. herbicola* pv. *gypsophilae*, pv. *betae*	Plasmid, transposable element	VALINSKY et al. 1998
psvA	*P. syringae* pv. *eriobotryae*	Plasmid, transposable element	KAMIUNTEN 1999
pthG	*E. herbicola* pv. *gypsophilae*	Plasmid	EZRA et al. 2000
virPphA	*P. syringae* pv. *phaseolicola*	Plasmid, PAI	JACKSON et al. 1999
avrBs3[a]	*X. campestris* pv. *vesicatoria*	Plasmid, inverted repeat	BONAS et al. 1989
avrXv4	*X. campestris* pv. *vesicatoria*	Bacteriophage	GenBank accession no. AF221058

[a] Members of the *avrBs3* family of virulence/avirulence genes are widely distributed, usually in multiple copies, among pathovars of *Xanthomonas* species (LEACH and WHITE 1996).
[b] References that suggest the association of specific gene with mobile sequence elements, not necessarily original reports of each gene.

cally linked to *hrp* genes (BONAS and VAN DEN ACKERVEKEN 1999; WHITE et al. 2000). Instead, many *avr* genes are located in different chromosomal loci or are plasmid-borne, and there is an abundance of evidence that they are associated with mobile DNA and have been horizontally transferred between bacteria (Table 2; LEACH and WHITE 1996; KIM et al. 1998a; GABRIEL 1999).

3.2 *P. syringae avr* Genes Often Accumulate to Form Unstable Clusters of Pathogenicity Islets

Most of the cloned *avr* genes of *P. syringae* have significantly lower G + C contents (40%–52%) than those of the *P. syringae* genome (59%–61%) and are associated with plasmids or sequences similar to bacteriophages or transposable elements IS*51*, IS*801*, and Tn*501*, suggesting relatively recent introduction and frequent lateral transfer (KIM et al. 1998a). For example, the 154-kb plasmid pAV511 in *P. syringae* pv. *phaseolicola* race 7 strain 1449B contains three known *avr* genes (*avrD*, *avrPphC*, and *avrPphF*), and three potential virulence genes (*vir*) in a 30-kb region (JACKSON et al. 1999). Because there were also IS*100* and Tn*501* sequences in the vicinity and a G + C content lower than expected for *P. syringae*, the researchers described this as a plasmid-borne PAI (JACKSON et al. 1999). Interestingly, one of the *vir* genes within the PAI, *virPphA*, is capable of suppressing the HR induced by resident Avr proteins, which was revealed when typically susceptible plants became resistant when infected with a *P. s. phaeolicola virPphA* mutant (JACKSON et al. 1999). Another *avr* gene in this PAI, *avrPphF*, acts as an avirulence gene on certain plants when the bacterial strain lacks another *avr* gene, *avrPphC*, normally on the pAV511 plasmid (TSIAMIS et al. 2000). Because *avrPphC* encodes an "antidote" of sorts that prevents recognition of the *avrPphF* gene product in plants that can normally perceive it, it makes evolutionary sense that these two virulence genes would be horizontally transferred together.

There have been several examples of rapid conversion of an avirulent strain into a virulent one due to inactivation of an *avr* gene or loss of a host plasmid (LEACH and WHITE 1996). Race change may also occur due to a deletion of a chromosomally encoded *avr* gene. An intriguing example of this is the sponta-neous loss of a region ca. 40kb containing *avrPphB* in *P. syringae* pv. *phaseolicola* race 4 strain 1302A, which resulted in an extended host range (JACKSON et al. 2000). Sequence analysis of the junctions of the deleted region indicated that the region in strain 1302A was inserted into a tRNA^{Lys} gene (JACKSON et al. 2000). Another recent example of the mobility/instability of *avr* genes is *avrPpiA1*, which is an unstable *avr* gene present in certain races of *P. s. pisi* and is flanked by sequences with similarity to bacteriophages and transposases (ARNOLD et al. 2000). The EEL of the *P. syringae* Hrp PAI is another region of the genome associated with *avr* genes that appears to be a hot spot for recombination (ALFANO et al. 2000). These loci begin immediately downstream of the conserved *hrpK* gene and are dissimilar among closely related strains of *P. syringae*. The EEL encode diverse candidate effector genes, including *hopPsyA* (*hrmA*) in

P. s. syringae 61 and homologs of *avrPphE* and the *avrB/avrC* and *avrRxv/yopJ* in *P. s. syringae* B728a.

3.3 The *avrBs3/pthA* Family of *avr* Genes in *Xanthomonas* Species

avr genes of the large *avrBs3* family of *Xanthomonas* spp. are frequently flanked by repeat elements immediately outside of the coding region and are reminiscent of gene cassettes (RECCHIA and HALL 1995). The *avrBs3* family genes tend to accumulate in a single location, possibly either by repeated duplication or homologous recombination between the repeat elements and may undergo frequent rearrangement. A notable example is *avrBs3* homologs in *X. campestris* pv. *malvacearum* strain H. In this strain, at least six genes are tightly linked on a 90-kb plasmid (DE FEYTER and GABRIEL 1991), and spontaneous race-change mutants with deleted *avr* genes have been isolated (DE FEYTER et al. 1993).

4 Phytotoxin Gene Clusters

4.1 Phytotoxins Are Virulence Factors that Induce Chlorotic or Necrotic Symptoms

Phytotoxins are products of plant pathogens that influence the course of disease development or symptom production and are generally thought of as virulence factors. Most bacterial phytotoxins lack host specificity and often increase disease severity. Among the best-characterized phytotoxins are those produced by *P. syringae*. The most intensively studied *P. syringae* phytotoxins include the lipodepsipeptide toxins syringomycin and syringopeptin, coronatine (COR), phaseolotoxin, and tabtoxin (BENDER et al. 1999). Lipodepsipeptide toxins form pores in the plasma membrane causing necrotic lesions; COR functions partly as a mimic of the phytohormone methyl jasmonate, a compound that acts as an inducer of the wound-inducible octadecanoid signaling pathway; phaseolotoxin functions by inhibiting ornithine carbamoyltransferase, a critical enzyme in the urea cycle and tabtoxin acts by inhibiting glutamine synthetase, which prevents the assimilation of ammonia by the plant (BENDER et al. 1999). COR, tabtoxin, and phaseolotoxin are examples of phytotoxins that produce chlorotic symptoms. Most bacterial toxins are secondary metabolites of common metabolic pathways. For example, tabtoxin is made from byproducts of the lysine biosynthetic pathway. Thus, many of the genes required for phytotoxin production are housekeeping genes not likely to be horizontally transferred. However, the clustering of the genes involved in syringomycin, syringopeptin, and coronative biosynthesis would allow them to be horizontally transferred if a mechanism for mobility was available. The coronatine biosynthesis gene cluster is associated with IS elements and is carried on a self-transmissible plasmid in several pathovars of *P. syringae* (ALARCÓN-CHAIDEZ et al. 1999). Recent progress on research on the gram-positive plant pathogenic *Streptomyces* species indicate that they carry a cluster of genes that encodes for the production of a cyclic dipeptide phytotoxin, called thaxtomin, which appears to be horizontally transferred (HEALY et al. 1999). The coronatine and thaxtomin gene clusters are described in more detail in Sects. 4.2 and 4.3.

4.2 The Phytotoxin Coronatine PAI of *P. syringae* Carried on a Virulence Plasmid

COR consists of two distinct structural components: (1) the polyketide coronafacic acid (CFA) and (2) coronamic acid (CMA), an ethylcyclopropyl amino acid derived from isoleucine (BENDER et al. 1999). In *P. syringae* pv. *glycinea* PG4180, the COR biosynthetic genes are carried on a 90-kb plasmid designated p4180A. The 32.8-kb COR gene cluster contains two distinct regions, which encode the structural genes for CMA and CFA biosynthesis, and are separated by a 3.4-kb regulatory region. Two lines of evidence suggest that the COR gene cluster present on p4180A may be a PAI: Multiple IS elements including IS*51*, IS*801*, IS*870*, and IS*1240* flank the COR gene cluster (ALARCÓN-CHAIDEZ et al. 1999); and the COR gene cluster may also be chromosomally encoded in *P. syringae* pv. *maculicola* (CUPPELS and AINSWORTH 1995). The acquisition of the CMA and CFA structural gene clusters probably occurred independently, since the G+C content in these regions differ (55% for CFA vs. 65% for CFA) and IS*870*-like elements that flank them show little nucleotide identity (ALARCÓN-CHAIDEZ et al. 1999).

4.3 The *nec1* and Thaxtomin Gene Clusters of Plant Pathogenic *Streptomyces* Appear to be Horizontally Transferred

Streptomyces spp. are gram-positive soil inhabitants that produce a wide array of secondary metabolites. Out of the hundreds of *Streptomyces* spp. described, four are recognized to be pathogenic to plants (LORIA et al. 1997). A gene from pathogenic *S. scabies* called *nec1* enables non-pathogen *S. lividans* to colonize and necrotize potato tubers. *nec1* is linked to a transposase pseudogene and to a functional IS element and is also present in other plant-pathogenic *Streptomyces* spp. (BUKHALID and LORIA 1997; BUKHALID et al. 1998; HEALY et al. 1999). The G+C content of *nec1*, together with the atypical codon bias, suggests that this gene was introduced from another taxon. Genes required for synthesis of the phytotoxin thaxtomin have been cloned from *S. acidiscabies*, where they are linked to a copy of IS*1629*, suggesting a role for IS*1629* in the horizontal transfer of these virulence genes (HEALY et al. 2000).

5 Genes for Synthesis of Plant Hormones

5.1 *Agrobacterium* Virulence Plasmids and Interkingdom Gene Transfer

It has been known for over 20 years that the bacterial plant pathogen *Agrobacterium tumefaciens* can deliver bacterial DNA into plant cells, where it stably integrates into the genome (CHILTON et al. 1977). By incorporating DNA fragments into plant chromosomes, *Agrobacterium* spp. transform plant cells into "mini-factories" that synthesize an *Agrobacterium*-preferred carbon source called opines and, in doing so, cause the plant to form neoplastic growths called crown galls (WINANS 1992; ZAMBRYSKI 1992). Interestingly, *A. tumefaciens* has recently been shown to be capable of stably transforming several types of human cells (KUNIK et al. 2001). The genetic element responsible for transformation is an extra-chromosomal element called the Ti (for tumor-inducing) plasmid. The Ti plasmid carries a segment of DNA that is transferred into plant cells called transferred DNA (T-DNA), which encodes proteins required for phytohormone and opine synthesis genes. The Ti plasmid also carries the *vir* region, which encodes all the proteins needed for T-DNA processing and translocation, *tra/trb* genes for conjugal plasmid transfer, and gene sets for opine catabolism and uptake (ZHU et al. 2000a). T-DNA transfer is carried out by a protein-delivery system (type IV secretion; CHRISTIE 1997), which is encoded by the *virB* operon, which resembles conjugal transfer systems. The region containing the *vir* genes and T-DNA has sequences similar to various IS elements indicating recombination has occurred in these regions, possibly introducing new genes to the plasmid. One indication that the Ti plasmid has acquired additional genes via horizontal transfer is that an opine-catabolic plasmid from non-pathogenic *A. radiobacter* strains lacks detectable homology with *vir* genes or T-DNA (CLARE et al. 1990). These features suggest that the *vir* region of the Ti plasmid may constitute a PAI. There is precedence for type IV genes existing within PAIs given that they are located in the *cag* PAI in *Helicobacter pylori* (COVACCI et al. 1999).

5.2 Phytohormone Genes of *P. syringae* and *E. herbicola* Are Often Plasmid-Borne and Linked to Transposable Elements

Certain bacteria have the ability to produce plant hormones. The plant-growth regulator indole-3-acetic acid (IAA; auxin) is produced by many plant-associated bacteria (COSTACURTA and VANDERLEYDEN 1995; PATTEN and GLICK 1996), and it has a role in virulence in some pathogenic strains of *P. syringae* and *E. herbicola* (SILVERSTONE et al. 1993; SOBY et al. 1994; MANULIS et al. 1998). These bacteria also occasionally carry genes for synthesis of cytokinins that induce the hyperplasia associated with gall production. Production of another hormone, ethylene, by several pathovars of *P. syringae* has been established (WEINGART and VÖKSCH 1997). Several features of the phytohormone genes in *P. syringae* and *E. herbicola* suggest that they appear to have undergone horizontal transfer and that some of them may be viewed as PAIs. For example, the genes for synthesis of IAA and cytokinin in *P. syringae* and *E. herbicola* are highly similar to the corresponding genes in *A. tumefaciens* (YAMADA et al. 1985; POWELL and MORRIS 1986; LICHTER et al. 1995). Moreover, the genes for IAA synthesis or modification enzymes can be either plasmid-borne or chromosomally encoded (GLICKMANN et al. 1998). Finally, sequences similar to transposable elements often flank bacterial genes that encode proteins involved in plant hormone biosynthesis (J.F. Kim, unpublished observation). Thus, the apparent mobility of these gene clusters, their location on either plasmids or chromosomes, and their association with mobile DNA suggest that they have been exchanged between bacteria via horizontal transfer.

5.3 A Linear Plasmid from *Rhodococcus fascians* Carries a Cytokinin Synthesis Gene

The gram-positive bacterium *Rhodococcus fascians* incites the proliferation of plant growth, causing the plant to develop various malformations or fasciations. The most typical malformation is the horizontal spreading of short roots at the soil interface of infected plants known as leafy galls (VEREECKE et al. 2000). Genes involved in pathogenicity of *R. fascians* strain D188 were shown to be located on a large, conjugative, linear plasmid pFiD188 (CRESPI et al. 1992). Random mutagenesis of the pFiD188 plasmid identified three virulence loci called *fas* loci for *fas*ciation (GOETHALS et al. 2001). The best-characterized *fas* locus consists of a six-gene operon. The key genes in the operon are a cytochrome P450 gene and an isopentenyl transferase (*ipt*) gene. The *ipt* gene is homologous to *ipt* genes of other plant pathogens and involved in the biosynthesis of a cytokinin precursor (CRESPI et al. 1992, 1994). Two other virulence loci located on the plasmid are *hyp* and *att*: mutations in the *hyp* locus result in hypervirulent mutants, whereas mutants with mutations in the *att* locus display attenuated virulence phenotypes. A regulatory gene, *fasR*, which encodes a positive regulatory protein belonging to the AraC family, is required for *fas* gene expression (TEMMERMAN et al. 2000).

6 Pathogenicity Genes in the *Xylella fastidiosa* Genome

Xylella fastidiosa is a fastidious vascular pathogen, which causes citrus variegated chlorosis, a serious disease in citrus, and a variety of other diseases on grapevine, oleander, almond and many other plants. The pathogen is transmitted and introduced into plants by leafhopper insects. The 2.7-Mb genome sequence of a citrus pathogenic clone *X. fastidiosa* 9a5c has been recently completed, marking the first time a plant pathogenic bacterial genome has been sequenced (SIMPSON et al. 2000; home page: http://aeg.lbi.ic.unicamp.br/xf/). Although closely related to the genus

Xanthomonas, the bacterium does not have a type III secretion system encoded by *hrp/hrc* genes. However, the genome does contain numerous genes implicated in pathogenicity. For example, genes encoding type I and type II secretion systems and expolysaccharide production are present. The recent reviews by Dow and DANIELS (2000) and KEEN et al. (2000) nicely cover the implications the *Xylella* genome sequence has on plant pathogenicity. Several other strains of *Xylella* have also been sequenced, providing an opportunity to compare complete genomes of the same bacterial species for insights into the different diseases caused by this pathogen.

7 Conclusions

It is an exciting time for scientists who are studying evolution of bacterial plant pathogenicity. During the last few years, numerous cases of pathogenicity or virulence genes residing in PAIs have been reported for bacterial plant pathogens. It is becoming clear that the number of identified PAIs will increase as more genes are sequenced and characterized. Indeed, the discovery of PAIs will accelerate as more genome projects are completed for plant pathogenic bacteria. Further efforts on elucidating mechanisms, host-ranges, and frequencies of horizontal transfer of PAIs and virulence plasmids, as well as detailed analysis of the contribution of each pathogenicity factor to virulence, would help reconstruct the evolutionary events that allowed plant pathogenicity to develop. Moreover, by combining molecular biological techniques with the new functional genomic technologies, scientists have an excellent opportunity to make major strides in understanding the nature of bacterial pathogenicity of plants with the long-term goal of improving the ability of plants to defend themselves against bacteria.

Acknowledgement. We thank Steven V. Beer, Christian Boucher, Alan Collmer, David L. Coplin, Sunggi Heu, Ingyu Hwang, Byoung Keun Park for kindly providing the results of their work prior to publication. We regret that many of the significant papers are not discussed due to space limitation.

References

Agrios GN (1997) Plant Pathology. Academic Press, New York
Alarcón-Chaidez FJ, Penaloza-Vazquez A, Ullrich M, Bender CL (1999) Characterization of plasmids encoding the phytotoxin coronatine in *Pseudomonas syringae*. Plasmid 42:210–220
Aldon D, Brito B, Boucher C, Genin S (2000) A bacterial sensor of plant cell contact controls the transcriptional induction of *Ralstonia solanacearum* pathogenicity genes. EMBO J 19:2304–2314
Alfano JR, Collmer A (1996) Bacterial pathogens in plants: life up against the wall. Plant Cell 8: 1683–1698
Alfano JR, Collmer A (1997) The type III (Hrp) secretion pathway of plant pathogenic bacteria: trafficking harpins, Avr proteins, and death. J Bacteriol 179:5655–5662

Alfano JR, Kim H-S, Delaney TP, Collmer A (1997) Evidence that the *Pseudomonas syringae* pv. *syringae* *hrp*-linked *hrmA* gene encodes an Avr-like protein that acts in an *hrp*-dependent manner within tobacco cells. Mol Plant Microbe Interact 10:580–588

Alfano JR, Charkowski AO, Deng WL, Badel JL, Petnicki-Ocwieja T, van Dijk K, Collmer A (2000) The *Pseudomonas syringae* Hrp pathogenicity island has a tripartite mosaic structure composed of a cluster of type III secretion genes bounded by exchangeable effector and conserved effector loci that contribute to parasitic fitness and pathogenicity in plants. Proc Natl Acad Sci USA 97:4856–4861

Arlat M, Van Gijsegem F, Huet JC, Pernollet JC, Boucher CA (1994) PopA1, a protein which induces a hypersensitivity-like response on specific Petunia genotypes, is secreted via the Hrp pathway of *Pseudomonas solanacearum*. EMBO J 13:543–553

Arnold DL, Jackson RW, Vivian A (2000) Evidence for the mobility of an avirulence gene, *avrPpiA1*, between the chromosome and plasmids of races of *Pseudomonas syringae* pv. *pisi*. Mol Plant Pathol 1:195–199

Baker B, Zambryski P, Staskawicz B, Dinesh-Kumar SP (1997) Signaling in plant-microbe interactions. Science 276:726–733

Bender CL, Alarcon-Chaidez F, Gross DC (1999) *Pseudomonas syringae* phytotoxins: mode of action, regulation, and biosynthesis by peptide and polyketide synthetases. Microbiol Mol Biol Rev 63:266–292

Bogdanove AJ, Beer SV, Bonas U, Boucher CA, Collmer A, Coplin DL, Cornelis GR, Huang H-C, Hutcheson SW, Panopoulos NJ, Van Gijsegem F (1996) Unified nomenclature for broadly conserved *hrp* genes of phytopathogenic bacteria. Mol Microbiol 20:681–683

Bogdanove AJ, Kim JF, Wei Z, Kolchinsky P, Charkowski AO, Conlin AK, Collmer A, Beer SV (1998) Homology and functional similarity of an *hrp*-linked pathogenicity locus, *dspEF*, of *Erwinia amylovora* and the avirulence locus *avrE* of *Pseudomonas syringae* pathovar *tomato*. Proc Natl Acad Sci USA 95:1325–1330

Bonas U (1994) *hrp* genes of phytopathogenic bacteria. Curr Top Microbiol Immunol 192:79–98

Bonas U, Van den Ackerveken G (1999) Gene-for-gene interactions: bacterial avirulence proteins specify plant disease resistance. Curr Opin Microbiol 2:94–98

Bonas U, Stall RE, Staskawicz B (1989) Genetic and structural characterization of the avirulence gene *avrBs3* from *Xanthomonas campestris* pv. *vesicatoria*. Mol Gen Genet 218:127–136

Boucher CA, Gough CL, Arlat M (1992) Molecular genetics of pathogenicity determinants of *Pseudomonas solanacearum*, with special emphasis on *hrp* genes. Annu Rev Phytopathol 30:443–461

Bukhalid RA, Loria R (1997) Cloning and expression of a gene from *Streptomyces scabies* encoding a putative pathogenicity factor. J Bacteriol 179:7776–7783

Bukhalid RA, Chung SY, Loria R (1998) *nec1*, a gene conferring a necrogenic phenotype, is conserved in plant-pathogenic *Streptomyces* spp. and linked to a transposase pseudogene. Mol Plant Microbe Interact 11:960–967

Charkowski AO, Alfano JR, Preston G, Yuan J, He SY, Collmer A (1998) The *Pseudomonas syringae* pv. *tomato* HrpW protein has domains similar to harpins and pectate lyases and can elicit the plant hypersensitive response and bind to pectate. J Bacteriol 180:5211–5217

Chilton M-D, Drummond MH, Merlo DJ, Sciaky D, Montoya AL, Gordon MP, Nester EW (1977) Stable incorporation of plasmid DNA into higher plant cells: the molecular basis of crown gall tumorigenesis. Cell 11:263–271

Christie PJ (1997) *Agrobacterium tumefaciens* T-complex transport apparatus: a paradigm for a new family of multifunctional transporters in eubacteria. J Bacteriol 179:3085–3094

Clare BG, Kerr A, Jones DA (1990) Characteristics of the nopaline catabolic plasmid in *Agrobacterium* strains K84 and K1026 used for biological control of crown gall disease. Plasmid 23:126–137

Collmer A, Badel JL, Charkowski AO, Deng WL, Fouts DE, Ramos AR, Rehm AH, Anderson DM, Schneewind O, van Dijk K, Alfano JR (2000) *Pseudomonas syringae* Hrp type III secretion system and effector proteins. Proc Natl Acad Sci USA 97:8770–8777

Coplin DL, Frederick RD, Majerczak DR, Tuttle LD (1992) Characterization of a gene cluster that specifies pathogenicity in *Erwinia stewartii*. Mol Plant Microbe Interact 5:81–88

Cornelis GR, Van Gijsegem F (2000) Assembly and function of type III secretory systems. Annu Rev Microbiol 54:734–774

Costacurta A, Vanderleyden J (1995) Synthesis of phytohormones by plant-associated bacteria. Crit Rev Microbiol 21:1–18

Cournoyer B, Sharp JD, Astuto A, Gibbon MJ, Taylor JD, Vivian A (1995) Molecular characterization of the *Pseudomonas syringae* pv. *pisi* plasmid-borne avirulence gene *avrPpiB* which matches the R3 resistance locus in pea. Mol Plant Microbe Interact 8:700–708

Covacci A, Telford JL, Del Giudice G, Parsonnet J, Rappuoli R (1999) *Helicobacter pylori* virulence and genetic geography. Science 284:1328–1333

Crespi M, Messens E, Caplan AB, van Montagu M, Desomer J (1992) Fasciation induction by the phytopathogen *Rhodococcus fascians* depends upon a linear plasmid encoding a cytokinin synthase gene. EMBO J 11:795–804

Crespi M, Vereecke D, Temmerman W, Van Montagu M, Desomer J (1994) The *fas* operon of *Rhodococcus fascians* encodes new genes required for efficient fasciation of host plants. J Bacteriol 176:2492–2501

Cuppels DA, Ainsworth T (1995) Molecular and physiological characterization of *Pseudomonas syringae* pv. tomato and *Pseudomonas syringae* pv. *maculicola* strains that produce the phytotoxin coronatine. Appl Env Microbiol 61:3530–3536

Dangl JL (1994) The enigmatic avirulence genes of phytopathogenic bacteria. Curr Top Microbiol Immunol 192:99–118

De Feyter R, Gabriel DW (1991) At least 6 avirulence genes are clustered on a 90-kilobase plasmid in *Xanthomonas campestris* pv. *malvacearum*. Mol Plant Microbe Interact 4:423–432

De Feyter R, Yang Y, Gabriel DW (1993) Gene-for-genes interactions between cotton *R* genes and *Xanthomonas campestris* pv. *malvacearum avr* genes. Mol Plant Microbe Interact 6:225–237

Dow JM, Daniels MJ (2000) *Xylella* genomics and bacterial pathogenicity to plants. Yeast 17:263–271

Expert D, Enard C, Masclaux C (1996) The role of iron in plant host-pathogen interactions. Trends Microbiol 4:232–237

Ezra D, Barash I, Valinsky L, Manulis S (2000) The dual function in virulence and host range restriction of a gene isolated from the pPATH (Ehg) plasmid of *Erwinia herbicola* pv. *gypsophilae*. Mol Plant Microbe Interact 13:683–692

Freiberg C, Fellay R, Bairoch A, Broughton WJ, Rosenthal A, Perret X (1997) Molecular basis of symbiosis between *Rhizobium* and legumes. Nature 387:394–401

Gabriel DW (1999) Why do pathogens carry avirulence genes? Physiol Mol Plant Pathol 55:205–214

Galán JE, Collmer A (1999) Type III secretion machines: bacterial devices for protein delivery into host cells. Science 284:1322–1328

Genin S, Gough CL, Zischek C, Boucher CA (1992) Evidence that the *hrpB* gene encodes a positive regulator of pathogenicity genes from *Pseudomonas solanacearum*. Mol Microbiol 6:3065–3076

Gibbon MJ, Jenner C, Mur LAJ, Puri N, Mansfield JW, Taylor JD, Vivian A (1997) Avirulence gene *avrPpiA* from *Pseudomonas syringae* pv. *pisi* is not required for full virulence on pea. Physiol Mol Plant Pathol 50:219–236

Glickmann E, Gardan L, Jacquet S, Hussain S, Elasri M, Petit A, Dessaux Y (1998) Auxin production is a common feature of most pathovars of *Pseudomonas syringae*. Mol Plant Microbe Interact 11: 156–162

Goethals K, Vereecke D, Jaziri M, Van Montagu M, Holsters M (2001) Leafy gall formation by *Rhodococcus fascians*. Annu Rev Phytopathol 39:27–52

Gottfert M, Rothlisberger S, Kundig C, Beck C, Marty R, Hennecke H (2001) Potential symbiosis-specific genes uncovered by sequencing a 410-kb DNA region of the *Bradyrhizobium japonicum* chromosome. J Bacteriol 183:1405–1412

Gueneron M, Timmers AC, Boucher C, Arlat M (2000) Two novel proteins, PopB, which has functional nuclear localization signals, and PopC, which has a large leucine-rich repeat domain, are secreted through the *hrp*-secretion apparatus of *Ralstonia solanacearum*. Mol Microbiol 36:261–277

Ham JH, Bauer DW, Fouts DE, Collmer A (1998) A cloned *Erwinia chrysanthemi* Hrp (type III protein secretion) system functions in Escherichia coli to deliver *Pseudomonas syringae* Avr signals to plant cells and to secrete Avr proteins in culture. Proc Natl Acad Sci USA 95:10206–10211

Healy FG, Bukhalid RA, Loria R (1999) Characterization of an insertion sequence element associated with genetically diverse plant pathogenic *Streptomyces* spp. J Bacteriol 181:1562–1568

Healy FG, Wach M, Krasnoff SB, Gibson DM, Loria R (2000) The *txtAB* genes of the plant pathogen *Streptomyces acidiscabies* encode a peptide synthetase required for phytotoxin thaxtomin A production and pathogenicity. Mol Microbiol 38:794–804

Hinsch M, Staskawicz B (1996) Identification of a new *Arabidopsis* disease resistance locus, *RPS4*, and cloning of the corresponding avirulence gene, *avrRps4*, from *Pseudomonas syringae* pv. *pisi*. Mol Plant Microbe Interact 9:55–61

Hirano SS, Upper CD (2000) Bacteria in the leaf ecosystem with emphasis on *Pseudomonas syringae* – a pathogen, ice nucleus, and epiphyte. Microbiol Mol Biol Rev 64:624–653

Hueck CJ (1998) Type III protein secretion systems in bacterial pathogens of animals and plants. Microbiol Mol Biol Rev 62:379–433

Hugouvieux-Cotte-Pattat N, Condemine G, Nasser W, Reverchon S (1996) Regulation of pectinolysis in *Erwinia chrysanthemi*. Annu Rev Microbiol 50:213–257

Jackson RW, Athanassopoulos E, Tsiamis G, Mansfield JW, Sesma A, Arnold DL, Gibbon MJ, Murillo J, Taylor JD, Vivian A (1999) Identification of a pathogenicity island, which contains genes for virulence and avirulence, on a large native plasmid in the bean pathogen *Pseudomonas syringae* pathovar phaseolicola. Proc Natl Acad Sci USA 96:10875–10880

Jackson RW, Mansfield JW, Arnold DL, Sesma A, Paynter CD, Murillo J, Taylor JD, Vivian A (2000) Excision from tRNA genes of a large chromosomal region, carrying *avrPphB*, associated with race change in the bean pathogen, *Pseudomonas syringae* pv. *phaseolicola*. Mol Microbiol 38:186–197

Kamiunten H (1999) Isolation and characterization of virulence gene *psvA* on a plasmid of *Pseudomonas syringae* pv. *eriobotryae*. Ann Phytopathol Soc Jpn 65:501–509

Keen NT (1990) Gene-for-gene complementarity in plant-pathogen interactions. Annu Rev Genet 24:447–463

Keen NT, Korsi Dumenyo C, Yang CH, Cooksey DA (2000) From rags to riches: insights from the first genomic sequence of a plant pathogenic bacterium. Genome Biol 1:REVIEWS1019

Kim JF, Beer SV (1998) HrpW of *Erwinia amylovora*, a new harpin that contains a domain homologous to pectate lyases of a distinct class. J Bacteriol 180:5203–5210

Kim JF, Beer SV (2000) *hrp* genes and harpins of *Erwinia amylovora*: a decade of discovery. In: Vanneste JL (ed) Fire Blight and its Causative Agent, *Erwinia amylovora*. CAB International, Wallingford, UK

Kim JF, Charkowski AO, Alfano JR, Collmer A, Beer SV (1998a) Transposable elements and bacteriophage sequence flanking *Pseudomonas syringae* avirulence genes. Mol Plant Microbe Interact 11:1247–1252

Kim JF, Ham JH, Bauer DW, Collmer A, Beer SV (1998b) The *hrpC* and *hrpN* operons of *Erwinia chrysanthemi* EC16 are flanked by *plcA* and homologs of hemolysin/adhesin genes and accompanying activator/transporter genes. Mol Plant Microbe Interact 11:563–567

Kjemtrup S, Nimchuk Z, Dangl JL (2000) Effector proteins of phytopathogenic bacteria: bifunctional signals in virulence and host recognition. Curr Opin Microbiol 3:73–78

Kobayashi DY, Tamaki SJ, Keen NT (1989) Cloned avirulence genes from the tomato pathogen *Pseudomonas syringae* pv. *tomato* confer cultivar specificity on soybean. Proc Natl Acad Sci USA 86:157–161

Kunik T, Tzfira T, Kapulnik Y, Gafni Y, Dingwall C, Citovsky V (2001) Genetic transformation of HeLa cells by *Agrobacterium*. Proc Natl Acad Sci USA 98:1871–1876

Leach JE, White FF (1996) Bacterial avirulence genes. Annu Rev Phytopathol 34:153–179

Lee IM, Davis RE, Gundersen-Rindal DE (2000) Phytoplasma: phytopathogenic mollicutes. Annu Rev Microbiol 54:221–255

Lichter A, Barash I, Valinsky L, Manulis S (1995) The genes involved in cytokinin biosynthesis in *Erwinia herbicola* pv. *gypsophilae*: characterization and role in gall formation. J Bacteriol 177:4457–4465

Lindgren PB (1997) The role of *hrp* genes during plant-bacterial interactions. Ann Rev Phytopathol 35:129–152

Lorang JM, Keen NT (1995) Characterization of *avr* E from *Pseudomonas syringae* pv. *tomato*: a *hrp*-linked avirulence locus consisting of at least two transcriptional units. Mol Plant Microbe Interact 8:49–57

Loria R, Bukhalid RA, Fry BA, King RR (1997) Plant pathogenicity in the genus *Streptomyces*. Plant Dis 81:836–846

Manulis S, Haviv-Chesner A, Brandl MT, Lindow SE, Barash I (1998) Differential involvement of indole-3-acetic acid biosynthetic pathways in pathogenicity and epiphytic fitness of *Erwinia herbicola* pv. *gypsophilae*. Mol Plant Microbe Interact 11:634–642

Marenda M, Brito B, Callard D, Genin S, Barberis P, Boucher C, Arlat M (1998) PrhA controls a novel regulatory pathway required for the specific induction of *Ralstonia solanacearum hrp* genes in the presence of plant cells. Mol Microbiol 27:437–453

Meinhardt LW, Krishnan HB, Balatti PA, Pueppke SG (1993) Molecular cloning and characterization of a sym plasmid locus that regulates cultivar-specific nodulation of soybean by *Rhizobium fredii* USDA257. Mol Microbiol 9:17–29

Mor H, Manulis S, Zuck M, Nizan R, Coplin DL, Barash I (2001) Genetic organization of the *hrp* gene cluster and *dspAE/BF* operon in *Erwinina herbicola* pv. *gypsophilae*. Mol Plant Microbe Interact 14:431–436

Mudgett MB, Staskawicz BJ (1998) Protein signaling via type III secretion pathways in phytopatogenic bacteria. Curr Opin Microbiol 1:109–114

Mudgett MB, Staskawicz BJ (1999) Characterization of the *Pseudomonas syringae* pv. *tomato* AvrRpt2 protein: demonstration of secretion and processing during bacterial pathogenesis. Mol Microbiol 32:927–941

Mudgett MB, Chesnokova O, Dahlbeck D, Clark ET, Rossier O, Bonas U, Staskawicz BJ (2000) Molecular signals required for type III secretion and translocation of the *Xanthomonas campestris* AvrBs2 protein to pepper plants. Proc Natl Acad Sci USA 97:13324–13329

Mushegian AR, Fullner KJ, Koonin EV, Nester EW (1996) A family of lysozyme-like virulence factors in bacterial pathogens of plants and animals. Proc Natl Acad Sci USA 93:7321–7326

Nizan R, Barash I, Valinsky L, Lichter A, Manulis S (1997) The presence of *hrp* genes on the pathogenicity-associated plasmid of the tumorigenic bacterium *Erwinia herbicola* pv. *gypsophilae*. Mol Plant Microbe Interact 10:677–682

Patten CL, Glick BR (1996) Bacterial biosynthesis of indole-3-acetic acid. Can J Microbiol 42:207–220

Powell GK, Morris RO (1986) Nucleotide sequence and expression of a *Pseudomonas savastanoi* cytokinin biosynthetic gene: homology with *Agrobacterium tumefaciens tmr* and *tzs* loci. Nucleic Acids Res 14:2555–2565

Rainey PB (1999) Adaptation of *Pseudomonas fluorescens* to the plant rhizosphere. Environ Microbiol 1:243–257

Recchia GD, Hall RM (1995) Gene cassettes: a new class of mobile element. Microbiology 141:3015–3027

Rossier O, Wengelnik K, Hahn K, Bonas U (1999) The *Xanthomonas* Hrp type III system secretes proteins from plant and mammalian bacterial pathogens. Proc Natl Acad Sci USA 96:9368–9373

Rossier O, Van den Ackerveken G, Bonas U (2000) HrpB2 and HrpF from *Xanthomonas* are type III-secreted proteins and essential for pathogenicity and recognition by the host plant. Mol Microbiol 38:828–838

Shan L, He P, Zhou JM, Tang X (2000) A cluster of mutations disrupt the avirulence but not the virulence function of AvrPto. Mol Plant Microbe Interact 13:592–598

Silverstone SE, Gilchrist DG, Bostock RM, Kosuge T (1993) The 73-kb pIAA plasmid increases competitive fitness of *Pseudomonas syringae* subspecies *savastanoi* in oleander. Can J Microbiol 39:659–664

Simpson AJ, Reinach FC, Arruda P, Abreu FA, Acencio M, Alvarenga R, Alves LM, Araya JE, Baia GS, Baptista CS, Barros MH, Bonaccorsi ED, Bordin S, Bove JM, Briones MR, Bueno MR, Camargo AA, Camargo LE, Carraro DM, Carrer H, Colauto NB, Colombo C, Costa FF, Costa MC, Costa-Neto CM, Coutinho LL, Cristofani M, Dias-Neto E, Docena C, El-Dorry H, Facincani AP, Ferreira AJ, Ferreira VC, Ferro JA, Fraga JS, Franca SC, Franco MC, Frohme M, Furlan LR, Garnier M, Goldman GH, Goldman MH, Gomes SL, Gruber A, Ho PL, Hoheisel JD, Junqueira ML, Kemper EL, Kitajima JP, Marino CL (2000) The genome sequence of the plant pathogen *Xylella fastidiosa*. Nature 406:151–157

Soby S, Kirkpatrick B, Kosuge T (1994) Characterization of high-frequency deletions in the *iaa*-containing plasmid, pIAA2, of *Pseudomonas syringae* pv. *savastanoi*. Plasmid 31:21–30

Temmerman W, Vereecke D, Dreesen R, Van Montagu M, Holsters M, Goethals K (2000) Leafy gall formation is controlled by *fasR*, an AraC-type regulatory gene in *Rhodococcus fascians*. J Bacteriol 182:5832–5840

Tsiamis G, Mansfield JW, Hockenhull R, Jackson RW, Sesma A, Athanassopoulos E, Bennett MA, Stevens C, Vivian A, Taylor JD, Murillo J (2000) Cultivar-specific avirulence and virulence functions assigned to *avrPphF* in *Pseudomonas syringae* pv. *phaseolicola*, the cause of bean halo-blight disease. EMBO J 19:3204–3214

Valinsky L, Manulis S, Nizan R, Ezra D, Barash I (1998) A pathogenicity gene isolated from the pPATH plasmid of *Erwinia herbicola* pv. *gypsophilae* determines host specificity. Mol Plant Microbe Interact 11:753–762

van Dijk K, Fouts DE, Rehm AH, Hill AR, Collmer A, Alfano JR (1999) The Avr (effector) proteins HrmA (HopPsyA) and AvrPto are secreted in culture from *Pseudomonas syringae* pathovars via the Hrp (type III) protein secretion system in a temperature and pH-sensitive manner. J Bacteriol 181:4790–4797

Van Gijsegem F, Vasse J, Camus JC, Marenda M, Boucher C (2000) *Ralstonia solanacearum* produces *hrp*-dependent pili that are required for PopA secretion but not for attachment of bacteria to plant cells. Mol Microbiol 36:249–260

Vanneste JL (2000) Fire Blight and its Causative Agent, *Erwinia amylovora*. CAB International, Wallingford, UK

Vereecke D, Burssens S, Simon-Mateo C, Inze D, Van Montagu M, Goethals K, Jaziri M (2000) The *Rhodococcus fascians*-plant interaction: morphological traits and biotechnological applications. Planta 210:241–251

Vivian A, Gibbon MJ (1997) Avirulence genes in plant-pathogenic bacteria: signals or weapons? Microbiology 143:693–704

Wei Z-M, Beer SV (1995) hrpL activates Erwinia amylovora hrp gene transcription and is a member of the ECF subfamily of sigma factors. J Bacteriol 177:6201–6210

Wei Z-M, Laby RJ, Zumoff CH, Bauer DW, He SY, Collmer A, Beer SV (1992) Harpin, elicitor of the hypersensitive response produced by the plant pathogen Erwinia amylovora. Science 257:85–88

Weingart H, Vöksch B (1997) Ethylene production by Pseudomonas syringae pathovars in vivo and in planta. Appl Environ Microbiol 63:156–161

Wengelnik K, Bonas U (1996) HrpXv, an AraC-type regulator, activates expression of five of the six loci in the hrp cluster of Xanthomonas campestris pv. vesicatoria. J Bacteriol 178:3462–3469

White FF, Yang B, Johnson LB (2000) Prospects for understanding avirulence gene function. Curr Opin Plant Biol 3:291–298

Winans SC (1992) Two-way chemical signaling in Agrobacterium-plant interactions. Microbiol Rev 56:12–31

Winstanley C, Hales BA, Hart CA (1999) Evidence for the presence in Burkholderia pseudomallei of a type III secretion system-associated gene cluster. J Med Microbiol 48:649–656

Xiao Y, Heu S, Yi J, Lu Y, Hutcheson SW (1994) Identification of a putative alternate sigma factor and characterization of a multicomponent regulatory cascade controlling the expression of Pseudomonas syringae pv. syringae Pss61 hrp and hrmA genes. J Bacteriol 176:1025–1036

Yamada T, Palm CJ, Brooks B, Kosuge T (1985) Nucleotide sequences of the Pseudomonas savastanoi indoleacetic acid genes show homology with Agrobacterium tumefaciens T-DNA. Proc Natl Acad Sci USA 82:6522–6526

Yang B, Zhu W, Johnson LB, White FF (2000) The virulence factor AvrXa7 of Xanthomonas oryzae pv. oryzae is a type III secretion pathway-dependent nuclear-localized double-stranded DNA-binding protein. Proc Natl Acad Sci USA 97:9807–9812

Yucel I, Boyd C, Debnam Q, Keen NT (1994a) Two different classes of avrD alleles occur in pathovars of Pseudomonas syringae. Mol Plant Microbe Interact 7:131–139

Yucel I, Slaymaker D, Boyd C, Murillo J, Buzzell RI, Keen NT (1994b) Avirulence gene avrPphC from Pseudomonas syringae pv. phaseolicola 3121: a plasmid-borne homologue of avrC closely linked to an avrD allele. Mol Plant Microbe Interact 7:677–679

Zambryski P (1992) Chronicles from the Agrobacterium-plant cell DNA transfer story. Annu Rev Plant Physiol Plant Mol Biol 43:465–490

Zhang Y, Geider K (1999) Molecular analysis of the rlsA gene regulating levan production by the fireblight pathogen Erwinia amylovora. Physiol Mol Plant Pathol 54:187–201

Zhu J, Oger PM, Schrammeijer B, Hooykaas PJ, Farrand SK, Winans SC (2000a) The bases of crown gall tumorigenesis. J Bacteriol 182:3885–3895

Zhu W, MaGbanua MM, White FF (2000b) Identification of two novel hrp-associated genes in the hrp gene cluster of Xanthomonas oryzae pv. oryzae. J Bacteriol 182:1844–1853

Genome Structure of Pathogenic Fungi

G. Köhler[1,3], J. Morschhäuser[1], and J. Hacker[2]

1 Introduction

Fungal organisms form a polyphyletic group in the domain Eucarya. They are typical eukaryotes with nuclear membranes, the main difference to Bacteria and Archea. While fungi are in several kingdoms, including Chromista and Protozoa or Fungi, human pathogenic and opportunistic fungi are mostly found in the phylum Oomycota of the Chromista and in the phyla Zygomycota, Ascomycota and Basidiomycota of the Fungi (see Table 1). A recent detailed review published by Guarro and coauthors (Guarro et al. 1999) summarizes the taxonomy of clinically relevant fungi.

[1] Zentrum für Infektionsforschung, Universität Würzburg, Germany
[2] Institut für Molekulare Infektionsbiologie, Universität Würzburg, Germany
[3] Department of Stomatology, University of California San Francisco, 521 Parnassus, Room C-740, San Francisco, Calif. USA 94143-0422, USA

Table 1. Phyla of fungal pathogens in humans

Kingdom	Phylum	Most relevant human pathogenic genera/species
Chromista	Hyphochytriomycota	*Rhinosporidium seeberi*
	Labyrinthulomycota	
	Oomycota	*Phythium insidiosum*
Fungi	Ascomycota	*Pneumocystis carinii*
		Pseudallescheria boydii/Scedosporium spp.
		Sporothrix schenckii
		Chaetomium spp.
		Fusarium spp.
		Cladophialophora spp.
		Cladosporium spp.
		Exophiala spp.
		Phialophora spp.
		Aspergillus spp.
		Penicillium marneffei
		Blastomyces dermatitidis
		Coccidioides immitis
		Paracoccidioides brasiliensis
		Histoplasma capsulatum
		Trichophyton spp.
		Epidermophyton floccosum
		Microsporum spp.
		Candida spp.
	Basidiomycota	*Cryptococcus* spp.
		Trichosporon spp.
		Malassezia spp.
	Chytridiomycota	
	Zygomycota	*Absidia* spp.
		Rhizopus spp.
Protozoa	Acrasiomycota	
	Dictyosteliomycota	
	Myxomycota	
	Plasmodiophoromycota	

The number of fungal species that were accepted by 1995 was approximately 70,000 (HAWKSWORTH 1995); however, it has been estimated that only 5%–7% of the mycobiota have been discovered so far (HAWKSWORTH 1991; SAVAGE 1995). In contrast, only about 3,100 bacteria species are known (SAVAGE 1995). Only a few fungal species (about 150) are pathogens of humans and animals (KWON-CHUNG 1992), but the number of species causing opportunistic infections in immuno-compromised individuals has grown rapidly by a rate of 20 species annually (GUARRO et al. 1999). The emergence of these pathogens will probably continue parallel to the increase of fungal infections per se, due to the expanding population of immunocompromised hosts. Impairment of the host's immune system is not only a consequence of viral infections (e.g., HIV) and neoplastic diseases, it is also caused by intensive treatments and procedures in transplant and cancer patients in modern medicine.

Fungi have a cell wall and are nonmotile (with exceptions) similar to plant cells, however, they are achlorophyllous. Unicellular, multicellular to filamentous absorptive forms can be found that reproduce by sexual or asexual propagules or even by fission. Fungal modes of propagation in a sexual state (teleomorph) and one or more asexual states (anamorphs) have led to a dual nomenclature of fungi because very often the teleomorph and anamorph(s) develop under different conditions with different morphology. For instance, the perfect (teleomorphic) state of the pathogenic fungus *Blastomyces dermatitidis* is *Ajellomyces dermatitidis*. In many cases, however, the teleomorphs of pathogenic fungi have not been discovered, partially due to the fact that they are rarely seen in clinical material, or they have been lost during evolution. Such "fungi imperfecti" are currently classified in the form phylum Deuteromycota, with the majority representing anamorphs of ascomycetous fungi with missing sexual states. In general, classification and identification of fungi have been based on morphological criteria, rather than on biochemical or physiological properties as in bacteria. This phenotypic approach is still very powerful, especially in the clinical setting. Nevertheless, recent cladistic and molecular methods like sequence determination and comparison of ribosomal RNAs are necessary to address the open questions of fungal systematics (e.g., finding teleomorphs) and phylogeny. One noticeable example is the taxonomic position of the opportunistic pathogen *Pneumocystis carinii*, which shares morphological and structural features with both fungi and protozoa. Recent molecular data confirm that *P. carinii* indeed groups with the Ascomycota (EDMAN et al. 1988; TAYLOR et al. 1994). Certainly, molecular approaches will not only help us to draw a natural phylogenetic tree of fungal life, but also have a major impact on the identification of medically and agriculturally important fungi.

With the advent of genome research, molecular studies of physiological, biochemical and especially virulence properties of pathogenic (micro)organisms have entered a new dimension. The genome of the fungus *Saccharomyces cerevisiae* was the first eukaryotic genome sequence to be completed in 1996. Still, this is the only fungal genome sequence publicly available, although the sequence of the opportunistic pathogen *Candida albicans* will be published soon. Many other genome sequences of fungi should follow, since fungi have one trait in common: They are exceptionally diverse with a wide range of metabolic and genetic capabilities encoded in their genomes. This review tries to summarize our current knowledge of the genome structure of pathogenic fungi with special emphasis on the organisms causing infections in humans.

2 *Saccharomyces cerevisiae*: the Apathogenic Paradigm?

2.1 Introduction to *Saccharomyces cerevisiae*

The yeast *Saccharomyces cerevisiae* has been associated with mankind for more than 7,000 years (MORTIMER 2000) because it has been an important component in baking, brewing, distilling and wine making. Typically, this yeast propagates asexually by budding cells with multilateral bud formation (blastoconidia). The sexual life cycle is characterized by the presence of an ascus and ascospore formation; therefore, this fungus is grouped in the Ascomycetes. Under conditions of nitrogen starvation so-called pseudohyphae may be formed, which are filaments of elongated and unseparated blastoconidia (GIMENO et al. 1992). Often the cell-to-cell attachment points in pseudohyphae are constricted.

Despite a few reports on *S. cerevisiae* causing infections in severely immuno-compromised humans, the fungus is generally considered apathogenic (ORIOL et al. 1993; SETHI et al. 1988; TAWFIK et al. 1989).

2.2 The Yeast Genome

Starting in the 1930s, major research activities focused on the genetics of *S. cerevisiae* as a model eukaryotic microorganism. Vast scientific knowledge on eukaryotic cell biology, on cell cycle, signal transduction, gene expression and regulation, as well as genetic manipulation, has been accumulated by studying "the yeast". In 1996 with the publication of the yeast genome, the first eukaryotic genome sequenced to completion, the "genomic revolution" had been initiated. Since then *S. cerevisiae* is the "workhorse" of many ambitious and successful projects in functional genomics (GOFFEAU 2000).

The genome of *S. cerevisiae* (strain αS288 C) is comprised of 13,392-kb nuclear DNA in a haploid set of 16 chromosomes with sizes ranging from 200 to 2,200-kb (MEWES et al. 1997) and 86-kb of mitochondrial DNA (FOURY et al. 1998) (see Fig. 1). Three main databases harboring information on the genome and proteome of this yeast are publicly available on the Internet:

– The MIPS Yeast Genome Database (http://www.mips.biochem.mpg.de/desc/yeast/) at the Munich Information Center for Protein Sequences (MIPS), Munich, Germany (MEWES et al. 1999).
– The *Saccharomyces* Genome Database (http://genome-www.stanford.edu/Saccharomyces/) at Stanford University, Calif., USA.
– The YPD *Saccharomyces cerevisiae* Proteome Databases (http://www.proteome.com/databases/index.html) from Proteome, Inc., Beverly, Mass., USA.

In November 2000 MIPS estimated the number of open reading frames (ORFs) in the nuclear genome of *S. cerevisiae* to be 6,340 and 28 in the mitochondrial genome; 4,363 of these ORFs were known by biochemistry, genetics or homology, and 1,551 were unknown and 448 "questionable". Numbers on ORFs of known or unknown function vary between the aforementioned databases because of different definitions in the sequence annotation process. For instance, YPD counted a total of 6,145 proteins of which 3,751 had been characterized by biochemistry or genetics, 568 were known by homology and 1,826 remained unknown.

Repetitive DNA and Retroelements. The genome of *S. cerevisiae* strain S288c contains several regions with repeated sequences with a total of about 1-Mb. The 100 copies of the 9-kb ribosomal DNA (rDNA) repeat on chromosome XII form the major part, and the rest is constituted of smaller repeats like the Y' elements. Retrotransposons of the five Ty classes are present in copy numbers of 1 (Ty5) to 33

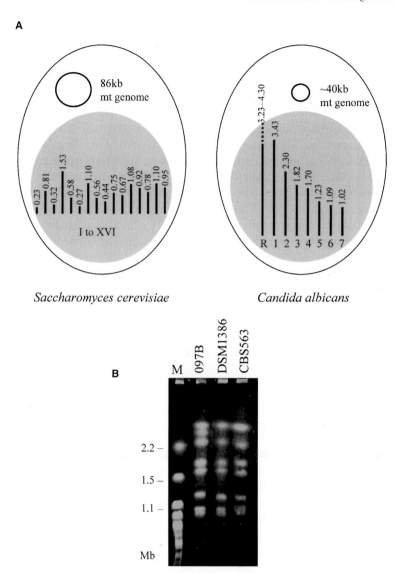

Fig. 1A,B. Comparison of the genomes of *S. cerevisiae* and *C. albicans*. **A** The haploid set of chromosomes in each microorganism and the respective mitochondrial genome is depicted. Vertical numbers show the (rounded) sizes of the chromosomes. The approximately 1-Mb of repeat sequences in *S. cerevisiae* (mainly rDNA repeats on chromosome XII) are not indicated. In *C. albicans* considerable size variation is possible in the R sister chromosomes, which carry the rDNA repeats. **B** Karyotype analysis of three *C. albicans* strains. The chromosomes were separated on a CHEF gel. Strain 097B shows R chromosome size variation. *S. cerevisiae* chromosomes were used as chromosome size markers (*M*). The 2.2-Mb band is chromosome XII containing rDNA repeats. (CHEF analysis courtesy of Axel Lischewsky)

(Ty1) in the αS288 C genome (HANI and FELDMANN 1998). With the exception of chromosome XI, all chromosomes carry Ty elements, which amount to 300-kb of occupied sequence. Long flanking direct repeats, the so-called long terminal repeats (LTRs), are characteristic for retrotransposons of the Ty classes. Former transposition/excision events leave "solo" LTRs in the genome, which lost their function in retrotransposition. These remnants – 268 have been located in the *S. cerevisiae* genome – may modulate adjacent gene expression or may affect genome organization, although probably not to the same extent as the intact retroelements could.

Genome Variation. Intraspecies strain variation has been reported from many fungal species; *S. cerevisiae* is no exception (BALEIRAS COUTO et al. 1996; MORTIMER 2000). Although the genome of this yeast may be relatively stable during laboratory conditions (GASENT-RAMIREZ 1999), genetic recombination events are inherent in mating or might be caused directly or indirectly by the presence of retroelements and repetitive DNA. Recessive heterozygosities in homothallic diploids could be expressed in the new diploids generated by sporulation and mating leading to "genome renewal" (see MORTIMER 2000). The formation of interspecific hybrids in the genus *Saccharomyces* has also been reported. Haploid spores or cells of closely related species are able to mate with each other and form viable zygotes. Even sporulation of these zygotes has been observed; however, the spores are sterile. Interspecific combination may lead to altered ploidy, e.g. hybrids turn tetraploid or aneuploid. In hybrids of phylogenetically less related species, though, one parental chromosome set predominates and only small fragments of the other are retained (MARINONI et al. 1999). If settings are favorable in nature, horizontal gene transfer as the outcome of hybrid formation among *Saccharomyces* species could be an important mechanism in the evolution of this fungus.

2.3 Apathogenic vs. Pathogenic

S. cerevisiae is the best studied eukaryotic organism. Therefore, this yeast's genome sequence is certainly paradigmatic for research on other fungal genomes. However, the probability of extensive gene loss in *S. cerevisiae* during evolution has to be considered as reported by Braun and coworkers (BRAUN et al. 2000), who compared the complete genome sequence of *S. cerevisiae* with sequence data on the more complex ascomycete *Neurospora crassa*. Nevertheless, comparison of the genome of the apathogenic yeast *S. cerevisiae* with genomes of a closely related pathogenic fungus like *Candida albicans* will be important for defining what makes the difference in pathogenicity.

3 *Candida* Species

3.1 Introduction to *Candida*

The complex genus *Candida* is comprised of 163 anamorphic species with teleomorphs in about 13 genera (KURTZMAN and FELL 1998). Nearly 20 species are clinically relevant, *Candida albicans* being the most prominent, followed by *C. glabrata*, *C. tropicalis*, *C. parapsilosis* and *C. krusei*. With the exception of *C. krusei*, all of the aforementioned *Candida* species have no known teleomorph; therefore, they are placed in the Deuteromycetes (LATOUCHE et al. 1997).

3.2 Medical Relevance of *Candida*

Infections in patients with impaired immune systems caused by species of the genus *Candida* have been on the rise since the onset of the AIDS epidemic in the 1980s and the increase of intensive medical care in oncology and transplantation wards. Though the most important fungal pathogen in general is *Candida albicans*, a recent study on nosocomial bloodstream infections showed that other *Candida* species like *C. glabrata*, *C. parapsilosis* and *C. tropicalis* account for 46.8% of the candidemias (EDMOND et al. 1999). This study conducted in 49 U.S. hospitals also shows that *Candida* spp. are the fourth leading cause of nosocomial bloodstream infections, surpassed only by Coagulase-negative staphylococci, *Staphylococcus aureus* and Enterococci.

Most research on the genus *Candida* has been done on *C. albicans*, the most frequently isolated fungal pathogen. In general, *C. albicans* is considered an opportunist, which causes weak to severe infections, depending on the host's immune status. In many normal individuals, this species is commensal and, therefore, does not cause damage. However, a certain predisposition, for example, temporarily acquired by an antibiotic therapy, can lead to (vaginal) candidiasis in hosts with normal immune responses. Much higher prevalence of candidiasis is seen in hosts with impaired immune defenses. The disease spectrum ranges from superficial candidiasis, e.g., oropharyngeal infections and vulvovaginitis, mainly in HIV infected individuals, to deep candidiasis, localized in the gastrointestinal or urinary tract or hematogeneously disseminated, which is a major complication in cancer or transplant patients (KWON-CHUNG and BENNETT 1992; ODDS 1988). Therapeutic intervention against *C. albicans* has been increasingly hampered by the occurrence of resistance to the main antimycotic fluconazole and the lack of alternatives thereof.

3.3 The Genome of *C. albicans*

C. albicans presents some molecular genetic features that have slowed the progress of genetic manipulation and study of this fungus: First, the non-canonical decoding of the CUG codon to serine rather than leucine (SANTOS et al. 1993; SANTOS and TUITE 1995; WHITE et al. 1995) has been a hurdle for heterologous gene expression. Second, because of the absence of a (known) haploid phase of the diploid *C. albicans* gene inactivation procedures have to be repeated to "knock-out" both alleles of a gene. Third, the existence of sexual reproduction has remained elusive in this fungus, although *C. albicans* homologs of genes involved in sexual reproduction of *S. cerevisiae* were identified. Recently, two groups described mating in *C. albicans* under the prerequisite of homozygosity in the mating-type-like (MTL) locus (HULL et al. 2000; MAGEE and MAGEE 2000). Though evidence for meiosis has not been found.

Nevertheless, powerful tools for molecular genetic studies on the pathogenicity of *C. albicans* have been developed (reviewed in DE BACKER et al. 2000). These include transformation and selection systems (FONZI and IRWIN 1993; KÖHLER et al. 1997; MORSCHHÄUSER et al. 1999; WIRSCHING et al. 2000a,b), reporter genes (SRIKANTHA et al. 1996; CORMACK et al. 1997; MORSCHHÄUSER et al. 1998), a tetracycline-regulatable promoter system (NAKAYAMA et al. 2000) and an in vivo expression technology (STAIB et al. 1999, 2000a,b).

After completion of the *Candida* Sequencing Project carried out at the Stanford Genome Center (http://www-sequence.stanford.edu/group/candida/), the genomic sequence will become publicly available with ten-fold coverage. A proprietary version of the genome with 3.2-fold coverage is owned by Incyte Pharmaceuticals, Inc., Palo Alto, Calif., USA. Now, the critical tools for functional genomics have to be developed to overcome the aforementioned difficulties confronting molecular and genetic approaches to *C. albicans*.

With approximately 16 million base pairs in size, the *C. albicans* genome is ∼25% larger than that of *S. cerevisiae* (see Fig. 1A,B). Eight pairs of homologous chromosomes, ranging in size from 1.03-Mb to ∼4.3-Mb, have been identified by pulsed-field gel electrophoresis (PFGE). The largest chromosome is numbered 1, the smallest 7. The chromosome carrying the ribosomal DNA (rDNA) repeats varies in size in different strains; it has been assigned the letter R. Chromosome R size variation is probably caused by unequal crossing-over between the homologs. This results in different positions of R homologs in electrophoretic karyotypes of some *C. albicans* strains: One R homolog is larger than chromosome 1 (3.43-Mb) in some strains; in others, one homolog is smaller than chromosome 2 (2.6-Mb). In general, clinical isolates show relatively high variability in their karyotypes, rearranged chromosomes and length polymorphisms of homologs are found more often in these strains than in laboratory strains. Chromosome translocations seem to take place in the major repeat sequence (MRS), a middle repetitive element ranging in size from 10 to 100-kb, that is present on all *C. albicans* chromosomes (CHU et al. 1993; NAVARRO-GARCIA et al. 1995). Differences in the copy number of the 2-kb repeated sequence element in the MRS (IWAGUCHI et al. 1992) could account for the homolog length polymorphisms. Aneuploidy is another variation of the karyotype, which can be induced by environmental stresses such as growth on sorbose or the antifungal fluconazole (RUSTCHENKO et al. 1997; PEREPNIKHATKA et al. 1999). These aneuploids tend to return to euploidy. A stable aneuploid strain was characterized by MAGEE and MAGEE (1997). Genomic variation among *C. albicans* strains is also detectable at the level of gene sequences, repeat numbers and microsatellites. Considerable allelic variation can be found in different strains, and even in single strains some genes are heteroallelic. Besides point mutations and slippage events, retroelements are possible causes for some of these sequence differences. Transposition or transposon excision generate heterogeneity among strains or sister chromosomes. The *C. albicans* genome harbors 34 distinct LTR-retrotransposon families, a much larger number than the genome of *S. cerevisiae* (GOODWIN and POULTER 2000). However, few of the *Candida* retrotransposons seem to be intact and fully functional because their copy numbers are in general lower than those of the Ty elements in yeast. Nevertheless, many solo LTRs and LTR fragments remain as remnants from former transposition and recombination events.

Recently, Seoighe and coworkers (SEOIGHE et al. 2000) compared the gene order in the available genome sequence data from *C. albicans* with the *S. cerevisiae* genome sequence. They came to the conclusion that the gene order of the two species, which diverged 140–330 million years ago, is not well-conserved. Only 9% of gene pairs found in one species are in the same arrangement in the other species. The main pathway for rearrangements in gene order seems to be inversion of small DNA regions with less than ten genes by an uncharacterized mechanism.

With the completion of the *Candida albicans* genome sequence, we will be a step closer toward the elucidation of candidal pathogenicity. DNA arrays for expression analysis as well as proteomics will be invaluable tools for functional characterization of the 8,000 to 9,000 genes in *C. albicans*. Unfortunately, the powerful molecular genetic tools for functional genomics in *S. cerevisiae* are not readily applicable in *C. albicans* because of the disadvantage of diploidy and the lack of a "normal" sexual phase in this organism. New approaches, e.g., for genome-wide mutagenesis, still have to be developed.

4 Further Human-Pathogenic Fungi and their Genomes

Among the primary fungal pathogens for humans are many "opportunists" and few "true" or "obligate" pathogens, although the definitions of these two groups of microbial pathogens is a matter of discussion (CASADEVALL and PIROFSKI 1999, 2000). Opportunistic pathogens attack hosts with impaired immune functions, while "obligate" pathogens are able to cause disease in healthy individuals. However, a large inoculum or a specific virulence factor may enable an opportunistic pathogen to damage a normal host. Nevertheless, in the following we will hold on to the concept of opportunism and focus on the main fungal species considered to be opportunistic in this section. Besides *Candida* spp. there are the Aspergilli, *Cryptococcus neoformans* and *Pneumocystis carinii*. Information on their genomes is summarized in Table 2. Section 5 treats most of the important obligate fungal pathogens including *Blastomyces dermatidis*, *Histoplasma capsulatum*, *Coccidioides immitis*, *Paracoccidioides brasiliensis* and the dermatophytes.

4.1 Aspergilli

The genus *Aspergillus* is a rather complex genus among the Ascomycetes with approximately 180 species and a high diversity of associated teleomorphs. Of

Table 2. The most important opportunistic human pathogenic fungi and their genomes

Organism	Diseases	Haploid genome size	Genome structure
Candida albicans	Cutaneous, mucosal and gastrointestinal infections; vulvovaginitis; deep and disseminated candidiasis	~16-Mb	8 chromosomes (R, 1–7), 1.03 to ~4.3-Mb
Aspergillus fumigatus (*Neosartorya* spp.)[a]	Allergic bronchopulmonary aspergillosis, fungus ball, invasive aspergillosis	30 to 35-Mb	Probably 8 chromosomes
Cryptococcus neoformans var. *neoformans* (*Filobasidiella neoformans*)	Cryptococcosis: meningoencephalitis, pneumonia	~23-Mb	12 to 13 chromosomes, 0.77 to 3.87-Mb
Pneumocystis carinii	Pulmonary infections	~8-Mb	13 to 15 chromosomes

[a] Teleomorphs in parentheses.

medical or veterinarian interest, however, are only a few species: *A. fumigatus*, *A. flavus*, *A. terreus*, and, very rarely, *A. niger* or *A. nidulans*. The disease spectrum caused by these species, though, is wide, ranging from allergic to superficial to invasive aspergillosis. Furthermore, some species, e.g. *A. flavus*, are able to produce mycotoxins (aflatoxin). *Aspergillus* spores are ubiquitous in the environment due to the abundance of these saprophytic fungi in soil and decomposing organic materials. Therefore, especially immunocompromised individuals are at risk of contracting severe forms of aspergillosis from the environment. Patients with invasive aspergillosis have a mortality rate of 85% (DENNING 1998).

A. fumigatus is the most common mold causing infections in humans worldwide (LATGE 1999). There are probable multiple factors contributing to the virulence of this species: It grows very well at 37°C (up to 50°C) and its spores are very small, allowing them to be inhaled easily into the lung. Generation of gliotoxin, a substance with immunosuppressive activity, and the production of superoxid dismutases, catalases and mannitol as protectants from phagocytes may further contribute to virulence. Despite the role as a major pathogen, molecular genetic information on *A. fumigatus*, however, is scarce because most studies have been conducted on the genetically more easily tractable *A. nidulans* or on *A. niger*, which is important in the biotechnology industry (BROOKMAN and DENNING 2000). The genome structure of *A. fumigatus* is not well characterized. While earlier reports stated the presence of four bands on CHEF gels, a recent publication suggested eight chromosomes (AMAAR and MOORE 1998), the same number was found in *A. nidulans*, *A. niger* and *A. flavus*. The genome size of *A. fumigatus* and *A. nidulans* has been estimated at approximately 30-Mb (BROOKMAN and DENNING 2000). A physical genome map is available for the latter (PRADE 2000). Consistent with their analysis of gene density in a 38.8-kb region of the *A. nidulans* genome, Kupfer and coauthors (KUPFER et al. 1997) predicted that multi-cellular Ascomycetes harbor more than 8,000 genes in their genomes. In contrast to the *S. cerevisiae* genome, which has a higher gene density, the genomes of multicellular fungi seem to have a higher portion of non-coding regions (e.g., introns), and, therefore, a lower gene density. Nonetheless, the genomes of multicellular fungi such as *A. nidulans* or *Neurospora crassa* are larger and more complex than the genomes of unicellular Ascomycetes like *S. cerevisiae*. Multiple mechanisms of spatial and temporal cell differentiation, as well as extensive metabolic capabilities, certainly are mirrored in a higher genome content.

Comparative analysis of the genome of the most pathogenic *Aspergillus* species *A. fumigatus* with the genome of *A. nidulans* will help us identify determinants of fungal virulence, which is certainly multifactorial. Distinct virulence factors such as exoenzymes or toxins may play a role in pathogenicity and certain structural or metabolic properties (e.g., pigmentation or size of the spores) may enable one species to infect and damage the host easier and faster than the other. An initial study by Tsai and coworkers (TSAI et al. 1999) demonstrated that the conidial pigment biosynthesis genes, which are involved in virulence, are clustered in *A. fumigatus*. In *A. nidulans* the *wA* and *yA* genes of the pigment formation pathway are not linked.

4.2 *Cryptococcus*

The Basidiomycete *Cryptococcus neoformans* (teleomorph: *Filobasidiella neoformans*) is a pathogenic yeast that causes pneumonia and meningoencephalitis in humans with an impaired immune system. Cryptococcosis is one of the most common life-threatening infections in AIDS-patients (KWON-CHUNG and BENNETT 1992). Two varieties have been described as the etiological agents of cryptococcosis: *C. neoformans* var. *neoformans* and *C. neoformans* var. *gatti*. The latter variety is rarely involved in AIDS-related disease, since it is only prevalent in regions with *Eucalyptus camaldulensis*, the natural source of these fungi. Many patients infected in these regions have no obvious predisposing factors. Exposure to avian excreta and soil is the main route to developing an infection by var. *neoformans*.

Two genome sequencing projects have been started on this important fungal pathogen:

- The *Cryptococcus neoformans* Genome Project at the Stanford Genome Technology Center (http://www-sequence.stanford.edu/group/C.neoformans/index.html)
- The *Cryptococcus neoformans* cDNA Sequencing (http://www.genome.ou.edu/cneo.html)

As of December 2000 1,400 cDNA clones, the 33,199-bp circular mitochondrial genome and the nuclear genome with 2.8 coverage (12.9-Mb, 3,900 contigs) have been sequenced in these projects.

Electrophoretic karyotypes, with an average of 12 chromosomes in the *neoformans* variety and 13 in the *gattii* variety, were detected in multiple isolates of *C. neoformans* (WICKES et al. 1994). The genome size was estimated to be approximately 23-Mb.

4.3 *Pneumocystis carinii*

The classification of *Pneumocystis carinii* as fungi, and not as protozoa, has been confirmed very recently by morphological and molecular studies. *P. carinii* probably represents an early divergent line in the kingdom Fungi with affinities to the Ascomycetes (GUARRO et al. 1999). The taxon, however, probably still includes several species that originate from different hosts.

AIDS patients frequently suffer from pulmonary infections caused by *P. carinii*, and the occurrences of these infections are now considered indicative of the disease.

The haploid genome of *P. carinii* (formae specialis *carinii*) appears to be about 8-Mb in size, and it is divided into 13 to 15 linear chromosomes. Genes in this microorganism usually are interrupted by up to nine, typically rather small, introns less than 50-bp in length (STRINGER and CUSHION 1998). A *P. carinii* genome-sequencing project is currently under way (for further information see http://biology.uky.edu/Pc/).

5 Obligate Pathogenic Fungi

Most true pathogenic fungi belong to two groups in the Ascomycetes (order Onygenales), dimorphic fungi and dermatophytes (GUARRO et al. 1999). Dimorphic fungi grow at 25°C as filamentous forms and at 37°C in yeast-like forms. The major pathogens in this group are *Blastomyces dermatitidis*, *Coccidioides immitis*, *Histoplasma capsulatum* and *Paracoccidioides brasiliensis*. All are endemic to certain areas where subclinical and clinical infections are detected (GALGIANI 1999; RETALLACK and WOODS 1999; HOGAN et al. 1996; KWON-CHUNG and BENNETT 1992). The mycoses usually start as pulmonary infections, which can progress, albeit infrequently, to disseminated and fatal infections. Data on the organization of the genomes of these fungi are summarized in Table 3.

Dermatophytes are a monophyletic group of anthropophilic, zoophilic and geophilic pathogenic fungi in the three anamorphic genera *Microsporum*, *Epidermophyton* and *Trichophyton* (GUARRO et al. 1999; WEITZMANN and SUMMERBELL 1995). To our knowledge, only the mitochondrial genome of *T. rubrum* is being sequenced so far (DE BIEVRE and DUJON 1999); further information on genome sequencing is not available.

6 Fungal Plant Pathogens

Most of the numerous fungal pathogens of plants belong either to the phyla Oomycota, Ascomycota or Basidiomycota. Many species cause diseases of

Table 3. The most important obligate human pathogenic fungi and their genomes

Organism	Diseases	Main endemic regions	Haploid genome size	Genome structure
Blastomyces dermatitidis (*Ajellomyces dermatitidis*)[a]	Blastomycosis: infection of the lung; dissemination possible	Ohio-Mississippi river valley, Eastern US, Central America, Africa	n.a.[b]	n.a.
Coccidioides immitis	Coccidioidomycosis: infection of the lung; dissemination possible	Southwestern US, Latin America	28.2 ± 2.6-Mb (PAN and COLE 1992)	4 chromosomes
Paracoccidioides brasiliensis	Paracoccidioidomycosis: infection of the lung; dissemination possible	Continental Latin America: Central Mexico to northeastern Argentina	23 to 27.6-Mb (NOGUEIRA CANO et al. 1998)	4 chromosomes
Histoplasma capsulatum (*Ajellomyces capsulatum*)	Histoplasmosis: intracellular infection of the monocyte-macrophage system; often pulmonary infections; dissemination	Eastern US, Latin America, Asia, Africa	23-Mb (32-Mb in aneuploid or partially diploid strain; see CARR and SHEARER 1998)	3, 4 or 7 chromosomes (strain dependent; see STEELE et al. 1989)
Dermatophytes: *Trichophyton* spp., *Microsporum* spp., *Epidermophyton floccosum*	Dermatophytoses: Ringworm, Tinea, Dermatomycoses	Worldwide	n.a.	n.a.

n.a., not available;
[a] Teleomorphs in parentheses.

economic concern in agricultural plant production. We will focus on a selection of phytopathogenic fungi, which are major pathogens and have been genetically well characterized.

Phytophtora infestans is an Oomycete that causes the late blight disease of potato and tomato (JUDELSON 1997). The best-known example of crop losses due to *P. infestans* is the Irish potato famine of the 1840s. An initiative for the characterization of the genomes of this fungus and another related species, *P. sojae*, has already been started (for further information see http://www.ncgr.org/pgc/index.html). The 65-Mb *P. sojae* genome will be sequenced. Efforts on the *P. infestans* genome will be restricted to sequencing of expressed sequence tags (ESTs) because of its large size of 250-Mb. *P. infestans* seems to be diploid with nine to ten chromosomes; however, substantial differences in ploidy have been observed among natural isolates. In general, as in many other fungal species, genetic variability is extensive, probably caused by multiple mechanisms involving epigenetic processes and mobile elements.

Magnaporthe grisea is a heterothallic Ascomycete that causes rice blast, one of the most devastating diseases of rice in all regions where this cereal is grown. The fungus is a model organism with well-studied biology and genetics for investigations on plant-pathogen interaction. Its genome is 40-Mb to 50-Mb in size with seven chromosomes separable by pulsed-field gel electrophoresis. A physical map of the smallest chromosome, the 4.2-Mb chromosome 7, was constructed by Zhu and coworkers (ZHU et al. 1999). Interestingly, while expressed genes are distributed relatively evenly along the chromosome, various repetitive elements tend to cluster, sometimes in gene-rich regions, which might be more accessible as transposition targets.

Ustilago hordei, a Basidomycete, causes the covered smut disease on small-grain cereals like barley and oats. Its genome was estimated to be 18.4 to 25.9-Mb in size with a haploid set of 16 to 21 chromosomes (MCCLUSKEY and MILLS 1990). In these fungi, sex and pathogenicity are interdependent: The sexual phase of the life cycle is only completed when infection of the host plant occurs via a filamentous dikaryon, which is formed from mated cells with opposite mating-types. A 500-kb region controlling mating-type (*MAT* locus) and pathogenicity has been identified on the largest chromosome of *U. hordei* (LEE et al. 1999). Interesting features of the *MAT* locus include recombination suppression and regions of nonhomology between the opposite mating-types. These characteristics, together with the sex-determining genes on this chromosome, are reminiscent of dimorphic sex chromosomes (X/Y systems), which may also have evolved in these fungi.

Nectria haematococca, an ascomycete fungus that causes disease in peas, presents a noteworthy example of genetic variability in fungal genomes: Certain isolates of *N. haematococca* mating population (MP) VI harbor a 1.6-Mb chromosome, which is conditionally dispensable (MIAO et al. 1991). This supernumerary chromosome is not essential for saprophytic growth. However, if it gets lost during sexual reproduction, the virulence of *N. haematococca* on chickpea plants is diminished because genes coding for phytoalexin detoxifying enzymes are located on this chromosome (COVERT et al. 1996; ENKERLI et al. 1998; REIMMANN and

VANETTEN 1994). A physical map of the chromosome was constructed recently by Enkerli and coworkers (ENKERLI et al. 2000), and the chromosome breakpoints generated during sexual reproduction of several isolates were determined. Location and quantity of repetitive DNA and/or hotspots of recombination could contribute to the meiotic instability of the conditionally dispensable chromosome.

7 Concluding Remarks

This review represents a snapshot on the constantly increasing field of genome research in pathogenic fungi. Naturally, due to their larger genome sizes and the sheer number of species of biological, medical or economical importance, few fungal genomes have been characterized in detail. The availability of the total genome sequence of the yeast *S. cerevisiae* and the almost completed genome sequence of the pathogenic yeast *C. albicans* present paradigmatic steps toward further characterization of fungal biology and pathogenicity. Current information on the genome organization of fungi reveals a high degree of plasticity and complexity. Genetic variability generated by intrachromosomal and heterochromosomal recombination, rDNA chromosome size polymorphism and even horizontal transfer of genetic material stands in apparent contrast to the relatively low frequency of karyotypic changes during mitotic growth. A hypermutable state probably caused by environmental stresses in both asexual and sexual fungi as well as meiotic recombination in sexual fungi could lead to the sometimes dramatic changes in the genomes of these microorganisms. In some species, regions on chromosomes or entire chromosomes are dispensable. With the progress of genome, transcriptome and proteome analysis in fungi, we will be able to define fungal pathogenicity and to study what role the mechanisms of genome variation play in virulence.

Acknowledgement. We thank Hilde Merkert for editorial help and Axel Lischewsky for providing the CHEF gel image of Fig. 1B.

References

Amaar YG, Moore MM (1998) Mapping of the nitrate-assimilation gene cluster (crnA-niiA-niaD) and characterization of the nitrite reductase gene (niiA) in the opportunistic fungal pathogen *Aspergillus fumigatus*. Curr Genet 33:206–215

Baleiras Couto MM, Eijsma B, Hofstra H, Huis in't Veld JH, van der Vossen JM (1996) Evaluation of molecular typing techniques to assign genetic diversity among *Saccharomyces cerevisiae* strains. Appl Environ Microbiol 62:41–46

Braun EL, Halpern AL, Nelson MA, Natvig DO (2000) Large-scale comparison of fungal sequence information: mechanisms of innovation in *Neurospora crassa* and gene loss in *Saccharomyces cerevisiae*. Genome Res 10:416–430

Brookman JL, Denning DW (2000) Molecular genetics in *Aspergillus fumigatus* (In Process Citation). Curr Opin Microbiol 3:468–474

Casadevall A, Pirofski LA (1999) Host-pathogen interactions: redefining the basic concepts of virulence and pathogenicity. Infect Immun 67:3703–3713

Casadevall A, Pirofski LA (2000) Host-pathogen interactions: basic concepts of microbial commensalism, colonization, infection, and disease (In Process Citation). Infect Immun 68:6511–6518

Chu WS, Magee BB, Magee PT (1993) Construction of an SfiI macrorestriction map of the Candida albicans genome. J Bacteriol 175:6637–6651

Cormack BP, Bertram G, Egerton M, Gow NA, Falkow S, Brown AJ (1997) Yeast-enhanced green fluorescent protein (yEGFP)a reporter of gene expression in *Candida albicans*. Microbiology 143: 303–311

Covert SF, Enkerli J, Miao VP, VanEtten HD (1996) A gene for maackiain detoxification from a dispensable chromosome of *Nectria haematococca*. Mol Gen Genet 251:397–406

De Backer MD, Magee PT, Pla J (2000) Recent developments in molecular genetics of *Candida albicans* (In Process Citation). Annu Rev Microbiol 54:463–498

de Bievre C, Dujon B (1999) Organisation of the mitochondrial genome of *Trichophyton rubrum* III. DNA sequence analysis of the NADH dehydrogenase subunits 1, 2, 3, 4, 5 and the cytochrome b gene. Curr Genet 35:30–35

Denning DW (1998) Invasive aspergillosis. Clin Infect Dis 26:781–803; quiz 804–805

Edman JC, Kovacs JA, Masur H, Santi DV, Elwood HJ, Sogin ML (1988) Ribosomal RNA sequence shows *Pneumocystis carinii* to be a member of the fungi. Nature 334:519–522

Edmond MB, Wallace SE, McClish DK, Pfaller MA, Jones RN, Wenzel RP (1999) Nosocomial bloodstream infections in United States hospitals: a three-year analysis (see comments). Clin Infect Dis 29:239–244

Enkerli J, Bhatt G, Covert SF (1998) Maackiain detoxification contributes to the virulence of *Nectria haematococca* Mp VI on chickpea. Mol Plant Microbe Interact 11:317–326

Enkerli J, Reed H, Briley A, Bhatt G, Covert SF (2000) Physical map of a conditionally dispensable chromosome in *Nectria haematococca* mating population VI and location of chromosome break-points. Genetics 155:1083–1094

Fonzi WA, Irwin MY (1993) Isogenic strain construction and gene mapping in *Candida albicans*. Genetics 134:717–728

Foury F, Roganti T, Lecrenier N, Purnelle B (1998) The complete sequence of the mitochondrial genome of *Saccharomyces cerevisiae*. FEBS Lett 440:325–331

Galgiani JN (1999) Coccidioidomycosis: a regional disease of national importance. Rethinking approaches for control. Ann Intern Med 130:293–300

Gasent-Ramirez JM, Castrejon F, Querol A, Ramon D, Benitez T (1999) Genomic stability of *Saccharomyces cerevisiae* baker's yeasts. Syst Appl Microbiol 22:329–340

Gimeno CJ, Ljungdahl PO, Styles CA, Fink GR (1992) Unipolar cell divisions in the yeast *S. cerevisiae* lead to filamentous growth: regulation by starvation and RAS. Cell 68:1077–1090

Goffeau A (2000) Four years of post-genomic life with 6,000 yeast genes. FEBS Lett 480:37–41

Goodwin TJ, Poulter RT (2000) Multiple LTR-retrotransposon families in the asexual yeast *Candida albicans*. Genome Res 10:174–191

Guarro J, Gene J, Stchigel AM (1999) Developments in fungal taxonomy. Clin Microbiol Rev 12:454–500

Hani J, Feldmann H (1998) tRNA genes and retroelements in the yeast genome. Nucleic Acids Res 26:689–696

Hawksworth DL (1991) The fungal dimension of biodiversity: magnitude, significance, and conservation. Mycol Res 84:641–655

Hawksworth DL (1995) Steps along the road to a harmonized bionomenclature. Taxon 44:447–456

Hogan LH, Klein BS, Levitz SM (1996) Virulence factors of medically important fungi. Clin Microbiol Rev 9:469–488

Hull CM, Raisner RM, Johnson AD (2000) Evidence for mating of the "asexual"; yeast *Candida albicans* in a mammalian host (see comments). Science 289:307–310

Iwaguchi S, Homma M, Chibana H, Tanaka K (1992) Isolation and characterization of a repeated sequence (RPS1) of *Candida albicans*. J Gen Microbiol 138:1893–1900

Judelson HS (1997) The genetics and biology of *Phytophthora infestans*: modern approaches to a historical challenge. Fungal Genet Biol 22:65–76

Köhler GA, White TC, Agabian N (1997) Overexpression of a cloned IMP dehydrogenase gene of *Candida albicans* confers resistance to the specific inhibitor mycophenolic acid. J Bacteriol 179:2331–2338

Kupfer DM, Reece CA, Clifton SW, Roe BA, Prade RA (1997) Multicellular ascomycetous fungal genomes contain more than 8,000 genes. Fungal Genet Biol 21:364–372

Kurtzman CP, Fell JW (1998) The yeasts, a taxonomic study. Elsevier Science B.V., Amsterdam, The Netherlands

Kwon-Chung KJ, Bennet JE (1992) Medical Mycology. Lea & Febiger, Malvern, Pa., USA

Latge JP (1999) *Aspergillus fumigatus* and aspergillosis. Clin Microbiol Rev 12:310–350

Latouche GN, Daniel HM, Lee OC, Mitchell TG, Sorrell TC, Meyer W (1997) Comparison of use of phenotypic and genotypic characteristics for identification of species of the anamorph genus *Candida* and related teleomorph yeast species. J Clin Microbiol 35:3171–3180

Lee N, Bakkeren G, Wong K, Sherwood JE, Kronstad JW (1999) The mating-type and pathogenicity locus of the fungus *Ustilago hordei* spans a 500-kb region. Proc Natl Acad Sci USA 96:15026–15031

Magee BB, Magee PT (1997) WO-2, a stable aneuploid derivative of *Candida albicans* strain WO-1, can switch from white to opaque and form hyphae. Microbiology 143:289–295

Magee BB, Magee PT (2000) Induction of mating in *Candida albicans* by construction of MTLa and MTLalpha strains (see comments). Science 289:310–313

Marinoni G, Manuel M, Petersen RF, Hvidtfeldt J, Sulo P, Piskur J (1999) Horizontal transfer of genetic material among *Saccharomyces* yeasts. J Bacteriol 181:6488–6496

McCluskey K, Mills D (1990) Identification and characterization of chromosome length polymorphisms among strains representing fourteen races of *Ustilago hordei*. Mol Plant Microbe Interact 3:366–373

Mewes HW, Albermann K, Bahr M, Frishman D, Gleissner A, Hani J, Heumann K, Kleine K, Maierl A, Oliver SG, Pfeiffer F, Zollner A (1997) Overview of the yeast genome (published erratum appears in Nature 1997 Jun 12;387(6634):737). Nature 387:7–65

Mewes HW, Heumann K, Kaps A, Mayer K, Pfeiffer F, Stocker S, Frishman D (1999) MIPS: a database for genomes and protein sequences. Nucleic Acids Res 27:44–48

Miao VP, Covert SF, VanEtten HD (1991) A fungal gene for antibiotic resistance on a dispensable ("B") chromosome. Science 254:1773–1776

Morschhäuser J, Michel S, Hacker J (1998) Expression of a chromosomally integrated, single-copy GFP gene in *Candida albicans*, and its use as a reporter of gene regulation. Mol Gen Genet 257:412–420

Morschhäuser J, Michel S, Staib P (1999) Sequential gene disruption in *Candida albicans* by FLP-mediated site-specific recombination. Mol Microbiol 32:547–556

Mortimer RK (2000) Evolution and variation of the yeast (*Saccharomyces*) genome (published erratum appears in Genome Res 2000 Jun;10(6):891). Genome Res 10:403–409

Nakayama H, Mio T, Nagahashi S, Kokado M, Arisawa M, Aoki Y (2000) Tetracycline-regulatable system to tightly control gene expression in the pathogenic fungus *Candida albicans* (In Process Citation). Infect Immun 68:6712–6719

Navarro-Garcia F, Perez-Diaz RM, Magee BB, Pla J, Nombela C, Magee P (1995) Chromosome reorganization in *Candida albicans* 1001 strain. J Med Vet Mycol 33:361–366

Odds FC (1988) *Candida* and candidosis. Bailliere Tindall, Philadelphia, Pa., USA

Oriol A, Ribera JM, Arnal J, Milla F, Batlle M, Feliu E (1993) *Saccharomyces cerevisiae* septicemia in a patient with myelodysplastic syndrome (letter). Am J Hematol 43:325–326

Perepnikhatka V, Fischer FJ, Niimi M, Baker RA, Cannon RD, Wang YK, Sherman F, Rustchenko E (1999) Specific chromosome alterations in fluconazole-resistant mutants of *Candida albicans*. J Bacteriol 181:4041–4049

Prade RA (2000) The reliability of the *Aspergillus nidulans* physical map. Fungal Genet Biol 29:175–185

Reimmann C, VanEtten HD (1994) Cloning and characterization of the PDA6–1 gene encoding a fungal cytochrome P-450, which detoxifies the phytoalexin pisatin from garden pea. Gene 146:221–226

Retallack DM, Woods JP (1999) Molecular epidemiology, pathogenesis, and genetics of the dimorphic fungus *Histoplasma capsulatum*. Microbes Infect 1:817–825

Rustchenko EP, Howard DH, Sherman F (1997) Variation in assimilating functions occurs in spontaneous *Candida albicans* mutants having chromosomal alterations. Microbiology 143:1765–1778

Santos MA, Tuite MF (1995) The CUG codon is decoded in vivo as serine and not leucine in *Candida albicans*. Nucleic Acids Res 23:1481–1486

Santos MA, Keith G, Tuite MF (1993) Non-standard translational events in *Candida albicans* mediated by an unusual seryl-tRNA with a 5'-CAG-3' (leucine) anticodon. EMBO J 12:607–616

Savage JM (1995) Systematics and the biodiversity crisis. BioScience 45:673–679

Seoighe C, Federspiel N, Jones T, Hansen N, Bivolarovic V, Surzycki R, Tamse R, Komp C, Huizar L, Davis RW, Scherer S, Tait E, Shaw DJ, Harris D, Murphy L, Oliver K, Taylor K, Rajandream MA, Barrell BG, Wolfe KH (2000) Prevalence of small inversions in yeast gene order evolution. Proc Natl Acad Sci USA 97:14433–14437

Sethi N, Mandell W (1988) *Saccharomyces fungemia* in a patient with AIDS. N Y State J Med 88:278–279

Srikantha T, Klapach A, Lorenz WW, Tsai LK, Laughlin LA, Gorman JA, Soll DR (1996) The sea pansy *Renilla reniformis* luciferase serves as a sensitive bioluminescent reporter for differential gene expression in Candida albicans. J Bacteriol 178:121–129

Staib P, Kretschmar M, Nichterlein T, Köhler G, Michel S, Hof H, Hacker J, Morschhäuser J (1999) Host-induced, stage-specific virulence gene activation in *Candida albicans* during infection. Mol Microbiol 32:533–546

Staib P, Kretschmar M, Nichterlein T, Hof H, Morschhäuser J (2000a) Differential activation of a *Candida albicans* virulence gene family during infection. Proc Natl Acad Sci USA 97:6102–6107

Staib P, Kretschmar M, Nichterlein T, Köhler G, Morschhäuser J (2000b) Expression of virulence genes in *Candida albicans*. Adv Exp Med Biol 485:167–176

Stringer JR, Cushion MT (1998) The genome of *Pneumocystis carinii*. FEMS Immunol Med Microbiol 22:15–26

Tawfik OW, Papasian CJ, Dixon AY, Potter LM (1989) *Saccharomyces cerevisiae* pneumonia in a patient with acquired immune deficiency syndrome. J Clin Microbiol 27:1689–1691

Taylor JW, Swann FC, Berbee ML (1994) Molecular evolution of ascomycete fungi: phylogeny and conflict. In: Hawksworth DL (ed) Ascomycete systematics: problems and perspectives in the nineties. Plenum Press, New York, NY, pp 201–212

Tsai HF, Wheeler MH, Chang YC, Kwon-Chung KJ (1999) A developmentally regulated gene cluster involved in conidial pigment biosynthesis in *Aspergillus fumigatus*. J Bacteriol 181:6469–6477

Weitzman I, Summerbell RC (1995) The dermatophytes. Clin Microbiol Rev 8:240–259

White TC, Andrews LE, Maltby D, Agabian N (1995) The "universal" leucine codon CTG in the secreted aspartyl proteinase 1 (SAP1) gene of *Candida albicans* encodes a serine in vivo. J Bacteriol 177:2953–2955

Wickes BL, Moore TD, Kwon-Chung KJ (1994) Comparison of the electrophoretic karyotypes and chromosomal location of ten genes in the two varieties of *Cryptococcus neoformans*. Microbiology 140:543–550

Wirsching S, Michel S, Köhler G, Morschhäuser J (2000a) Activation of the multiple drug resistance gene MDR1 in fluconazole-resistant, clinical *Candida albicans* strains is caused by mutations in a trans-regulatory factor. J Bacteriol 182:400–404

Wirsching S, Michel S, Köhler G, Morschhäuser J (2000b) Activation of the multiple drug resistance gene MDR1 in fluconazole-resistant, clinical *Candida albicans* strains is caused by mutations in a trans-regulatory factor. J Bacteriol 182:400–404

Zhu H, Blackmon BP, Sasinowski M, Dean RA (1999) Physical map and organization of chromosome 7 in the rice blast fungus, *Magnaporthe grisea*. Genome Res 9:739–750

Impact of Integrons and Transposons on the Evolution of Resistance and Virulence

D.A. Rowe-Magnus[1], J. Davies[2], and D. Mazel[1]

1 Introduction

At first glance, antibiotic resistance and virulence in human and animal pathogens can be seen as adaptive functions in response to selective pressures in the same ecological niche. Indeed, the hosts are identical and bacterial colonization implies circumvention of their immune or chemical defenses. As for many other bacterial adaptive traits (DE LA CRUZ and DAVIES 2000; OCHMAN et al. 2000), it is now clearly established that virulence and resistance development proceeds mainly

[1] Unite de Programmation Moleculaire et Toxicologie Genetique, CNRS URA 1444, Departement des Biotechnologies, Institut Pasteur, 25 rue du Dr Roux, 75724, Paris, France
[2] Department of Microbiology and Immunology, University of British Columbia, 6174 University Boulevard, Vancouver, B.C., Canada, V6T 1Z3

through the acquisition of exogenous genetic loci. In most cases, these loci are delivered by disseminating genetic structures, such as conjugative or mobilizable plasmids, bacteriophages and transposons.

A major difference lies in the evolutionary time-scale of virulence and resistance development in human and animal pathogens. Contemporary pathogens can be seen as the product of a constant co-evolutionary race between the escape attempts of the hosts and bacterial innovation, which has been on going for millions of years, whereas chemical anti-microbial threat in humans is a 6-decades-old phenomenon.

Transposons have been involved in the spread of a large number of functions. Their contributions to the development of multi-drug and metal resistance and their role in the conveyance of many catabolic and pathogenicity traits have been firmly established.

The integrons per se do not belong to the mobile DNA element family. Instead, they comprise a family of natural genetic engineering elements. Integrons are able to stockpile selectable genes, structured in a highly mobile form, at a specific site. Through their gene-capture ability integrons have been randomly selected as components of many transposons and their impact on the development of multi-drug resistance has been considerable. They were first identified in the enterobacteria and Pseudomonads as part of several transposons gathering resistance genes. Recently, their importance as a general evolutionary apparatus in bacteria has been expanded by the discovery of another type of integron, the super-integron, naturally present in the genome of several genera of the γ-proteobacteria.

This review will emphasize the involvement of transposons and integrons in the development of antibiotic resistance and, to a lesser extent, virulence, in light of the recent discovery of the chromosomal super-integrons.

2 Antibiotic Resistance Development: a Transposon Affair?

All available evidence suggests that the acquisition and dissemination of antibiotic resistance genes in human pathogens and commensal strains has occurred during the past 50 years. The best support for this recent invasion comes from studies of Hughes and Datta (DATTA and HUGHES 1983; HUGHES and DATTA 1983), who examined the "Murray Collection", a collection of (mainly) Gram-negative pathogens obtained from clinical specimens in the pre-antibiotic era, for their antibiotic resistance and conjugative plasmid content. None of these strains, isolated between 1917 and 1952, was resistant to any of the antibiotics in current use. Notably, these isolates were also found to harbor plasmids from the same compatibility groups as those found to carry resistance genes (the R factors) a few years later.

Resistance has been encountered as an impediment to antibiotic therapy for as long as antibiotics have been used. With only a few exceptions, antibiotic resistance in bacterial pathogens was identified soon after the introduction of antibiotics into clinical practice, illustrating the genetic flexibility of bacteria. This was first seen in development of resistance to sulfonamides (Su) and penicillinase in *pneumococci* in the late '30s (MACLEAN et al. 1939) and streptomycin resistance mutations in *mycobacteria* in 1948. Between 1949 and 1951 in Japan, the Su resistance in *Shigella* isolates rose from 10% to almost 90%. Multi-drug resistance was never anticipated, since the co-appearance of multiple mutations conferring such phenotypes was considered to be beyond the evolutionary potential of a given bacterial population. However, in 1955 in Japan, 5 years after the quasi-concomitant introduction of streptomycin (Sm), tetracycline (Tc) and chloramphenicol (Cm) in medicine and massive production of these antibiotics, the first cases of resistance were reported (MITSUHASHI et al. 1961) (Fig. 1). In 1956 in Japan, increasing numbers of *Shigella dysenteriae* strains were isolated that were resistant to up to four antibiotics simultaneously (Tc, Cm, Sm, Su). It became clear that the emergence of multiple resistant strains could not be attributed to mutation alone. Furthermore, both sensitive and resistant *Shigella* could be isolated from a single patient, and *Shigella* spp. and *Escherichia coli* obtained from the same patients often exhibited the same multiple resistance patterns (AKIDO et al. 1960; WATANABE 1963). This was the time when transposons, and with them integrons, appeared in the human pathogen and commensal bacterial population as factors in resistance gene dissemination by

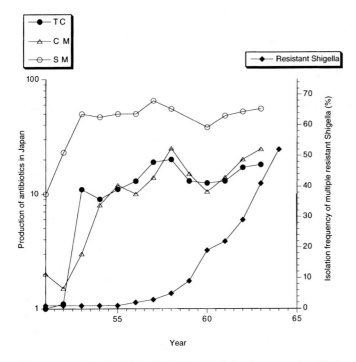

Fig. 1. Production of antibiotics in Japan and isolation frequency of antibiotics resistant *Shigella* strains. *TC*, tetracycline; *CM*, chloramphenicol; *SM*, streptomycin

hitchhiking on conjugative plasmids. Indeed, early mapping of R-plasmids showed the presence of resistance islands (see for example MITSUHASHI 1965, 1969), while inter-specific conjugative transfer of resistance was demonstrated (AKIDO et al. 1960). At the same time, the first insertion sequences (IS) were discovered to be the cause of auxotrophic mutations in *E. coli* (JORDAN et al. 1968; SHAPIRO 1969). The link between such elements and the demonstrated mobility of several resistance determinants (DATTA et al. 1971; RICHMOND and SYKES 1972) soon led to the first characterizations of resistance encoding transposons (Tn) (BERG et al. 1975; HEDGES and JACOB 1974). Integrons were discovered in the late '80s through the observation that Tns with different antibiotic resistance spectra shared the same backbone and differed only in the resistance genes they harbored (MARTINEZ and DE LA CRUZ 1990; OUELLETTE et al. 1987; STOKES and HALL 1989; SUNDSTRÖM et al. 1988). It is clear, however, that they were definitely part of the first multi-drug resistance outbreaks in the '50s, as attested by the involvement of Tn21, an integron-containing transposon, in the very first events (LIEBERT et al. 1999; NAKAYA et al. 1960).

3 Impact of Transposons in Resistance and Virulence Gene Flow

3.1 Transposons and Antibiotic Resistance Dissemination

It has been amply demonstrated that most resistance genes are carried by transposons in both Gram-negative and Gram-positive species. The public-health problems raised by the general development of resistance has led to such an accumulation of data that it certainly places the dissemination of resistance genes within the bacterial population as the paradigm for horizontal gene transfer (HGT). Since their discovery in the late 1970s, resistance transposons have been the subject of numerous reviews. Many of their biological characteristics have been discussed, and for many, their mechanisms of propagation, their regulatory circuits and their coding capacities have been studied in depth (see for example BERG and HOWE 1989; EVERS et al. 1996; KLECKNER et al. 1996; LIEBERT et al. 1999; SKURRAY and FIRTH 1997). Resistance transposons belong to the four classes of transposons: composite transposons (Class I; e.g., Tn5, Tn9, Tn10, …), cointegrative transposons (Class II; e.g., Tn3, Tn21, …), integrative transposons (Class III, e.g., Tn7, Tn554) and conjugative transposons (Class IV); as defined in the mobile element nomenclature (MAHILLON 1998). There is apparently no bias in the type of resistance genes that can be propagated, as all types of resistance genes have been found in these structures. Complex resistance phenotypes, such as those requiring sequential and or co-expression of several genes or operons, are also found encoded in transposons. This is the case for the vancomycin-teicoplanin resistance transposon Tn1546 that carries nine genes organized in six transcriptional units (EVERS et al. 1996).

Among the resistance disseminating transposons, the conjugative transposons have specific characteristics that distinguish them from the three other classes of transposons and places them somewhere between prophage-like elements and classical transposons. First detected in gram-positive cocci, they are now known to be present in a variety of clinically important groups of gram-positive and gram-negative bacteria. They were originally identified when the transfer of antibiotic resistance determinants occurred in the absence of plasmids (FRANKE and CLEWELL 1981; GAWRON-BURKE and CLEWELL 1982; SHOEMAKER et al. 1980). Conjugative transposons are discrete elements that are normally integrated into a bacterial genome. Their transposition and transfer is thought to start by an excision event and the formation of a covalently closed circular intermediate, which can either integrate elsewhere in the same cell or into the genome of a recipient cell following self-transfer by conjugation. In contrast to conjugative plasmids, their propagation through integration in the host genome emancipates transposons from the constraint of a compatible replication system.

Conjugative transposons are not considered typical transposons, as they have a covalently closed circular transposition intermediate, and they do not duplicate the target site when they integrate (SALYERS et al. 1995; SCOTT 1992). At the present time, five different families of conjugative transposons have been established (HOCHHUT et al. 1997; HOCHHUT and WALDOR 1999; SALYERS and SHOEMAKER 1997; SALYERS et al. 1995; WALDOR et al. 1996):

1. The Tn916 family (originally found in *Streptococci* but now known also to occur in Gram-negative bacteria, such as *Campylobacter*)
2. The *S. pneumoniae* family (Tn5253)
3. The *Bacteroides* family
4. CTnscr94, a conjugative transposon found in enterobacteria
5. The SXT element found in *V. cholerae*

Two other mobile elements are also conjugative elements that integrate rather than replicate and behave like conjugative transposons (MURPHY and PEMBROKE 1995; RAVATN et al. 1998). The size of the different conjugative transposons ranges from 15kb to 150kb, and all but Ctnscr94 have been identified through their capacity to transfer resistance genes. In addition to other resistance genes, most encode tetracycline resistance determinants (e.g., Tn916 encodes the TetM determinant, and the TetQ determinant is found on the conjugative transposons from the *Bacteroides* group (NIKOLICH et al. 1994; SALYERS et al. 1995), while the SXT element encodes resistance to sulfamethoxazole, trimethoprim, chloramphenicol and streptomycin (WALDOR et al. 1996). These transposons use integration machinery similar to that of lambdoid phages, and all characterized elements carry an *int* gene. However, the target specificity for their integration varies considerably; Tn916 behaves more like a real transposon, i.e., with a poor specificity, while other elements behave more like lambdoid phages and have a higher specificity. For example, *Bacteroides* elements show a preference for three to seven sites (SALYERS et al. 1995). Ctnscr94 integration is restricted to two sites (HOCHHUT et al. 1997), and one unique site of integration has been identified for SXT (HOCHHUT and WALDOR 1999).

3.2 Transposons and Virulence Determinant Propagation

Transposons encoding pathogenicity determinants have been studied to a lesser extent than their counterparts carrying resistance genes or catabolic pathways. Thus, it is still very difficult to precisely measure their importance. Indeed, many, if not most, characterized chromosomal PAIs seem to be, or to have been in the past, structurally embodied in a prophage-like structure (see, for example, reviews GROISMAN and OCHMAN 1996, 1997; HACKER et al. 1997; MARCUS et al. 2000). However, there are several clear exceptions, and many pathogenicity genes found on virulence plasmids are or have been components of transposons. ISs or remnants of ISs are found at the border of several loci involved in pathogenesis, suggesting that these loci were at one time part of composite transposons. This might be the case with the EspC islet found in EPEC (Enteropathogenic *E. coli*), with part of the LEE locus (KAPER et al. 1999) or with part of SPI-3 in *Salmonella* (GROISMAN et al. 1999). In *Yersiniae pestis*, the 102-kb *pgm* locus, which encompasses the prophage-like HPI, is organized as a Tn, while its borders are defined by two copies of IS100. However, although deletion of this locus through homologous recombination between the two IS100 copies has been observed (FETHERSTON and PERRY 1994; FETHERSTON et al. 1992), propagation of this element as a transposon has yet to be demonstrated. Many of the loci carried on virulence plasmids from enterobacteria are also surrounded by ISs or ISs remnants (GROISMAN et al. 1999; IRIARTE and CORNELIS 1999; KAPER et al. 1999; PARSOT and SANSONETTI 1999). In gram-positive bacteria, such as *Staphylococci*, many of the resistance genes are part of composite Tns, and among those found in *S. aureus*, a large number are based on IS256 insertions (SKURRAY and FIRTH 1997). Only one PAI has been characterized so far in *S. aureus*, which is structurally related to and seems to behave as a prophage-like element (SaPI1) (LINDSAY et al. 1998).

The only virulence determinants that have been shown to be carried by active transposons are the heat-stable enterotoxin STa gene of Tn1681 (So et al. 1979) and the heat-stable enterotoxin STb gene of Tn4521 (LEE et al. 1985). The Tn1621 transposon consists mainly of the STa gene flanked by two IS1 copies (So and MCCARTHY 1980), while Tn4521 is a 9-kb composite transposon based on two IS2 sequences. Interestingly, other enterotoxin determinants are encoded in transposon remnants, such as the heat-stable enterotoxin *eltAB* operon, which is abutted by truncated copies of IS91 (SCHLOR et al. 2000). Notably, another heat-stable enterotoxin gene (*astA2*) might also be encoded in the smallest transposon ever characterized. Indeed, this gene is entirely located within a larger ORF, which is highly similar to an IS transposase and is flanked by a 30bp-long imperfect inverted repeat (MCVEIGH et al. 2000). This structure has been named IS1414, but initial attempts to show its translocation were unsuccessful (MCVEIGH et al. 2000).

3.3 Transposon Encoded Functions: Better Resistance than Virulence?

It is notable that most resistance genes are found in active transposons while pathogenicity determinants are usually associated with prophage-like structures.

Conversely, bacteriophages rarely carry resistance genes. Indeed, only two cases of natural bacteriophages encoding a resistance gene have ever been reported (PEM-BERTON and TUCKER 1977; SMITH 1972). What is the reason for these observed discrepancies? A major difference lies in the evolutionary time – scale of virulence and resistance development in animal pathogens. As mentioned in the introduction, contemporary pathogens are the refined product of a long co-evolution with their hosts, whereas the anti-microbial threat in humans is a six-decades-old phenome-non. Virulence is often due to the co-expression of several complex functions in the same bacteria and from an anthropomorphic point of view, phage or prophage structures have many advantages for this purpose. Indeed, they allow the simul-taneous delivery of large clusters of genes inside the same species or among very closely related species. Their narrow host range limits genetic transfer to bacteria that are already adapted to the expression of such complex and integrated functions (as seen, for example, in *V. cholerae* with CTXΦ infection and expression of the cholera toxin being dependent on previous integration of VPIΦ into the genome). On the other hand, transposons, through hitchhiking on broad-host range conju-gative plasmids, are able to convey simple functions to a large number of different hosts. They provide bacteria with a very rapid reaction system.

A crucial question is how do transposons acquire these resistance genes? The answer has been found for two types of transposons: composite transposons (class I of mobile elements) found in both Gram-positive and -negative species, and transposons harboring an integron (see Sect. 4). Composite transposons can be constructed by random insertion of an insertion sequence (IS) on either side of any gene or cluster of genes. Most of these mobile elements carry only one or two resistance loci (e.g., Tn9, Tn10, Tn903, Tn1546, ...) and rarely more (e.g., three in Tn5). Most of the transposons carrying other functions, for example catabolic genes, also correspond to composite Tn and belong to class I Tn (TAN 1999).

Several other types of contemporary resistance Tns, such as Tn21 and Tn7 from classes II and III of the mobile element classification, owe their resistance encoding capacities to the presence of an integron in the structure. As integrons do not rely on random processes, they offer more flexibility, and their participation in multi-resistance outbreaks is a common clinical problem.

4 Integrons and Resistance Gene Flow

Integrons are natural cloning and expression systems that incorporate open-reading frames and convert them to functional genes (COLLIS et al. 1993; DE LA CRUZ and GRINSTED 1982; MARTINEZ and DE LA CRUZ 1988, 1990; STOKES and HALL 1989; WIEDEMANN et al. 1986; for review see HALL and COLLIS 1995; ROWE-MAGNUS and MAZEL 1999). The integron platform (Fig. 2) codes for an integrase (*intI*) that mediates recombination between a proximal primary recombination site (*attI*) and a secondary target called an *attC* site (or 59-base elements [59be]). The *attC* site is

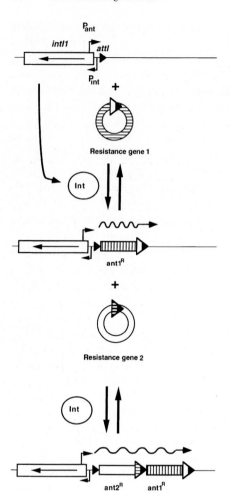

Fig. 2. Integron-mediated gene capture and the model for cassette exchange. Outline of the process, by which circular antibiotic resistance gene cassettes (antR) are repeatedly inserted at the specific *attI* site in a class1 integron downstream of the strong promoter Pant. *intI1*, integrase encoding gene; *Int*, integrase IntI1

normally found associated with a single open reading frame (ORF) and the ORF-*attC* structure is termed a gene cassette (HALL and STOKES 1993; RECCHIA and HALL 1995; STOKES et al. 1997; SUNDSTROM 1998). Insertion of the cassette at the *attI* site, which is located downstream of a resident promoter internal to the *intI* gene, drives expression of the encoded proteins (LEVESQUE et al. 1994).

Most of the *attC* sites of the integron cassettes identified to date are unique. Their length and sequence vary considerably (from 57 to 141bp), and their similarities are primarily restricted to their boundaries, which correspond to the inverse core-site (ICS; RYYYAAC) and the core site (CS; G↓TTRRRY; ↓, recombination point (COLLIS et al. 1998; STOKES et al. 1997)) (Fig. 2). More than 60 different antibiotic resistance genes, covering most antimicrobials presently in use, have been characterized in cassette structures (MAZEL and DAVIES 1999). The stockpiling of exogenous genetic loci to create multi-resistant integrons (MRIs) has contributed substantially to the current crisis in the treatment of infectious disease (DAVIES 1994; HALL and COLLIS 1998; JONES et al. 1997; MAZEL and DAVIES 1999; ROWE-MAGNUS and MAZEL 1999) as MRIs harboring up to five different resistance cassettes have been described (POIREL et al. 2000). The situation is exacerbated further by the formation of resistance gene clusters. Several resistance islands have been identified that are comprised of two integron structures in close proximity or a juxtaposition of IS-integron structures (for review, see ROWE-MAGNUS and MAZEL 1999).

Many different mechanisms exist to counteract the activity of antimicrobial compounds. Efflux systems, alterations in cell surface expression to decrease binding/permeability, enzymatic inactivation and cytoplasmic binding molecule paradigms have all been described (for review see DAVIES 1994; NIKAIDO 1994; SPRATT 1994). By selecting those resistance determinants that are encoded by single genes rather than more complex systems (MAZEL and DAVIES 1999), the integron/cassette assembly is apparently optimized to provide the required adaptive function to the host while minimizing potential incompatibility and transfer barriers.

The integron platform itself is defective for self-transposition, but this defect is often complemented through association with transposons and/or conjugative plasmids that can serve as vehicles for the intra- and inter-species transmission of genetic material. The Tn21 and Tn7 families provide examples of this. The potency of a highly efficient gene-capture and expression system in combination with broad-host range mobility is confirmed by the marked differences in codon usage among cassettes within the same integron, indicating that the antibiotic resistance determinants are of diverse origins. Furthermore, multi-resistance integrons are no longer restricted to the Gram-negative bacteria. A truncated integron in *M. tuberculosis* (MARTIN et al. 1990) and a complete and functional class 1 integron in another Gram-positive bacterium, *Corynebacterium glutamicum* (NESVERA et al. 1998) have also been found.

4.1 Big Brother: the *V. cholerae* Super-Integron

Had the full potential of integron-mediated bacterial evolution been realized with the discovery of MRIs? This was doubtful, as several initial observations suggested that the integron system had likely played an extended role in the evolution of bacteria that we only recently recognized due to the nature in which its activity became manifested. First, three classes of MRI-integrases have been characterized. The degree of homology between them (45%–58%) suggested that their evolutionary divergence had extended over a longer period than the 50 years of the antibiotic era. Second, the largest MRIs identified may have only contained eight cassettes, but the integron system has an apparently limitless capacity to exchange and stockpile cassettes. Thus, the only size limitation would be that of plasmid mobility and integron-harboring conjugative plasmids from 90–150Kb have been identified (DALSGAARD et al. 2000; FALBO et al. 1999). Third, the bias toward the propagation of resistance gene cassettes by MRIs was likely due to the selective pressure of antibiotic therapy regimes driving the specific capture of resistance cassettes. Despite the fact that only a handful of cassettes not related to antibiotic resistance have been found within MRIs, the presence of ORFs of unknown function implied that cassette genesis was not restricted to resistance determinants. Potentially any gene could be structured as a cassette, and integrons were likely to function as a general gene-capture mechanism in bacterial evolution.

The discovery of a new type of integron in the *Vibrio cholerae* genome (MAZEL et al. 1998) supported this notion in a convincing manner. The *V. cholerae* genome was found to contain repeated sequences (VCRs, *Vibrio cholerae* repeats) in clusters that mirrored the gene cassette arrays typically found in MRIs (RECCHIA and HALL 1997) (Fig. 3). They were first identified flanking the genes coding for two pathogenicity determinants in *V. cholerae* O:1 and non-O:1 isolates, the heat-stable toxin gene, *sto* (OGAWA and TAKEDA 1993) and the mannose-fucose-resistant hemagglutinin, *mrhA* (BARKER et al. 1994; BLAKE et al. 1980; VAN DONGEN et al. 1987). Like the *attC* sites of MRI cassettes: the VCRs were sequences of imperfect dyad symmetry that began with an ICS and ended with a CS identical to the integron-cassette consensus GTTRRRY; the ICS was always complementary to the CS of the upstream VCR; within these clusters, the VCRs were separated from one another by no more than two ORFs, and in most cases, they abutted a single ORF. Unlike the *attC* sites of MRIs, the VCRs were of uniform length (121–126bp) and were highly related (they shared >92% overall identity).

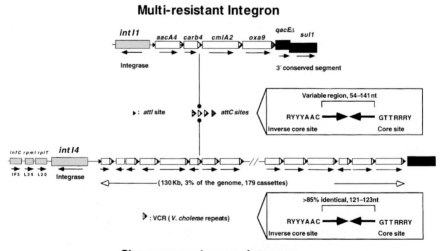

Fig. 3. Structural comparison of a "classical" multi-resistant integron and the *V. cholerae* N16961 super-integron. *Top*, schematic representation of In40; the various resistance genes are associated with different *attC* sites (see text). Antibiotic resistance cassettes confer resistance to the following compounds: *aacA4*, aminoglycosides; *cmlA2*, chloramphenicol; *qac*, quarternary ammonium compounds; *oxa9*, β-lactams. The *sul* gene, which provides resistance to sulfonamides, is not a gene cassette. *Bottom*, the ORFs are separated by highly homologous sequences, the VCRs

Mazel and co-workers (MAZEL et al. 1998) found a specific, but related, integrase gene, *intI4*, associated with the VCR cluster in the same structural organization as the one observed for MRIs. Furthermore, the activity of IntI4 was identical to that of IntI1, an MRI-integrase (ROWE-MAGNUS et al. 2001), and the gene-VCR structures could be directed to the *attI* site of a MRI by IntI1 (MAZEL et al. 1998). The *V. cholerae* integron element spans 126Kb and gathers at least 179 cassettes (HEIDELBERG et al. 2000; ROWE-MAGNUS et al. 1999) in a single structure termed a super-integron (SI), dwarfing previously identified MRIs. The resident genes were of diverse origins, as attested to by the wide variation in their base composition and codon usage. Although most of the cassettes were of undetermined function, those with identifiable activities were linked to adaptive functions and appeared to be mainly of bacterial origin. Considering the contribution of bacteria to the global biomass and that an estimated 99% of these species are unculturable, such a bias in origin and limited knowledge regarding their function was hardly surprising. However, the sole homologues of some of the cassettes were unassigned ORFs of viral or eukaryotic origin. Genetic transfer between kingdoms may not be as rampant as within the bacterial radiation, but the sequence data suggests that inter-kingdom genetic transfers have occurred (ROWE-MAGNUS et al. 1999).

4.2 The Integron Is an Ancient Evolutionary Apparatus that Is Prominent among Proteobacterial Genomes

If SI cassettes encode mostly adaptive functions, then the establishment of chromosomal super-integron islands can contribute significantly to, and radically change, the genetic makeup and evolution of the host bacterium. Their potential effect on bacterial evolution could be estimated if the distribution of SIs could be established. The extent to which this structure has impacted genome evolution has emerged with the discovery of SIs in several diverse proteobacterial genera (ROWE-MAGNUS et al. 2001) (Fig. 4). These include the Vibrionaceae, Shewanella, Xanthomonads, Pseudomonads and Nitrosomonads. A robust phylogenetic congruence between the 16s rRNA and *intI* trees was observed for the distribution of the SI-containing species. The extent of divergence between the *intI* genes was found to adhere to the line of descent among the bacterial species. Consequently, the integrases partitioned in genus-specific clades. The congruence of these dendrograms argued for the presence of an integron in the ancestral organism of each genus, and perhaps the γ-proteobacterial radiation itself, over the independent acquisition of integron platforms (i.e., the *intI* gene and the *attI* site) within each lineage. Furthermore, no evidence was found that the super-integron platforms were mobile. Thus integrons are ancient structures that have been steering the evolution of bacterial genomes for hundreds of millions of years, as the substitution rates calculated by Ochman and Wilson estimate that the *Vibrio* and *Pseudomonas/Xanthomonas* genera separated some 300–800 million years ago (OCHMAN and WILSON 1987).

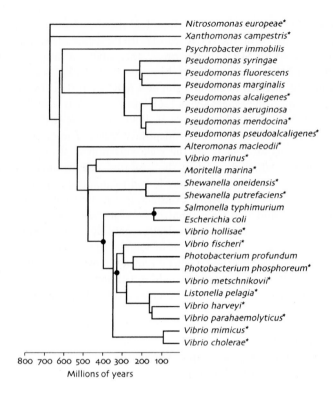

Nitrosomonas europeae*
Xanthomonas campestris*
Psychrobacter immobilis
Pseudomonas syringae
Pseudomonas fluorescens
Pseudomonas marginalis
Pseudomonas alcaligenes*
Pseudomonas aeruginosa
Pseudomonas mendocina*
Pseudomonas pseudoalcaligenes*
Alteromonas macleodii*
Vibrio marinus*
Moritella marina*
Shewanella oneidensis*
Shewanella putrefaciens*
Salmonella typhimurium
Escherichia coli
Vibrio hollisae*
Vibrio fischeri*
Photobacterium profundum
Photobacterium phosphoreum*
Vibrio metschnikovii*
Listonella pelagia*
Vibrio harveyi*
Vibrio parahaemolyticus*
Vibrio mimicus*
Vibrio cholerae*

800 700 600 500 400 300 200 100
Millions of years

Fig. 4. Tentative time scale for the evolution of eubacteria. *Asteriks* mark bacterial species known or believed to harbor an SI. *Circles* refer to calibrated branch points. Adapted from OCHMAN and WILSON 1987

5 The Adaptive Gene Pool Reservoir and Cassette Genesis

5.1 The Genetic Wealth of SI Cassette Reservoirs

The SIs identified to date collectively equal a small genome (ROWE-MAGNUS et al. 1999). The cassettes examined thus far appear to be unique to the host species, suggesting that the process of cassette genesis is constant and efficient. A precise inventory of the functions encoded by the cassettes remains to be established; however, a preliminary study indicates that many of the SI cassettes should encode adaptive functions, *sensu lato*, beyond pathogenicity and antibiotic resistance. The determination of the metabolic activities, other than antibiotic resistance and virulence, of three SI cassettes (ROWE-MAGNUS et al. 2001) confirms that integrons operate as a general gene-capture system in bacterial adaptation. Genes with homology to DNA methylases, immunity proteins, restriction endonucleases, dNTP triphophoshydrolases, periplasmic sulphate binding proteins and 8-oxoguanine triphosphatases (MutT), among others, have been found (ROWE-MAGNUS et al. 1999). Although a known antibiotic-resistance gene cassette has not yet been identified within an SI, several potential progenitor cassettes with significant homology to aminoglycoside, phosphinotricin, fosfomycin, streptothricin and chloramphenicol resistance genes were identified. If each bacterial species harboring an SI has its own cassette pool, the resource, in terms of gene cassette availability, will be immense, and the functions of the encoded genes have fantastic potential from both genetic and biotechnology standpoints.

5.2 The Process

But how is it that genes and *attC* sites become associated to form cassettes? The characteristics of SIs may yield important clues. Rowe-Magnus et al. (ROWE-MAGNUS et al. 2001) reported that the repeats of an individual SI were highly related to one another, yet they were species-specific, since they were distinct from those of other bacterial species. It was proposed that each distinct resistance cassette *attC* site of MRIs represents a specific SI; that the process of cassette genesis, in particular the mechanism of XXR propagation, occurs within bacteria possessing an SI; and that there is an initial directional flow of cassettes from SIs to MRIs. The virtually identity of numerous MRI cassette *attC* sites to SI repeats supports this notion (Fig. 5). It has been noted that XXRs occur exclusively in intergenic regions. Hall and colleagues proposed a model for the formation of cassettes through a reverse transcription mechanism (HALL 1997). While it is conceivable that an *attC* sequence could act as a primer for a reverse transcriptase (RT), the efficiency of transcription of DNA from a plethora of foreign sources (the gene cassettes can be of vastly different origins) is likely to be severely compromised in situ, limiting the substrate for the RT enzyme. Furthermore, some cassettes have their own promoter and/or are in the opposite orientation, compared to the *attC* site, characteristics incongruent with a *attC*-primer/RT model. The homogeneous yet distinctive nature of the XXRs is an attribute that may reflect enzymatic or gene-conversion events governing their propagation. However, the mechanics of this process remain a mystery.

5.3 The Sources

Where are all these resistance genes coming from? Determination of a definitive source for a particular resistance marker will be difficult, except in cases involving a recent exchange event, since differences in evolutionary rates and the passage of genes through intermediates will have created highly divergent descendants. However, many antibiotics are of bacterial origin, implying the existence of protective mechanisms in producer organisms and thus a potential source for resistance genes. Now there is evidence to support the trafficking of resistance genes from intrinsically resistant or antibiotic-producing organisms to clinical isolates. For example, the VanA and VanB proteins of the vancomycin-resistance gene cluster of *Enterococci* are more closely related to the dipeptide ligases of the glycopeptide-producing

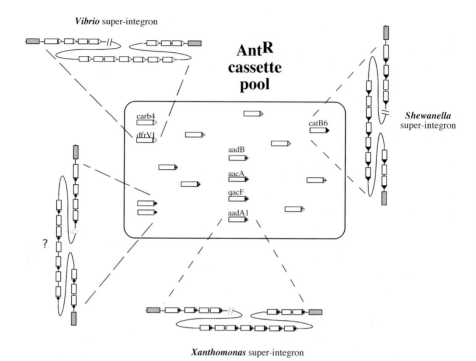

Fig. 5. A model for super-integrons as the source of the resistance gene cassettes of multi-resistant integrons. The pool of MRI gene cassettes is depicted as being derived from the reservoirs of SIs. Known resistance gene cassettes with *attC* sites that are highly related to those of known SI *attC* sites are show

organisms *Streptomyces toyocaensis* and *Amycolatopsis orientalis* (MARSHALL et al. 1997, 1998) than the dipeptide ligases of intrinsically resistant organisms (DUTKA-MALEN et al. 1990; EVERS et al. 1994, 1996). In addition, the potential recruitment of general housekeeping genes can provide an alternate route for the evolution of resistance determinants. Enzymes whose activities are not directly related to antibiotic resistance, such as aminoglycoside acetyltransferases and β-lactamases, have been found in the chromosomes of many bacteria including *Serratia*, *Providencia*, *Streptomyces*, *Klebsiella*, *Vibrio*, *Xanthomonas* and *Mycobacterium* spp. (for review see AINSA et al. 1996, 1997; CHOURY et al. 1999; FOURNIER et al. 1999; ROWE-MAGNUS and MAZEL 1999; SHAW et al. 1993; WENG et al. 1999).

6 Integrons and Virulence Gene Flow

6.1 Can Integrons Be Considered Pathogenicity Islands?

The best studied bacterial evolutionary transformations are those concerning antibiotic resistance and virulence development. The progression to virulence has been found to depend on both the pre-disposition of a bacterial species to become pathogenic (i.e., the ability to survive both within and outside of the host environment) and the subsequent acquisition of virulence-specific traits. Generally, the virulence phenotype is due to the concerted action of clusters of genes or operons grouped into PAIs. PAIs can vary considerably in size and are usually associated mobile DNA that may reside on extrachromosomal elements or become integrated into the host genome. Thus, in a single event, a bacterial species can be transformed from benign to pathogenic, the basis of evolution in quantum leaps. Phages are notorious for their role in establishing virulence loci. This type of virulence evolution is known to have occurred in, among others, *E. coli, Salmonella* and *Yersinia* (for review see GROISMAN and OCHMAN 1996; HACKER et al. 1997 and chapters in this volume). *V. cholerae* is known to have at least two phage-derived PAIs: CTXΦ (WALDOR and MEKALANOS 1996), which encodes cholerae toxin (CT), and VPIΦ (KARAOLIS et al. 1999), which encodes the toxin co-regulated pilus (TCP). Infection of *V. cholerae* by CTXΦ is dependent on the production of its cellular receptor, the TCP of VPIΦ, in essence creating a phage-on-phage dependence for establishment of virulence in *V. cholerae* (KARAOLIS et al. 1999).

Although PAIs often contain clusters of genes, only a subset of these may be required for the virulence phenotype. In fact, a single gene may be sufficient to cause disease symptoms, as is the case with CT (for review, see KAPER et al. 1995). Either way, interaction of newly acquired systems with the host genome must occur. CT provides an example, where the toxin encoded by a mobile element (CTXΦ) gains release from the cell via the host-encoded *eps* type II secretion system (SANDKVIST et al. 1997).

Do integrons fit into the scheme of a PAI? Like the encoded virulence factors of PAIs, the activity of integron cassettes offers a fast-track to bacterial innovation. But what defines a virulence factor? Wren wrote, "In the strict sense, it is a determinant that causes damage to the host cell (for example, an enterotoxin). In the broader sense, a determinant required for the survival of the pathogen in the host (for example, the ability to acquire iron)" (WREN 2000). By this broader definition, cannot resistance genes be considered virulence factors? This question aside, it is clear that CT and TCP are not the only virulence factors in *V. cholerae*. The heat-stable enterotoxin, NAG-ST, coded by the *sto* gene is able to cause cholerae-like disease symptoms in man (for review, see KAPER et al. 1995). This enterotoxin is processed and secreted by the host-encoded signal peptidase and general secretion pathway (SANDKVIST et al. 1997; STATHOPOULOS et al. 2000; TAKAO et al. 1985). Other functions are known to play a role in this organism's ability to colonize the small intestine, such as the adhesin MFRHA, encoded by the mannose-fucose resistant hemagglutinin gene (*mrhA*). Both the *mrhA* and *sto* genes are structured as cassettes. Thus, the single gene structure of cassettes does not necessarily compromise their pathogenic potential, particularly if the display of their protein products on the cell surface or their secretion can be brought about by host-encoded systems. Thus, integrons clearly have the capacity to participate in the establishment of virulence and, as such, the *V. cholerae* SI could be considered a PAI.

6.2 Using SIs to Track Bacterial Evolution in Real Time

Tracing the evolution of pathogenic microbes has entailed identifying the causative transforming agent(s). In events of lateral gene transfer, this means detailing the transmission mechanics and function(s) of the newly acquired gene(s). Can the cassette array order of SIs reveal the recent evolutionary path the host has followed? Scrutiny of the information garnered in such a way is, of course, paramount, since integron cassettes will be subject to episodic selection. The sheer size of SIs, together with the ancient and dynamic nature of the system, is a reminder that the cassettes that currently occupy the SI represent only a fraction of those that may have participated in the evolution of the host. Furthermore, specific alterations in cassette order are difficult to assess because we have not yet deciphered most of their functions. However, the maintenance of cassettes that provide the host with an adaptive advantage is expected as long as selective pressures persist. Thus, comparison of SI organization from recent and earlier isolates, as well as between recent isolates from different geographical locations, may yet tell us something. For example, can cassettes be mobilized in clusters? The SI organization of two *V. cholerae* strains suggests they can; the cassettes in positions 1–4 of the SI of strain 569B are found in the same order in the SI of strain N16961, but they occupy positions 79 to 82 (a displacement of more than 40Kb). This has also been seen for other cassettes (CLARK et al. 2000). These observations could represent a true group mobilization event or simply temporal differences in cassette acquisition. But there is evidence that not all repeated sequences are equally functional (HANSSON et al. 1997); some are known to contain mutations or deletions within the CS that could render them non-functional (D.A. Rowe-Magnus, A.-M. Guerout and D. Mazel, unpublished results). Therefore, their movement would have to be coordinated with those of other cassettes. Collis and Hall demonstrated that integron gene cassettes are excised as covalently closed circles and observed differences in the resulting recombination products (COLLIS and HALL 1992). Some cassettes could be mobilized as individual units while others could only be excised in tandem with another cassette. Whether such cassette hitchhiking is by design to ensure simultaneous transmission of genes or is just a matter of happenstance is not known.

What is the benefit of cassette array re-arrangement? Most gene cassettes do not contain a promoter, and their expression, therefore, depends on their integrating downstream of one in the proper orientation. Within MRIs it has been shown that the *attI* site is the preferred recombination point over the *attC* sites for incoming gene cassettes (HANSSON et al. 1997; MARTINEZ and DE LA CRUZ 1990). This places the cassette immediately downstream of an outward-oriented functional promoter internal to the *intI* gene. Cassettes closest to the *attI* site are more highly expressed than distal cassettes (COLLIS and HALL 1995; LEVESQUE et al. 1994). This feature may force the displacement of proximal cassettes that prevent expression of distal cassettes or force the re-integration of distal cassettes at other positions within the integron (downstream of a cassette containing a promoter, for example).

7 A Model for the Evolution of Integrons

The origin of the integron platform is not known. Although integrons lack the typical characteristics of temperate bacteriophages, the similarity of these systems at the level of the integrase gene, the attachment sites and the large number of ORFs of unassigned function is intriguing. Defective phages lack a fully functional mechanism to govern their propagation and, consequently, can become fixed in the chromosome. Deletions can then lead to the loss of many of the recognizable phage functions that remain (CAMPBELL 1996). Two naturally occurring defective pro-phages exemplify this. Like the integron platform, a λ-related defective prophage element of *E. coli* K-12, e14, shows no homology to other lambdoid phages aside from its attachment sites and putative integrase gene (CAMPBELL 1996). If e14 lysogenized *E. coli* K-12 as a fully active phage, then its small size of 14kB (compared to 49Kb for phage λ) must be due to the loss of considerable amounts of its once-functional genome. Likewise, the preferred chromosomal attachment site for bacteriophage P2 in *E. coli* K12 is occupied by a 639-bp defective remnant of P2 (BARREIRO and HAGGARD-LJUNGQUIST 1992). This remnant is proposed to have arisen in a lysogenic ancestor by a recombination event between the *attL* site (within a 27-nt core sequence) and a homologous region of 14 nts within a centrally located phage gene (the *D* gene), leaving behind an attachment site and residual phage DNA. Since the core sequence of the *attL* and *attR* sites is identical, re-combination in the opposite sense (that is between the *attR* site and the D gene) could occur, generating an integron-like prophage remnant containing an integrase gene, an attachment site and residual phage DNA. It is tempting to speculate that the ancestral integron was an immobilized prophage. If so, the integron and phage systems could have diverged to the extent that their functions no longer share any overlap, except the recombination machinery itself. The sequential phage infection process in the establishment of *V. cholerae* pathogenicity along with the antiquity and possible phage origin of the integron platform presents the intriguing possibility that the establishment of the *V. cholerae* SI through possible phage-related events was a prerequisite for VPIΦ, and subsequently CTXΦ, infection.

The current state of knowledge suggests that the integron platform is an ancient, defective prophage remnant comprised of an *intI* gene and its cognate *attI* site. The integrase activity allowed for rapid adaptation to the unpredictable flux of environmental niches by allowing the host to scavenge for foreign genes, in the form of cassettes, that could ultimately endow increased fitness, and the system was retained. MRIs likely evolved through the association of these remnants with mobile structures. Subsequently, the cassettes of MRIs were harvested from or exchanged with the many different kinds of SI cassette pools through multiple lateral transfers.

But SIs are not everywhere. Although retained among many extant proteo-bacterial genera, this system may have been lost in others (for example, the en-terobacteria). Genomes are dynamic, and ample opportunities exist for extensive changes in gene order and content to occur. These events can lead to deletion of non-essential genes. Integrons may not be essential systems since the SI cassettes examined to date seemingly encode adaptive rather than indispensable functions. Thus, loss of the integron may have occurred in certain genera or independently within species. Furthermore, other elements exist that allow bacteria to survive adaptive challenges and explore new niches. The participation of bacteriophages in this regard is well documented. Although their origin remains elusive, the presence of integrons among diverse Gram-positive and -negative clinical and environmental isolates establishes the quintessential role of integrons in adaptive bacterial evolution.

Acknowledgements. We would especially like to thank Professor Maurice Hofnung, Chef de l'Unité PMTG, for his support. This work was supported by the Natural Sciences and Engineering Research Council of Canada and the Canadian Bacterial Diseases Network (J.D.), the European Molecular Biology Organization (D.R.-M.), the Institut Pasteur, the Centre Nationale de la Recherche Scientifique and the Programme de Recherche Fondamentale en Microbiologie et Maladies Infectieuses et Parasitaires from the MENRT (D.M.).

References

Ainsa JA, Martin C, Gicquel B, Gomez-Lus R (1996) Characterization of the chromosomal aminoglycoside 2'-N-acetyltransferase gene from *Mycobacterium fortuitum*. Antimicrob Agents Chemother 40:2350–2355

Ainsa JA, Perez E, Pelicic V, Berthet FX, Gicquel B, Martin C (1997) Aminoglycoside 2'-*N*-acetyltransferase genes are universally present in mycobacteria: characterization of the aac(2')-Ic gene from *Mycobacterium tuberculosis* and the aac(2')-Id gene from *Mycobacterium smegmatis*. Mol Microbiol 24:431–441

Akido T, Koyama K, Ishiki Y, Kimura S, Fukushima T (1960) On the mechanism of the development of multiple-drug-resistant clones of *Shigella*. Jpn J Microbiol 4:219–227

Barker A, Clark CA, Manning PA (1994) Identification of VCR, a repeated sequence associated with a locus encoding a hemagglutinin in *Vibrio cholerae* O1. J Bacteriol 176:5450–5458

Barreiro V, Haggard-Ljungquist E (1992) Attachment sites for bacteriophage P2 on the *Escherichia coli* chromosome: DNA sequences, localization on the physical map, and detection of a P2-like remnant in E. coli K-12 derivatives. J Bacteriol 174:4086–4093

Berg DE, Howe MM (1989) Mobile DNA. American Society for Microbiology, Washington DC

Berg DE, Davies J, Allet B, Rochaix JD (1975) Transposition of R factor genes to bacteriophage lambda. Proc Nat Acad Sci USA 72:3628–3632

Blake PA, Weaver RE, Hollis DG (1980) Diseases of humans (other than cholera) caused by vibrios. Annu Rev Microbiol 34:341–367

Campbell A (1996) Cryptic prophages. In: Neidhardt FC (ed) *Escherichia coli* and *Salmonella:* Cellular and Molecular Biology. ASMpress, Washington DC

Choury D, Aubert G, Szajnert MF, Azibi K, Delpech M, Paul G (1999) Characterization and nucleotide sequence of CARB-6, a new carbenicillin-hydrolyzing beta-lactamase from *Vibrio cholerae*. Antimicrob Agents Chemother 43:297–301

Clark CA, Purins L, Kaewrakon P, Focareta T, Manning PA (2000) The *Vibrio cholerae* O1 chromosomal integron. Microbiology 146, 2605–2612

Collis CM, Hall RM (1992) Gene cassettes from the insert region of integrons are excised as covalently closed circles. Mol Microbiol 6:2875–2885

Collis CM, Hall RM (1995) Expression of antibiotic resistance genes in the integrated cassettes of integrons. Antimicrob Agents Chemother 39:155–162

Collis CM, Grammaticopoulos G, Briton J, Stokes HW, Hall RM (1993) Site-specific insertion of gene cassettes into integrons. Mol Microbiol 9:41–52

Collis CM, Kim MJ, Stokes HW, Hall RM (1998) Binding of the purified integron DNA integrase IntI1 to integron- and cassette-associated recombination sites. Mol Microbiol 29:477–490

Dalsgaard A, Forslund A, Petersen A, Brown DJ, Dias F, Monteiro S, Molbak K, Aaby P, Rodrigues A, Sandstrom A (2000) Class 1 integron-borne, multiple-antibiotic resistance encoded by a 150-kilobase conjugative plasmid in epidemic *Vibrio cholerae* O1 strains isolated in guinea-bissau [In Process Citation]. J Clin Microbiol 38:3774–3779

Datta N, Hughes V (1983) Plasmids of the same Inc groups in Enterobacteria before and after the medical use of antibiotics. Nature 306:616–617

Datta N, Hedges RW, Shaw EJ, Sykes RB, Richmond MH (1971) Properties of an R factor from *Pseudomonas aeruginosa*. J Bacteriol 108:1244–1249

Davies JE (1994) Inactivation of antibiotics and the dissemination of resistance genes. Science 264: 375–382

de la Cruz F, Davies J (2000) Horizontal gene transfer and the origin of species: lessons from bacteria. Trends Microbiol 8:128–133

de la Cruz F, Grinsted J (1982) Genetic and molecular characterization of Tn21, a multiple resistance transposon from R100.1. J Bacteriol 151:222–228

Dutka-Malen S, Molinas C, Arthur M, Courvalin P (1990) The VANA glycopeptide resistance protein is related to D-alanyl-D-alanine ligase cell wall biosynthesis enzymes. Mol Gen Genet 224:364–372

Evers S, Reynolds PE, Courvalin P (1994) Sequence of the vanB and ddl genes encoding D-alanine: D-lactate and D-alanine:D-alanine ligases in vancomycin-resistant *Enterococcus faecalis* V583. Gene 140:97–102

Evers S, Casadewall B, Charles M, Dutka-Malen S, Galimand M, Courvalin P (1996) Evolution of structure and substrate specificity in D-alanine:D-alanine ligases and related enzymes. J Mol Evol 42:706–712

Evers S, Quintiliani R Jr. Courvalin P (1996) Genetics of glycopeptide resistance in enterococci. Microb Drug Resist 2:219–223

Falbo V, Carattoli A, Tosini F, Pezzella C, Dionisi AM, Luzzi I (1999) Antibiotic resistance conferred by a conjugative plasmid and a class I integron in *Vibrio cholerae* O1 El Tor strains isolated in Albania and Italy. Antimicrob Agents Chemother 43:693–696

Fetherston JD, Perry RD (1994) The pigmentation locus of *Yersinia pestis* KIM6+ is flanked by an insertion sequence and includes the structural genes for pesticin sensitivity and HMWP2. Mol Microbiol 13:697–708

Fetherston JD, Schuetze P, Perry RD (1992) Loss of the pigmentation phenotype in *Yersinia pestis* is due to the spontaneous deletion of 102kb of chromosomal DNA, which is flanked by a repetitive element. Mol Microbiol 6:2693–2704

Fournier B, Gravel A, Hooper DC, Roy PH (1999) Strength and regulation of the different promoters for chromosomal beta-lactamases of *Klebsiella oxytoca*. Antimicrob Agents Chemother 43:850–855

Franke AE, Clewell DB (1981) Evidence for a chromosome-borne resistance transposon (Tn916) in *Streptococcus faecalis* that is capable of "conjugal" transfer in the absence of a conjugative plasmid. J Bacteriol 145:494–502

Gawron-Burke C, Clewell DB (1982) A transposon in *Streptococcus faecalis* with fertility properties. Nature 300:281–284

Groisman EA, Ochman H (1996) Pathogenicity islands: bacterial evolution in quantum leaps. Cell 87:791–794

Groisman EA, Ochman H (1997) How *Salmonella* became a pathogen. Trends Microbiol 5:343–349

Groisman EA, Blanc-Potard A-B, Uchiya K (1999) Pathogenicity Islands and the evolution of *Salmonella* virulence. In: Kaper JB, Hacker J (eds) Pathogenicity Islands and other mobile virulence elements. American Society for Microbiology, Washington DC, pp 127–150

Hacker J, Blum-Oehler G, Muhldorfer I, Tschape H (1997) Pathogenicity islands of virulent bacteria: structure, function and impact on microbial evolution. Mol Microbiol 23:1089–1097

Hall RM (1997) Mobile gene cassettes and integrons: moving antibiotic resistance genes in gram-negative bacteria. Ciba Foundation Symposium 207:192–202, discussion 202–205

Hall RM, Collis CM (1995) Mobile gene cassettes and integrons: capture and spread of genes by site-specific recombination. Mol Microbiol 15:593–600

Hall RM, Collis CM (1998) Antibiotic resistance in gram-negative bacteria: the role of gene cassettes and integrons [Review]. Drug Resistance Updates 1:109–119

Hall RM, Stokes HW (1993) Integrons: novel DNA elements which capture genes by site-specific recombination. Genetica 90:115–132

186   D.A. Rowe-Magnus et al.

Hansson K, Skold O, Sundstrom L (1997) Non-palindromic attI sites of integrons are capable of site-specific recombination with one another and with secondary targets. Mol Microbiol 26:441–453

Hedges RW, Jacob AE (1974) Transposition of ampicillin resistance from RP4 to other replicons. Mol Gen Genet 132:31–40

Heidelberg JF, Eisen JA, Nelson WC, Clayton RA, Gwinn ML, Dodson RJ, Haft DH, Hickey EK, Peterson JD, Umayam L et al. (2000) DNA sequence of both chromosomes of the cholera pathogen *Vibrio cholerae*. Nature 406:477–483

Hochhut B, Waldor MK (1999) Site-specific integration of the conjugal *Vibrio cholerae* SXT element into *prfC*. Mol Microbiol 32:99–110

Hochhut B, Jahreis K, Lengeler JW, Schmid K (1997) CTnscr94, a conjugative transposon found in enterobacteria. J Bacteriol 179:2097–2102

Hughes VM, Datta N (1983) Conjugative plasmids in bacteria of the 'pre-antibiotic' era. Nature 302:725–726

Iriarte M, Cornelis GR (1999) The 70 kilobase virulence plasmid of *Yersiniae*. In: Kaper JB, Hacker J (eds) Pathogenicity Islands and other mobile virulence elements. American Society for Microbiology, Washington DC, pp 91–125

Jones ME, Peters E, Weersink AM, Fluit A, Verhoef J (1997) Widespread occurrence of integrons causing multiple antibiotic resistance in bacteria. Lancet 349:1742–1743

Jordan E, Saedler H, Starlinger P (1968) O[0] and strong-polar mutations in the gal operon are insertions. Mol Gen Genet 102:353–363

Kaper JB, Morris JG Jr, Levine MM (1995) Cholera. Clin Microbiol Rev 8:48–86

Kaper JB, Mellies JL, Nataro JP (1999) Pathogenicity Islands and other mobile genetic elements of diarrheagenic *Escherichia coli*. In: Kaper JB, Hacker J (eds) Pathogenicity Islands and other mobile virulence elements. American Society for Microbiology, Washington DC, pp 33–58

Karaolis DK, Somara S, Maneval DR Jr, Johnson JA, Kaper JB (1999) A bacteriophage encoding a pathogenicity island, a type-IV pilus and a phage receptor in cholera bacteria. Nature 399:375–379

Kleckner N, Chalmers RM, Kwon D, Sakai J, Bolland S (1996) Tn10 and IS10 transposition and chromosome rearrangements: mechanism and regulation in vivo and in vitro. Curr Top Microbiol Immunol 204:49–82

Lee CH, Hu ST, Swiatek PJ, Moseley SL, Allen SD, So M (1985) Isolation of a novel transposon which carries the *Escherichia coli* enterotoxin STII gene. J Bacteriol 162:615–620

Levesque C, Brassard S, Lapointe J, Roy PH (1994) Diversity and relative strength of tandem promoters for the antibiotic-resistance genes of several integrons. Gene 142:49–54

Liebert CA, Hall RM, Summers AO (1999) Transposon Tn21, flagship of the floating genome. Microbiol Mol Biol Rev 63:507–522

Lindsay JA, Ruzin A, Ross HF, Kurepina N, Novick RP (1998) The gene for toxic shock toxin is carried by a family of mobile pathogenicity islands in *Staphylococcus aureus*. Mol Microbiol 29:527–543

Maclean IH, Rogers K, Fleming A (1939) M and B 693 and pneumococci. Lancet 1:562–568

Mahillon J (1998) Transposons as gene haulers. APMIS Suppl 84:29–36

Marcus SL, Brumell JH, Pfeifer CG, Finlay BB (2000) *Salmonella* pathogenicity islands: big virulence in small packages. Microbes Infect 2:145–156

Marshall CG, Broadhead G, Leskiw BK, Wright GD (1997) D-Ala-D-Ala ligases from glycopeptide antibiotic-producing organisms are highly homologous to the enterococcal vancomycin-resistance ligases VanA and VanB. Proc Nat Acad Sci USA 94:6480–6483

Marshall CG, Lessard IA, Park I, Wright GD (1998) Glycopeptide antibiotic resistance genes in glycopeptide-producing organisms. Antimicrob Agents Chemother 42:2215–2220

Martin C, Timm J, Rauzier J, Gomez-Lus R, Davies J, Gicquel B (1990) Transposition of an antibiotic resistance element in mycobacteria. Nature 345:739–743

Martinez E, de la Cruz F (1988) Transposon Tn21 encodes a RecA-independant site-specific integration system. Mol Gen Genet 211:320–325

Martinez E, de la Cruz F (1990) Genetic elements involved in Tn21 site-specific integration, a novel mechanism for the dissemination of antibiotic resistance genes. EMBO J 9:1275–1281

Mazel D, Davies J (1999) Antibiotic resistance in microbes. Cell Mol Life Sci 56:742–754

Mazel D, Dychinco B, Webb VA, Davies J (1998) A distinctive class of integron in the *Vibrio cholerae* genome. Science 280:605–608

McVeigh A, Fasano A, Scott DA, Jelacic S, Moseley SL, Robertson DC, Savarino SJ (2000) IS1414, an *Escherichia coli* insertion sequence with a heat-stable enterotoxin gene embedded in a transposase-like gene. Infect Immun 68:5710–5715

Mitsuhashi S (1965) Transmissible drug-resistance factor R. Gunma J Med Sci 14:169–209

Mitsuhashi S (1969) The R factors. J Infect Dis 119:89–100

Mitsuhashi S, Harada K, Hashimoto H, Egawa R (1961) On the drug-resistance of enteric bacteria. Jpn J Exp Med 31:47–52

Murphy DB, Pembroke JT (1995) Transfer of the IncJ plasmid R391 to recombination deficient *Escherichia coli* K12: evidence that R391 behaves as a conjugal transposon. FEMS Microbiol Lett 134:153–158

Nakaya R, Nakamura A, Murata Y (1960) Resistance transfer agents in *Shigella*. Biochem Biophys Res Comm 3:654–659

Nesvera J, Hochmannova J, Patek M (1998) An integron of class 1 is present on the plasmid pCG4 from gram-positive bacterium *Corynebacterium glutamicum*. FEMS Microbiol Lett 169:391–395

Nikaido H (1994) Prevention of drug access to bacterial targets: permeability barriers and active efflux. Science 264:382–388

Nikolich MP, Shoemaker NB, Wang GR, Salyers AA (1994) Characterization of a new type of Bacteroides conjugative transposon, Tcr Emr 7853. J Bacteriol 176:6606–6612

Ochman H, Wilson AC (1987) Evolution in bacteria: evidence for a universal substitution rate in cellular genomes. J Mol Evol 26:74–86

Ochman H, Lawrence JG, Groisman EA (2000) Lateral gene transfer and the nature of bacterial evolution. Nature 405:299–304

Ogawa A, Takeda T (1993) The gene encoding the heat-stable enterotoxin of *Vibrio cholerae* is flanked by 123-base pair direct repeats. Microbiol Immunol 37:607–616

Ouellette M, Bissonnette L, Roy PH (1987) Precise insertion of antibiotic resistance determinants into Tn21-like transposons: nucleotide sequence of the OXA-1 beta-lactamase gene. Proc Nat Acad Sci USA 84:7378–7382

Parsot C, Sansonetti PJ (1999) The virulence plasmid of Shigellae: an archipelago of pathogenicity Islands? In: Kaper JB, Hacker J (eds) Pathogenicity Islands and other mobile virulence elements. American Society for Microbiology, Washington DC, pp 151–165

Pemberton JM, Tucker WT (1977) Naturally occurring viral R plasmid with a circular supercoiled genome in the extracellular state. Nature 266:50–51

Poirel L, Le Thomas I, Naas T, Karim A, Nordmann P (2000) Biochemical sequence analyses of *GES-1*, a novel class A extended-spectrum-lactamase, and the class 1 integron In52 from *Klebsiella pneumoniae*. Antimicrob Agents Chemother 44:622–632

Ravatn R, Studer S, Springael D, Zehnder AJ, van der Meer JR (1998) Chromosomal integration, tandem amplification, and deamplification in *Pseudomonas putida* F1 of a 105-kilobase genetic element containing the chlorocatechol degradative genes from *Pseudomonas* sp. Strain B13. J Bacteriol 180:4360–4369

Ravatn R, Studer S, Zehnder AJ, van der Meer JR (1998) Int-B13, an unusual site-specific recombinase of the bacteriophage P4 integrase family, is responsible for chromosomal insertion of the 105-kilobase clc element of *Pseudomonas* sp. Strain B13. J Bacteriol 180:5505–5514

Recchia GD, Hall RM (1995) Gene cassettes: a new class of mobile element. Microbiol 141:3015–3027

Recchia GD, Hall RM (1997) Origins of the mobile gene cassettes found in integrons. Trends Microbiology 5:389–394

Richmond MH, Sykes RB (1972) The chromosomal integration of a -lactamase gene derived from the P-type R-factor RP1 in *Escherichia coli*. Genet Res 20:231–237

Rowe-Magnus DA, Mazel D (1999) Resistance gene capture. Cur Opin Microbiol 2:483–488

Rowe-Magnus DA, Guerout A-M, Mazel D (1999) Super-Integrons. Res Microbiol 150:641–651

Rowe-Magnus DA, Guerout A-M, Ploncard P, Dychinco B, Davies J, Mazel D (2001) The evolutionary history of chromosomal super-integrons provides an ancestry for multi-resistant integrons. Proc Natl Acad Sci USA: Jan 16; 98(2):652–657

Salyers AA, Shoemaker NB (1997) Conjugative transposons. Genet Eng (New York) 19:89–100

Salyers AA, Shoemaker NB, Stevens AM, Li LY (1995) Conjugative transposons: an unusual and diverse set of integrated gene transfer elements. Microbiol Rev 59:579–590

Sandkvist M, Michel L, Hough L, Morales V, Bagdasarian M, Koomey M, DiRita V (1997) General secretion pathway (eps) genes required for toxin secretion and outer membrane biogenesis in *Vibrio cholerae*. J Bacteriol 179:6994–7003

Schlor S, Riedl S, Blass J, Reidl J (2000) Genetic rearrangements of the regions adjacent to genes encoding heat-labile enterotoxins (*eltAB*) of enterotoxigenic *Escherichia coli* strains. Appl Environ Microbiol 66:352–358

Scott JR (1992) Sex and the single circle: conjugative transposition. J Bacteriol 174:6005–6010

Shapiro JA (1969) Mutations caused by the insertion of genetic material into the galactose operon of *Escherichia coli.* J Mol Biol 40:93–105

Shaw KJ, Rather PN, Hare RS, Miller GH (1993) Molecular genetics of aminoglycoside resistance genes and familial relationships of the aminoglycoside-modifying enzymes. Microbiol Rev 57:138–163

Shoemaker NB, Smith MD, Guild WR (1980) DNase-resistant transfer of chromosomal cat and tet insertions by filter mating in *Pneumococcus.* Plasmid 3:80–87

Skurray RA, Firth N (1997) Molecular evolution of multiply-antibiotic-resistant staphylococci. Ciba Foundation Symposium 207:167–183; discussion 183–191

Smith HW (1972) Ampicillin resistance in *Escherichia coli* by phage infection. Nat New Biol 238:205–206

So M, McCarthy BJ (1980) Nucleotide sequence of the bacterial transposon Tn1681 encoding a heat-stable (ST) toxin and its identification in enterotoxigenic *Escherichia coli* strains. Proc Natl Acad Sci USA 77:4011–4015

So M, Heffron F, McCarthy BJ (1979) The *E. coli* gene encoding heat stable toxin is a bacterial transposon flanked by inverted repeats of IS1. Nature 277:453–456

Spratt BG (1994) Resistance to antibiotics mediated by target alterations. Science 264:388–393

Stathopoulos C, Hendrixson DR, Thanassi DG, Hultgren SJ, St Geme JW 3rd, Curtiss R 3rd (2000) Secretion of virulence determinants by the general secretory pathway in gram-negative pathogens: an evolving story. Microbes Infect 2:1061–1072

Stokes HW, Hall RM (1989) A novel family of potentially mobile DNA elements encoding site-specific gene-integration functions: integrons. Mol Microbiol 3:1669–1683

Stokes HW, O'Gorman DB, Recchia GD, Parsekhian M, Hall RM (1997) Structure and function of 59-base element recombination sites associated with mobile gene cassettes. Mol Microbiol 26:731–745

Sundström L (1998) The potential of integrons and connected programmed rearrangements for mediating horizontal gene transfer. APMIS Supplementum 84:37–42

Sundström L, Radström P, Swedberg G, Sköld O (1988) Site-specific recombination promotes linkage between trimethoprim- and sulfonamide-resistance genes. Sequence characterization of dhfrV and sulI and a recombination active locus of Tn21. Mol Gen Genet 213:191–201

Takao T, Shimonishi Y, Kobayashi M, Nishimura O, Arita M, Takeda T, Honda T, Miwatani T (1985) Amino acid sequence of heat-stable enterotoxin produced by *Vibrio cholerae* non-01. FEBS Lett 193:250–254

Tan HM (1999) Bacterial catabolic transposons. Appl Microbiol Biotechnol 51:1–12

van Dongen WM, vanVlerken WA, DeGraaf FK (1987) Nucleotide sequence of a DNA fragment encoding a *Vibrio cholerae* haemagglutinin. Mol Gen (Life Sci. Adv.) 6:85–91

Waldor MK, Mekalanos JJ (1996) Lysogenic conversion by a filamentous phage encoding cholera toxin. Science 272:1910–1914

Waldor MK, Tschape H, Mekalanos JJ (1996) A new type of conjugative transposon encodes resistance to sulfamethoxazole, trimethoprim, and streptomycin in *Vibrio cholerae* O139. J Bacteriol 178:4157–4165

Watanabe T (1963) Infective heredity of multiple resistance in bacteria. Bacteriol Rev 27:87–115

Weng SF, Chen CY, Lee YS, Lin JW, Tseng YH (1999) Identification of a novel beta-lactamase produced by *Xanthomonas campestris*, a phytopathogenic bacterium. Antimicrob Agents Chemother 43:1792–1797

Wiedemann B, Meyer JF, Zuhlsdorf MT (1986) Insertions of resistance genes into Tn21-like transposons. J Antimicrob Chemother 18:85–92

Wren BW (2000) Microbial genome analysis: insights into virulence, host adaptation and evolution. Nature Rev 1:30–39

Subject Index

Subject Index for Part I

Current Topics in Microbiology and Immunology

Volumes published since 1989 (and still available)

Vol. 220: **Rauscher, Frank J. III; Vogt, Peter K. (Eds.):** Chromosomal Translocations and Oncogenic Transcription Factors. 1997. 28 figs. XI, 166 pp. ISBN 3-540-61402-8

Vol. 221: **Kastan, Michael B. (Ed.):** Genetic Instability and Tumorigenesis. 1997. 12 figs.VII, 180 pp. ISBN 3-540-61518-0

Vol. 222: **Olding, Lars B. (Ed.):** Reproductive Immunology. 1997. 17 figs. XII, 219 pp. ISBN 3-540-61888-0

Vol. 223: **Tracy, S.; Chapman, N. M.; Mahy, B. W. J. (Eds.):** The Coxsackie B Viruses. 1997. 37 figs. VIII, 336 pp. ISBN 3-540-62390-6

Vol. 224: **Potter, Michael; Melchers, Fritz (Eds.):** C-Myc in B-Cell Neoplasia. 1997. 94 figs. XII, 291 pp. ISBN 3-540-62892-4

Vol. 225: **Vogt, Peter K.; Mahan, Michael J. (Eds.):** Bacterial Infection: Close Encounters at the Host Pathogen Interface. 1998. 15 figs. IX, 169 pp. ISBN 3-540-63260-3

Vol. 226: **Koprowski, Hilary; Weiner, David B. (Eds.):** DNA Vaccination/Genetic Vaccination. 1998. 31 figs. XVIII, 198 pp. ISBN 3-540-63392-8

Vol. 227: **Vogt, Peter K.; Reed, Steven I. (Eds.):** Cyclin Dependent Kinase (CDK) Inhibitors. 1998. 15 figs. XII, 169 pp. ISBN 3-540-63429-0

Vol. 228: **Pawson, Anthony I. (Ed.):** Protein Modules in Signal Transduction. 1998. 42 figs. IX, 368 pp. ISBN 3-540-63396-0

Vol. 229: **Kelsoe, Garnett; Flajnik, Martin (Eds.):** Somatic Diversification of Immune Responses. 1998. 38 figs. IX, 221 pp. ISBN 3-540-63608-0

Vol. 230: **Kärre, Klas; Colonna, Marco (Eds.):** Specificity, Function, and Development of NK Cells. 1998. 22 figs. IX, 248 pp. ISBN 3-540-63941-1

Vol. 231: **Holzmann, Bernhard; Wagner, Hermann (Eds.):** Leukocyte Integrins in the Immune System and Malignant Disease. 1998. 40 figs. XIII, 189 pp. ISBN 3-540-63609-9

Vol. 232: **Whitton, J. Lindsay (Ed.):** Antigen Presentation. 1998. 11 figs. IX, 244 pp. ISBN 3-540-63813-X

Vol. 233/I: **Tyler, Kenneth L.; Oldstone, Michael B. A. (Eds.):** Reoviruses I. 1998. 29 figs. XVIII, 223 pp. ISBN 3-540-63946-2

Vol. 233/II: **Tyler, Kenneth L.; Oldstone, Michael B. A. (Eds.):** Reoviruses II. 1998. 45 figs. XVI, 187 pp. ISBN 3-540-63947-0

Vol. 234: **Frankel, Arthur E. (Ed.):** Clinical Applications of Immunotoxins. 1999. 16 figs. IX, 122 pp. ISBN 3-540-64097-5

Vol. 235: **Klenk, Hans-Dieter (Ed.):** Marburg and Ebola Viruses. 1999. 34 figs. XI, 225 pp. ISBN 3-540-64729-5

Vol. 236: **Kraehenbuhl, Jean-Pierre; Neutra, Marian R. (Eds.):** Defense of Mucosal Surfaces: Pathogenesis, Immunity and Vaccines. 1999. 30 figs. IX, 296 pp. ISBN 3-540-64730-9

Vol. 237: **Claesson-Welsh, Lena (Ed.):** Vascular Growth Factors and Angiogenesis. 1999. 36 figs. X, 189 pp. ISBN 3-540-64731-7

Vol. 238: **Coffman, Robert L.; Romagnani, Sergio (Eds.):** Redirection of Th1 and Th2 Responses. 1999. 6 figs. IX, 148 pp. ISBN 3-540-65048-2

Vol. 239: **Vogt, Peter K.; Jackson, Andrew O. (Eds.):** Satellites and Defective Viral RNAs. 1999. 39 figs. XVI, 179 pp. ISBN 3-540-65049-0

Vol. 240: **Hammond, John; McGarvey, Peter; Yusibov, Vidadi (Eds.):** Plant Biotechnology. 1999. 12 figs. XII, 196 pp. ISBN 3-540-65104-7

Vol. 241: **Westblom, Tore U.; Czinn, Steven J.; Nedrud, John G. (Eds.):** Gastroduodenal Disease and Helicobacter pylori. 1999. 35 figs. XI, 313 pp. ISBN 3-540-65084-9

Vol. 242: **Hagedorn, Curt H.; Rice, Charles M. (Eds.):** The Hepatitis C Viruses. 2000. 47 figs. IX, 379 pp. ISBN 3-540-65358-9

Vol. 243: **Famulok, Michael; Winnacker, Ernst-L.; Wong, Chi-Huey (Eds.):** Combinatorial Chemistry in Biology. 1999. 48 figs. IX, 189 pp. ISBN 3-540-65704-5

Vol. 244: **Daëron, Marc; Vivier, Eric (Eds.):** Immunoreceptor Tyrosine-Based Inhibition Motifs. 1999. 20 figs. VIII, 179 pp. ISBN 3-540-65789-4

Vol. 245/I: **Justement, Louis B.; Siminovitch, Katherine A. (Eds.):** Signal Transduction and the Coordination of B Lymphocyte Development and Function I. 2000. 22 figs. XVI, 274 pp. ISBN 3-540-66002-X

Vol. 245/II: **Justement, Louis B.; Siminovitch, Katherine A. (Eds.):** Signal Transduction on the Coordination of B Lymphocyte Development and Function II. 2000. 13 figs. XV, 172 pp. ISBN 3-540-66003-8

Vol. 246: **Melchers, Fritz; Potter, Michael (Eds.):** Mechanisms of B Cell Neoplasia 1998. 1999. 111 figs. XXIX, 415 pp. ISBN 3-540-65759-2

Vol. 247: **Wagner, Hermann (Ed.):** Immunobiology of Bacterial CpG-DNA. 2000. 34 figs. IX, 246 pp. ISBN 3-540-66400-9

Vol. 248: **du Pasquier, Louis; Litman, Gary W. (Eds.):** Origin and Evolution of the Vertebrate Immune System. 2000. 81 figs. IX, 324 pp. ISBN 3-540-66414-9

Vol. 249: **Jones, Peter A.; Vogt, Peter K. (Eds.):** DNA Methylation and Cancer. 2000. 16 figs. IX, 169 pp. ISBN 3-540-66608-7

Vol. 250: **Aktories, Klaus; Wilkins, Tracy, D. (Eds.):** Clostridium difficile. 2000. 20 figs. IX, 143 pp. ISBN 3-540-67291-5

Vol. 251: **Melchers, Fritz (Ed.):** Lymphoid Organogenesis. 2000. 62 figs. XII, 215 pp. ISBN 3-540-67569-8

Vol. 252: **Potter, Michael; Melchers, Fritz (Eds.):** B1 Lymphocytes in B Cell Neoplasia. 2000. XIII, 326 pp. ISBN 3-540-67567-1

Vol. 253: **Gosztonyi, Georg (Ed.):** The Mechanisms of Neuronal Damage in Virus Infections of the Nervous System. 2001. approx. XVI, 270 pp. ISBN 3-540-67617-1

Vol. 254: **Privalsky, Martin L. (Ed.):** Transcriptional Corepressors. 2001. 25 figs. XIV, 190 pp. ISBN 3-540-67569-8

Vol. 255: **Hirai, Kanji (Ed.):** Marek's Disease. 2001. 22 figs. XII, 294 pp. ISBN 3-540-67798-4

Vol. 256: **Schmaljohn, Connie S.; Nichol, Stuart T. (Eds.):** Hantaviruses . 2001, 24 figs. XI, 196 pp. ISBN 3-540-41045-7

Vol. 257: **van der Goot, Gisou (Ed.):** Pore-Forming Toxins, 2001. 19 figs. IX, 166 pp. ISBN 3-540-41386-3

Vol. 258: **Takada, Kenzo (Ed.):** Epstein-Barr Virus and Human Cancer. 2001. 38 figs. IX, 233 pp. ISBN 3-540-41506-8

Vol. 259: **Hauber, Joachim, Vogt, Peter K. (Eds.):** Nuclear Export of Viral RNAs. 2001. 19 figs. IX, 131 pp. ISBN 3-540-41278-6

Vol. 260: **Burton, Didier R. (Ed.):** Antibodies in Viral Infection. 2001. 51 figs. IX, 309 pp. ISBN 3-540-41611-0

Vol. 261: **Trono, Didier (Ed.):** Lentiviral Vectors. 2002. 32 figs. X, 258 pp. ISBN 3-540-42190-4

Vol. 262: **Oldstone, Michael B.A. (Ed.):** Arenaviruses I. 2002, 30 figs. XVIII, 197 pp. ISBN 3-540-42244-7

Vol. 263: **Oldstone, Michael B. A. (Ed.):** Arenaviruses II. 2002, 49 figs. XVIII, 268 pp. ISBN 3-540-42705-8

Printing (Computer to Film): Saladruck Berlin
Binding: Stürtz AG, Würzburg